Human Anatomy Essentials

A Guide to Integrated Learning

Human Anatomy Essentials

A Guide to Integrated Learning

Ling Eng Ang
S.Thameem Dheen
George Yip Wai Cheong
Deepika Kandilya

World Scientific

NEW JERSEY • LONDON • SINGAPORE • BEIJING • SHANGHAI • HONG KONG • TAIPEI • CHENNAI • TOKYO

Published by

World Scientific Publishing Co Pte Ltd
5 Toh Tuck Link, Singapore 596224
USA office: 27 Warren Street, Suite 401-402, Hackensack, NJ 07601
UK office: 57 Shelton Street, Covent Garden, London WC2H 9HE

British Library Cataloguing-in-Publication Data
A catalogue record for this book is available from the British Library.

HUMAN ANATOMY ESSENTIALS
A Guide to Integrated Learning

ISBN 978-981-98-2726-8 (hardcover)
ISBN 978-981-98-2791-6 (paperback)
ISBN 978-981-98-2727-5 (ebook for institutions)
ISBN 978-981-98-2728-2 (ebook for individuals)

For any available supplementary material, please visit
https://www.worldscientific.com/worldscibooks/10.1142/14501#t=suppl

Printed in Singapore

FOREWORD

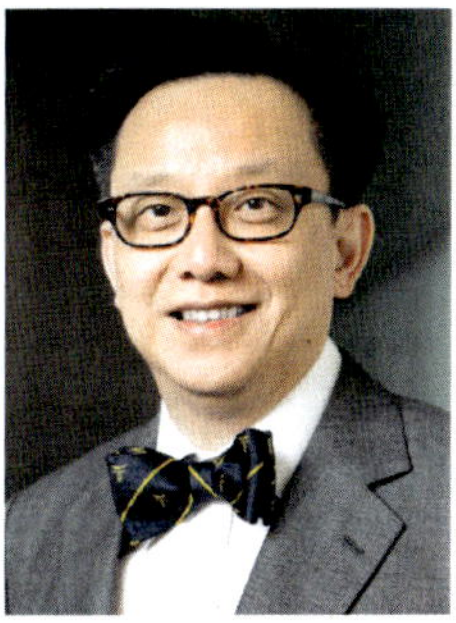

The year 2025 marks a significant milestone — the 120th anniversary of the Yong Loo Lin School of Medicine, National University of Singapore. The publication of 'Human Anatomy Essentials: A Guide to Integrated Learning' is especially timely, coinciding with the School's celebration of more than a century of excellence in teaching, led by outstanding educators.

Anatomy, one of the most ancient sciences, remains an integral part of the undergraduate medical curriculum, bridging theoretical knowledge and clinical skills. Established in 1922 within the King Edward VII College of Medicine (as the medical school was then known), the Department of Anatomy has earned a reputation as one of the leading anatomy departments in Asia in the training of medical, dental, nursing, allied health professional students, and surgical residents.

Over the years, the Department of Anatomy at NUS Medicine has trained generations of health sciences professionals and housed a number of eminent anatomists. In August 2023, the School of Medicine launched an enhanced medical curriculum focusing on technological advancements (AI, Digital Health) and medical humanities to better prepare future-ready doctors, dentists, nurses and allied health professionals. Additionally, students are introduced to clinical competencies during the preclinical years as part of an integrated training approach. In tandem, the anatomy curriculum and pedagogy have undergone substantial refinements to align with the objectives of the new enhanced medical curriculum.

The release of both print and electronic versions of this textbook marks another meaningful and apt milestone in the Department's continuing growth and development as a distinct and distinctive academic centre of anatomical teaching and research-oriented excellence within NUS Medicine. This textbook is the outcome of the dedicated efforts of eminent faculty members of the Department, reflecting decades of teaching experience and facilitates the integration of essential subspecialties within Anatomy. It closely aligns with the enhanced academic curriculum, beginning with foundational topics that are systematically followed by sections on systemic anatomy. The text is enriched with simplified yet conceptually integrated illustrations and histological images, including original, hand-drawn illustrations that has been digitised to elevate the learning experience of students at our School.

On behalf of all staff and students, past and present, I extend my heartiest congratulations and sincere appreciation to the book's contributors. I am confident that this book will serve as an invaluable resource for generations of learners.

Chong Yap Seng
Lien Ying Chow Professor in Medicine
Dean, Yong Loo Lin School of Medicine,
National University of Singapore

PREFACE

The teaching of Human Anatomy to students in the medical, dental, and allied health sciences has been the primary mission in medical education dating back to the then Faculty of Medicine, University of Singapore, Sepoy Lines campus in the 1970s. Over the past five decades, the curriculum for human anatomy and other preclinical science subjects at the Yong Loo Lin School of Medicine, National University of Singapore, has undergone periodic revisions, including in recent years.

In the traditional curriculum, first-year medical and dental students were required to learn a large volume of detailed anatomical information. Consequently, students often devoted considerable time to memorising medical terminology and factual anatomical content. Many students, and even some educators, relied heavily on mnemonics as a learning strategy without developing a thorough understanding of the underlying principles and fundamental concepts. As a result, human anatomy has often been perceived as a challenging and dry subject, which may diminish students' enthusiasm for learning and, in turn, affect the morale of educators.

Apart from the extensive anatomical detail, the traditional curriculum provided limited correlation between anatomy and its clinical applications, with minimal integration among its major subspecialties such as gross anatomy, histology, neuroanatomy, and embryology. These subjects were often taught in isolation, resulting in a fragmented understanding of the human body. For example, students examining the shoulder joint may understand its bony articulations and associated muscles but fail to connect these with the histology of articular cartilage, bone, capsule, and ligaments, or with the relevant innervation and its clinical implications in pain, inflammation, and arthritis. Similarly, the neuroanatomical basis of tendon reflexes, muscle tone, referred pain, and the functional components of peripheral nerves may not be readily appreciated during gross anatomy learning.

This challenge was further compounded by the substantial reduction in anatomy teaching hours, from more than 700 contact hours to fewer than 200 hours in recent years. With the expansion of the preclinical curriculum, teaching time has become increasingly constrained, necessitating the removal of less essential topics and the trimming of extraneous anatomical details. Although integration across subspecialties is widely recognised as essential, some integrative learning objectives have remained optional or have been left to students for self-integration. This approach assumes that students will independently develop a comprehensive and holistic understanding of anatomy.

Against this backdrop, there is a need for a comprehensive human anatomy resource that integrates the major anatomical subspecialties and highlights their clinical relevance. With this aim, we have compiled the current textbook to bring together the essential concepts of gross anatomy, histology, neuroanatomy, and embryology. We hope that this integrated resource will enrich students' learning experience and foster a deeper, more holistic understanding of human anatomy.

This textbook begins with the Foundation Topics on the structural organization of different primary tissues. We believe that a fuller understanding of the Foundation Topics along with some miscellaneous topics such as the skin, mammary gland, and lymph node, is essential to learning of the different body systems that are to follow. In this connection, simplified line diagrams were used to enhance student learning experience. All the diagrams were based on the original hand-drawn illustrations with colour chalks and more recently with colour pens and white board as adopted by Emeritus Professor Ling for the past five decades. Throughout this textbook, all the diagrams have been redrawn digitally by Dr Deepika for clarity and accuracy. Microscopic images, in colour, mostly stained with haematoxylin and eosin, and electron micrograph were used. The contents of this textbook follow the guiding learning objectives (practical classes and tutorials) prepared by the Department of Anatomy, NUS Medicine.

The Foundation Topics were followed sequentially by systemic anatomy beginning with the Respiratory System and the Cardiovascular System. Next to follow are the Renal System, Digestive System, Endocrine System, Reproductive System, Musculoskeletal System, Head & Neck, Back of Body, and Cranial nerves. For each system, the description begins with a general introduction. The explanation for each topic is reinforced with histological images and electron micrographs prepared by Emeritus Professor Ling; also, quizzes related to the applied and functional anatomy and clinical setting were included, where possible. All this are in line with the current system based curriculum.

It is important to emphasize that this textbook is far from being complete; it is, in fact, a preliminary version. Anticipated are some factual errors within its contents, but we are confident that these can be rectified and edited for improvement in future editions. The excellent technical, graphical, and secretarial assistance of Ms Bay Song Lin, Mr Yick Tuck Yong, Ms Catherine Ling, and former histological staff at the Department of Anatomy, NUS Medicine, is gratefully acknowledged.

Emeritus Professor Ling Eng Ang
Chief Editor

AUTHOR INFORMATION

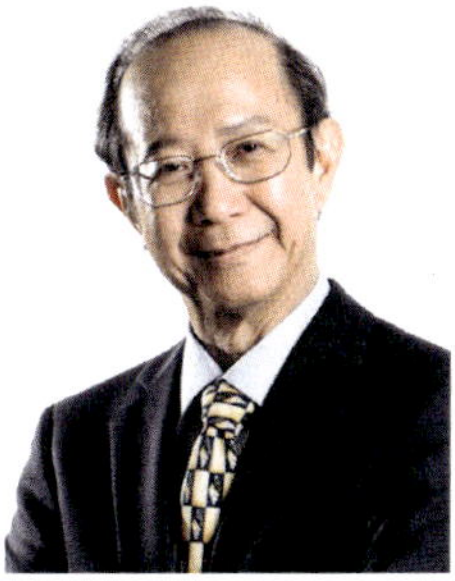

Emeritus Professor Ling Eng Ang (BSc, PhD, DSc)
Emeritus Professor Ling Eng Ang is a renowned academic in anatomy. With a career spanning five decades, he has become synonymous with his expertise and contributions to the field. He serves as the Chief Editor of this textbook, a testament to his extensive knowledge and expertise. His association with the Department of Anatomy at Yong Loo Lin School of Medicine dates back several decades. He has served as an Anatomy Educator for a remarkable fifty years, continuously imparting his knowledge and skills to students. His dedication to teaching has made a lasting impact on countless individuals in the field. He obtained his PhD in Cambridge under the supervision of Prof. E. Neville Willmer, an eminent British histologist. Subsequently, he did his post-doctoral fellowship in the laboratory of Prof. Charles Philippe Leblond, a renowned histologist and Canadian biologist. It was during this period that he developed a deep passion for histology and neuroanatomy, which later influenced his career path.

As Head of Anatomy at NUS from 1998 to 2008, he played a pivotal role in transforming the Department into a thriving center for human anatomy education. His vision and leadership guided the Department towards becoming a regional hub for human anatomy education in Asia. Among many notable contributions, one of which is developing the Anatomy Museum into one of the department's best learning resource centres.

Emeritus Professor Ling's dedication to anatomy and his unwavering commitment to excellence have earned him numerous accolades and recognition throughout his career. His expertise and passion for the field continue to inspire others, and his contributions have left an indelible mark on the field of anatomy.

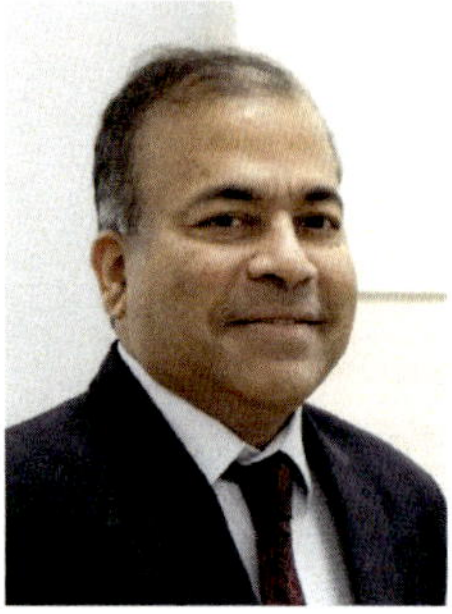

Professor S. Thameem Dheen (BSc, MSc, MPhil, PhD)
Professor S. Thameem Dheen is affiliated with the Department of Anatomy at the Yong Loo Lin School of Medicine, National University of Singapore. With over 20 years of experience in teaching anatomy, he has been deeply committed to educating students across various disciplines, including medicine, dentistry, nursing and allied health sciences. He is a strong advocate for the integration of digital tools in anatomy education.

Professor Dheen served as Head of the Department of Anatomy at NUS from 2016-2022. Under his leadership, the Department launched several digital platforms including the Anatomy e-Museum and the Human Anatomy Learning Resources (HALO). These initiatives offer interactive and immersive learning experiences, effectively bridging the gap between traditional anatomy teaching and evolving technological approaches. He believes that such initiatives not only enhance students' retention and comprehension but also foster a deeper appreciation of anatomy and its relevance to clinical practice.

As one of the editors of this textbook, Professor Dheen brings together his educational expertise, digital vision and academic leadership to deliver a resource that is aligned with the modern enhanced curriculum. This textbook reflects his commitment towards making anatomy more accessible, integrated and impactful for the next generation of healthcare professionals.

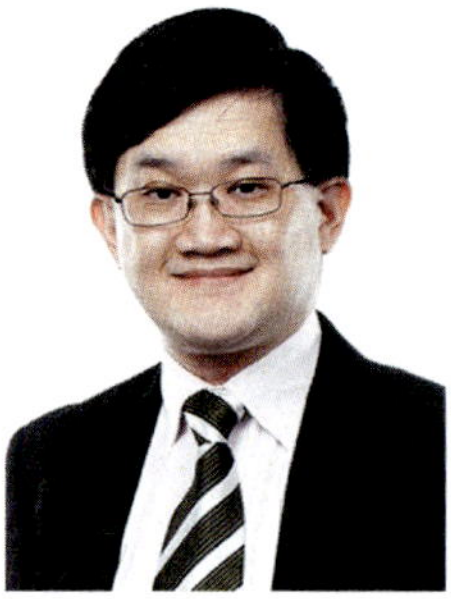

Associate Professor Yip Wai Cheong George (MBBS, PhD)
Associate Professor George Yip is the current Head of the Department of Anatomy at the Yong Loo Lin School of Medicine, National University of Singapore and is serving as one of the editors of this textbook. With extensive experience in teaching anatomy to undergraduate medical students and allied health professionals, Associate Professor Yip is deeply committed to advancing anatomy education. His teaching philosophy is anchored in the belief that anatomy forms the foundation of medical education, and he is dedicated to ensuring that students not only acquire knowledge of structures but also appreciate their clinical relevance.

His passion lies in developing innovative pedagogical approaches that enhance the students' learning experience. In particular, he has actively integrated technology into anatomy teaching, incorporating digital resources, interactive 3D models, and dynamic visualizations to deepen students' understanding of complex anatomical structures.

Beyond undergraduate education, Associate Professor Yip contributes actively to continuing education training initiatives within the School, supporting postgraduate residents across various medical disciplines in expanding their anatomical knowledge.

These initiatives underscore his commitment to lifelong learning and his recognition of the importance of anatomy across all stages of medical training. His efforts not only enhance the learning experience at NUS but also contribute to the broader advancement of medical education in the region.

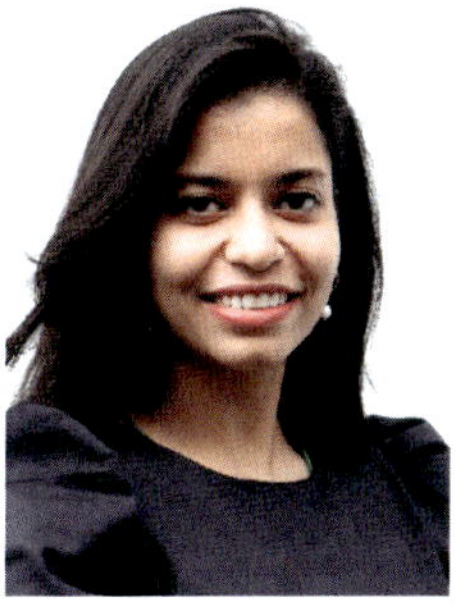

Dr. Deepika Kandilya (BSc, MSc, PhD)
Dr. Deepika Kandilya is a Lecturer in the Department of Anatomy, Yong Loo Lin School of Medicine, National University of Singapore. She is one of the editors of this textbook. She has passion for anatomy teaching and commitment to developing innovative pedagogies within the Department. Throughout the textbook, she has digitally redrawn all the hand-drawn illustrations originally created by Emeritus Professor Ling Eng-Ang. This collaborative effort has enhanced the accuracy and visual appeal of the illustrations. In addition to her artistic talents, Dr. Deepika has also played a significant role in formatting the final textbook using professional software. This journey has allowed her to further refine her pedagogy by considering the unique needs of a digital learning environment.

CONTENTS

Chapter 1

FOUNDATION TOPICS IN HUMAN ANATOMY

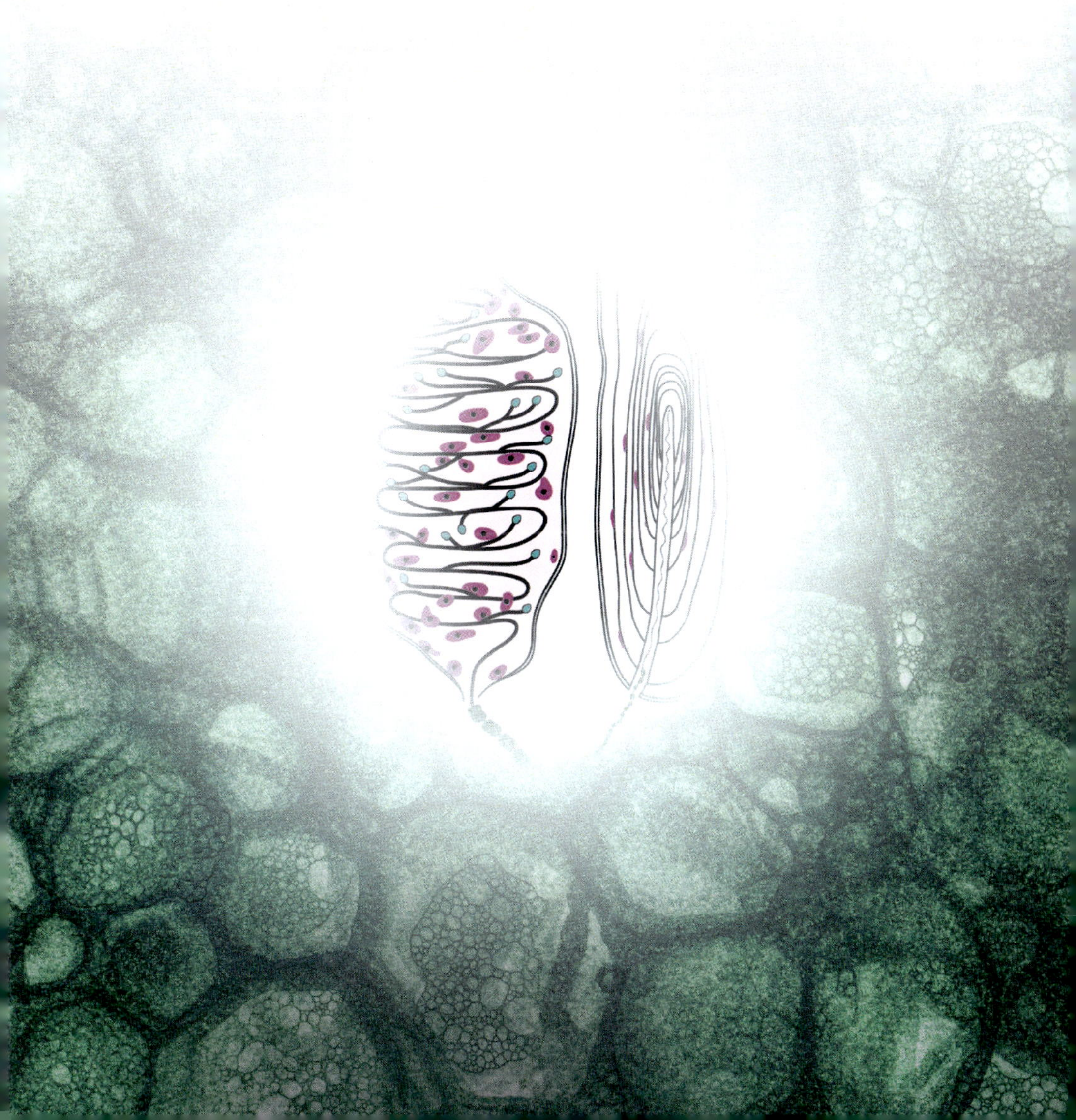

FOUNDATION TOPICS IN HUMAN ANATOMY

The human body is made up of multiple organ systems that are structurally and functionally interlinked. All these systems work together in synchrony to maintain normal physiological functions and execute physical activities.

Each system comprises various organs and structures which are built from primary tissues. The study of microscopic features of tissues and their physiological correlations is known as histology. A thorough understanding of the tissue organization is essential to the study of anatomy and physiology as all organs and body systems are formed from four basic types of primary tissues as follows:

1. Epithelial tissue
2. Connective tissue
3. Muscular tissue
4. Nervous tissue

EPITHELIAL TISSUE

The epithelial tissue or epithelium is a cellular membrane that lines the body surfaces (e.g., epidermis of the skin), body "tubes" (e.g., the lining of the respiratory passage and digestive tracts, and the endothelial lining of heart chambers and blood vessels) and body cavities (e.g., mesothelium (serous) lining of the pleural, pericardial, and peritoneal cavities). The epithelial tissue performs a variety of functions including protection, absorption, secretion, excretion, filtration and sensory functions. The epithelia are classified into different types based on their cell shapes: squamous (flattened), cuboidal or columnar, or number of cell layers: simple (single-layered) or stratified (multi-layered). All the epithelia rest on a supporting basement membrane, which separates the epithelium from the underlying connective tissue which provides structural support and contains blood vessels, lymphatic vessels, and nerves. A characteristic feature of epithelial tissue is that it is avascular (lack of blood vessels). Consequently, epithelial cells obtain oxygen and nutrients by diffusion from capillaries located in the underlying connective tissue across the basement membrane. Although the epithelium is avascular, terminal endings of sensory nerve fibers extend into epithelial layers. For example, free nerve endings responsible for pain sensation (nociception) are present within the epidermis of the skin.

Epithelial cells are tightly bound to one another by specialized intercellular junctions, including tight junctions, adherens junctions, desmosomes, gap junctions, and hemidesmosomes. These junctions maintain tissue integrity, facilitate communication between cells, and contribute to the specialized functions of different epithelia.

Types of Epithelia

A. Simple squamous epithelium (Fig. 1.1A, B, C; Fig. 1.2A, B)

It consists of single layer of thin, flattened cells whose nuclei bulge into the lumen or cavity. In a three-dimensional view, the cells appear as "fish scales". Because these cells are thin and flat, they facilitate the transport of ions, oxygen, metabolites, and glucose, across the tissue. Examples include the lining of blood and lymphatic vessels, known as the endothelium and the serous body cavities, such as peritoneal cavity, known as the mesothelium. In the heart chambers, the lining cells are called the endocardium. In the lungs, simple squamous epithelium forms the walls of the alveoli and plays an important role in gas exchange.

B. Stratified squamous epithelium (non-keratinized) (Fig. 1.1D; Fig. 1.2C)

It consists of multi-layered flattened cells.The lining cells are constantly sloughed off due to "wear and tear" and are continuously replenished by the new cells generated by proliferation. Examples include the lining epithelium of the oral cavity, oropharynx, esophagus, vagina, etc.

C. Stratified squamous epithelium (keratinized) (Fig. 1.1D; Fig. 1.2D)

It consists of multi-layered flattened cells with additional layer of keratin on top of the epithelium. An example is the skin. The epithelium provides protection against chemical and physical injuries.

D. Simple columnar epithelium (Fig. 1.1E; Fig. 1.2E)

It consists of the cells which have a prominent feature of striated or brush border (microvilli) for the absorption of water and nutrients. The height

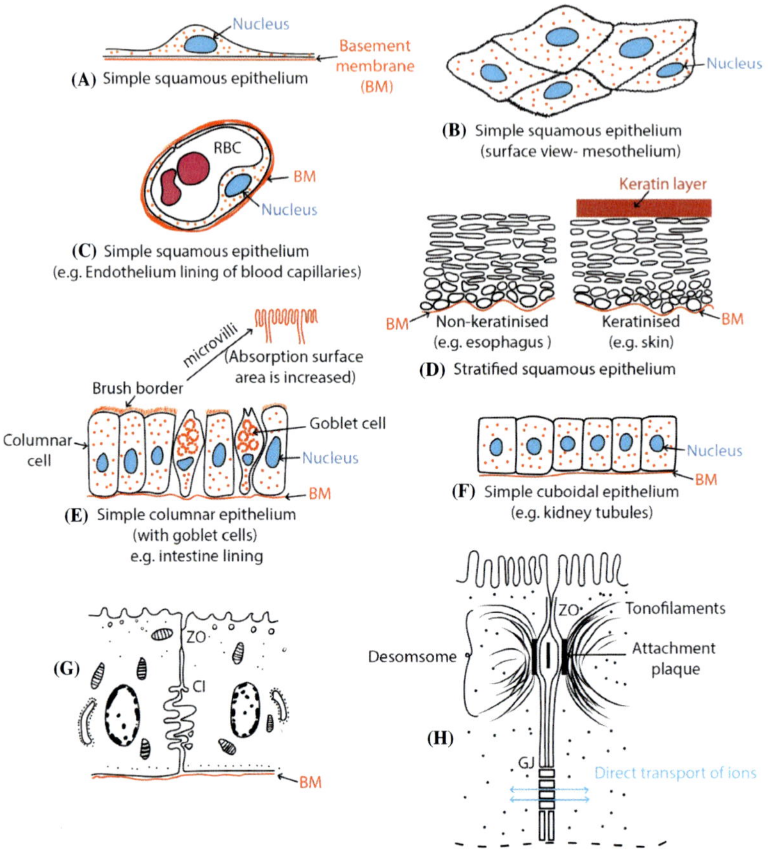

Cell junctions:

Epithelial cells are held togther by cell junctions.

1. Tight junctions - zona occludens (ZO) (tight seal) - Intercellular space is obliterated.
2. Cellular interdigitations (CI)
3. Desmosomes (macula adherens)
4. Gap junction (GJ) - nexus
   Direct communication between cells (e.g. intercalated discs in cardiac muscle)

Figure 1.1. Epithelial tissue. (A) Simple squamous epithelium. The flattened epithelium rests on a supporting basement membrane (BM). **(B)** Surface view of simple squamous epithelium, e.g., mesothelium lining the peritoneal cavity. **(C)** Simple squamous epithelium (endothelium) lines the lumen of the blood capillary. **(D)** Non-keratinized stratified squamous epithelium, e.g., esophagus, and keratinized squamous epithelium, e.g., skin. **(E)** Simple columnar epithelium rests on a layer of BM; an example of this is the lining of the intestines. Tall columnar cells and goblet cells make up the epithelium. **(F)** Simple cuboidal epithelium, e.g., lining epithelium of the renal tubules. **(G)** Intercellular digitations (CI) between two epithelial cells. **(H)** Desmosome. This holds two epithelial cells together with bundles of tonofilaments that are anchored to the attachment plaques. Showing also the gap junction (GJ) with microchannels that allow direct communication between cells (blue arrows).

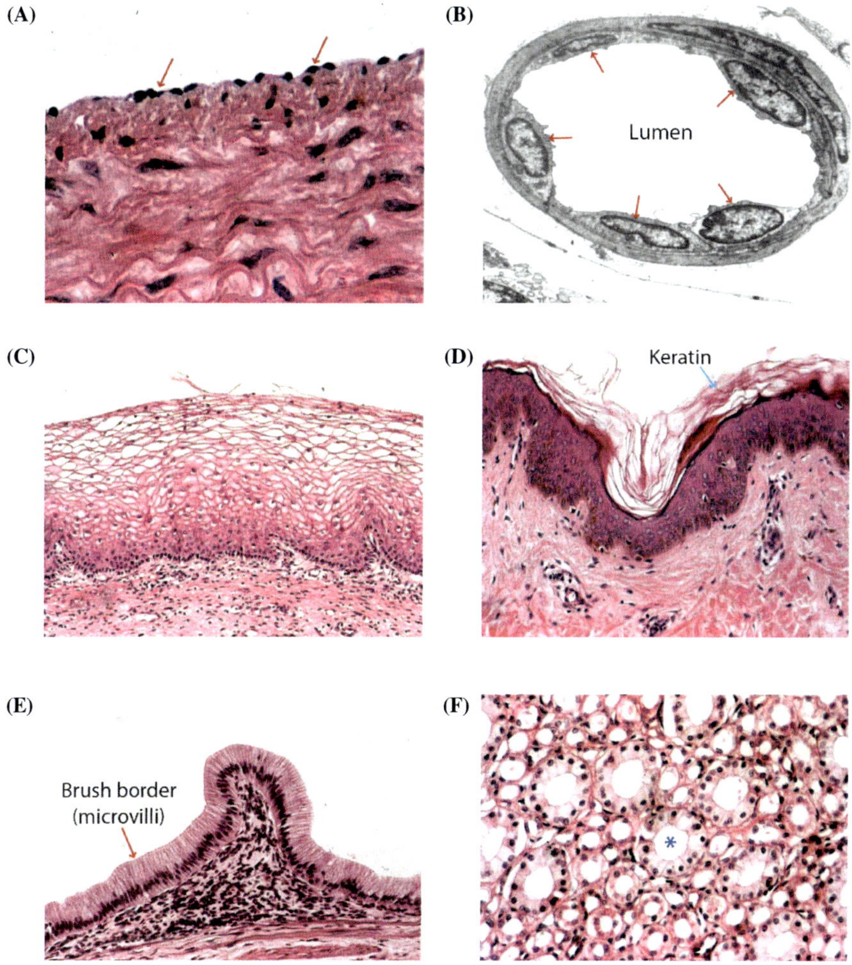

Figure 1.2. Epithelial tissue. (A) Simple squamous epithelium. The epithelial cells (arrows) line the lumen of a blood vessel. It is called the "endothelium." (Hematoxylin and eosin (H&E) stain.) **(B)** Electron micrograph showing the endothelial cells (arrows) lining the lumen of a blood vessel. Note the nucleus bulges into the vascular lumen. **(C)** Stratified squamous epithelium (non-keratinized). An example of this is the lining of the mucosa of the vagina. Note the flattened epithelial cells are multi-layered. (H&E stain.) **(D)** Stratified squamous epithelium (keratinized). The epithelium lines the thin skin. Note the keratin layer over the epithelium (arrow). (H&E stain.) **(E)** Simple columnar epithelium lines the mucosa of the gall bladder. Note that the lining cells possess a well-developed brush border (microvilli). (H&E stain.) **(F)** Simple cuboidal epithelium lines the renal tubules (collecting tubule) in the kidney (asterisk). (H&E stain.)

of the lining cells is greater than the width. Examples include the lining epithelium of the stomach, intestines, and gall bladder.

E. **Simple cuboidal epithelium (Fig. 1.1F; Fig. 1.2F)**

   It consists of cells which are cubical in shape. The luminal surface of the lining cells often shows a well-developed brush border or microvilli, which increases the surface area for absorption. An example of this includes the lining cells of the proximal convoluted tubule in the nephron.

F. **Pseudostratified ciliated columnar epithelium (Respiratory epithelium) (Fig. 1.3A, B, C; Fig. 1.4A)**

   It lines the respiratory passage and is known as the respiratory epithelium. The epithelium consists of the ciliated columnar cells, goblet cells which secrete mucous (glycoproteins), and basal cells located on the basement membrane. The basal cells are known to be germinative and undergo active proliferation to replace any cell loss. Examples include the lining epithelium of the nasal cavity, nasopharynx, trachea, and bronchus. The ciliated columnar cells present on the surface of the respiratory passage, propel the mucous and trapped dust particles or pathogens toward the pharynx, helping to keep the airways clear.

G. **Transitional epithelium (Urothelium) (Fig. 1.3D, E; Fig. 1.4B, C)**

   It lines the urinary system and is known as the urothelium, which is multi-layered. The surface cells facing the lumen are dome-shaped, referred to as the facet cells. The facet cells have specialized thickened plaques in the plasma membrane and help protect the cells against hyperosmotic urine. Examples include the renal pelvis, ureter, urinary bladder, and prostatic urethra. This epithelium also allows the stretching and relaxation of the bladder wall.

Types of Cell Junctions (Fig. 1.1G, H)

Epithelial cells are held together by cell junctions:

1. **Cellular interdigitations**

   This is the simplest configuration of cell junctions where finger-like projections of adjacent cell membranes interlock with each other and hold them together. This increases the surface area of contact and strengthen the cell junction. An example is the lining cells of the intestines.

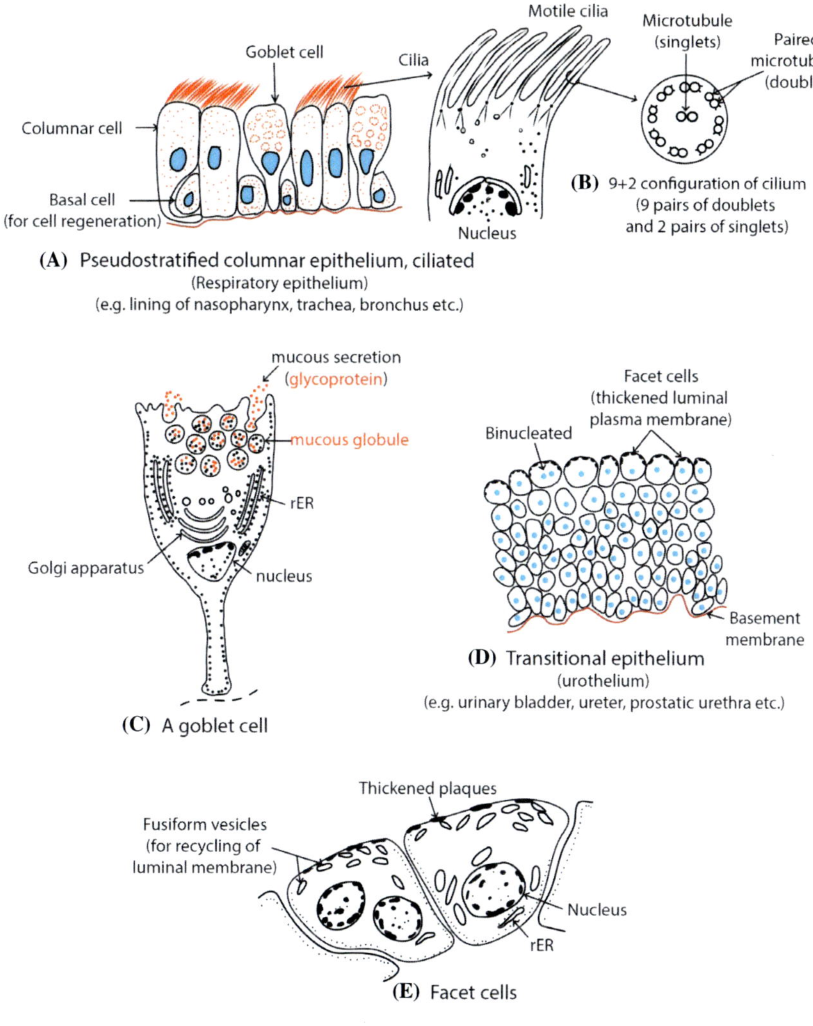

Figure 1.3. Epithelial tissue. (A) Pseudostratified columnar epithelium, ciliated (Respiratory epithelium), e.g., the lining of nasopharynx, trachea, and bronchus. It is composed of goblet cells, ciliated columnar cells, and basal cells. **(B)** Each cilium is composed of parallel arrays of microtubules (axoneme) arranged in nine peripheral doublets and two single singlets. **(C)** A goblet cell. It is filled with mucous globules (glycoprotein), which are discharged at the apical surface of the cell. **(D)** Transitional epithelium is also called the urothelium. It is confined mainly to the urinary system. **(E)** The top layer cells are called the "facet cells," which show thickened plaques in the luminal plasma membrane that protect against hyperosmotic urine.

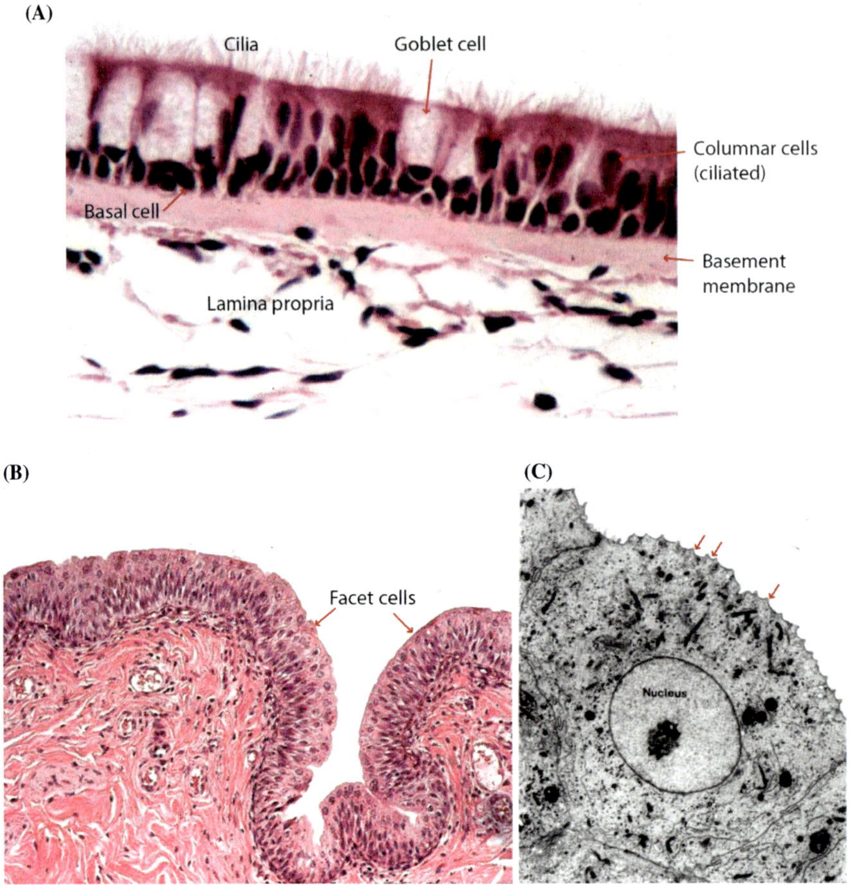

Figure 1.4. Epithelial tissue. (A) Pseudostratified columnar epithelium (ciliated). It lines the respiratory passage, e.g., the trachea, nasopharynx, and bronchus; hence, it is also called the respiratory epithelium. It is composed of columnar cells, goblet cells, and basal cells (stem cells). The epithelium rests on a layer of basement membrane overlying connective tissue bedding: lamina propria, which contains blood capillaries. (H&E stain.) **(B)** Transitional epithelium (urothelium). It lines the mucosa of the urinary bladder (also the ureter). Note that the epithelium is multi-layered. The top layer cells are dome-shaped and are called "facet cells" (arrows). (H&E stain.) **(C)** Electron micrograph showing a facet cell. The plasma membrane facing the lumen is thickened to form plaque-like structures (arrows) for protection against hypertonic urine.

2. Tight junctions (zonula occludens)

Tight junctions form a continuous belt around the apical region of adjacent epithelial cells. The outer leaflets of the apposed plasma membranes linked by sealing proteins, form a physical barrier preventing the passage or leakage of substances in the intercellular space. An example is the tight seal between the lining cells of the intestines.

3. **Desmosomes (macula adherens)**
   Desmosomes are spot-like adhesion junctions that provide strong mechanical attachment between adjacent cells. The intercellular space is wider than in tight junctions and contains adhesion proteins (cadherins). It has specialized features on the cytoplasmic surface of the plasma membrane where the dense attachment plaques anchor tonofilaments for structural support. Examples include the cardiac muscle cells.
4. **Gap junctions (Nexus)**
   Gap junctions consist of specialized protein channels (connexons) that directly connect the cytoplasm of adjacent cells. These channels allow the passage of ions and small molecules between cells. Example includes the cardiac muscle cells at the intercalated discs. In cardiac muscle, gap junctions allow rapid spread of depolarization from one myocyte to another, enabling coordinated contraction of the heart.

CONNECTIVE TISSUE

Connective tissue derives its name from its primary function of connecting, binding, and supporting other tissues and organs in the body. It provides the structural framework that maintains the shape and integrity of body structures.

Based on its structure and function, connective tissue can be classified into several types. Despite their differences, all connective tissues share a common basic structure consisting of cells embedded within an extracellular matrix composed of ground substance and fibers. Various types of intercellular fibers are distributed throughout this matrix. Although connective tissues share similar basic features, they differ in the types and numbers of cells present, the composition and arrangement of fibers, and the amount of ground substance. These variations allow connective tissues to perform specialized functions in different regions of the body.

The following sections describe the histological features of the various types of connective tissue.

(A) Loose Connective Tissue (Fig. 1.5; Fig. 1.6)

Loose connective tissue, also known as areolar tissue, is found in the dermis immediately beneath the epidermis. This tissue provides a supportive "bedding"

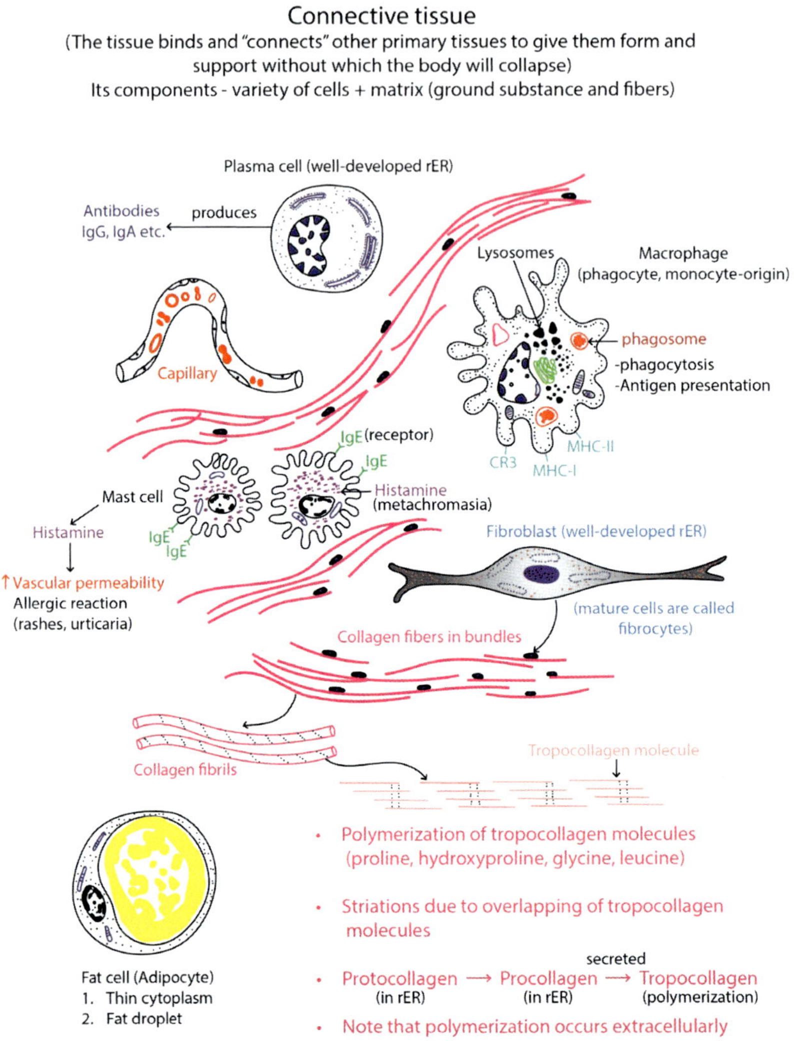

Figure 1.5. Connective tissue. Different cell types in the loose connective tissue: plasma cells, macrophages, mast cells, fat cells (adipocytes) and fibroblasts (fibrocytes), and intercellular matrix (collagen fibers and ground substance). The collagen fibers are produced by the fibroblast, which first synthesizes protocollagen in the cisternae of rER and procollagen. The procollagen molecules are released extracellularly as tropocollagen molecules, which then polymerize to form the collagen fibrils.

for the overlying epidermis and helps anchor tissues and organs in place. In addition, it serves several important functions, including thermoregulation, immune defense, and tissue repair. Loose connective tissue contains a variety of cell types, each contributing to specific functions within the tissue.

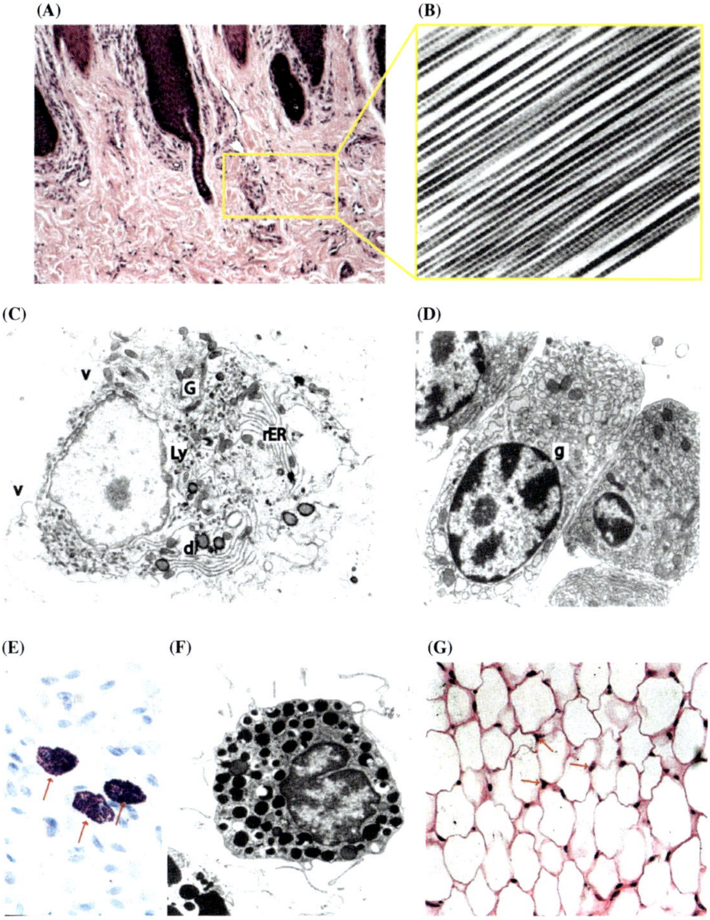

Figure 1.6. Connective tissue. (A) Loose connective tissue in the papillary layer of the skin (boxed area). Note the bundles of collagen fibers stained with eosin (pink). The small dense dots in between them are fibroblasts (fibrocytes). Their nuclei are stained with the hematoxylin stain. **(B)** Electron micrograph shows parallel arrays of collagen fibrils. Note the cross striations on each collagen fibril. **(C)** Electron micrograph shows a macrophage (phagocyte). Its cytoplasm is enriched with lysosomes (Ly), Golgi apparatus (g), lipid droplets (d), and cisternae of rough endoplasmic reticulum (rER). The nucleus exhibits margination of chromatin clumps. **(D)** Electron micrograph shows plasma cells. The cell shows a well-developed rough endoplasmic reticulum. The Golgi apparatus (g) is near the nucleus. Its nucleus is characterized by dense chromatin clumps (heterochromatin). **(E)** Three mast cells (arrows) stained with Toluidine blue. Note that the cytoplasm is laden with massive purple granules containing histamine. The preponderant light blue cells in the same field are fibroblasts (fibrocytes). **(F)** Electron micrograph shows a mast cell filled with dense granules. The cell surface shows microvillus projections. Its nucleus shows dense chromatin clumps (heterochromatin). **(G)** Adipose tissue. Note that the closely packed fat cells show a thin rim of cytoplasm (pink). The dense flattened nucleus (arrows) of the cells is compressed to the side. The fat contents of the cells were dissolved during tissue processing; hence, the cells appear empty. (H&E stain.)

Cell Types

1. **Fibroblasts/fibrocytes (Fig. 1.5; Fig. 1.6A, B)**
   They are the predominant cell type in the loose connective tissue. The cells are spindle-shaped (fusiform) and can undergo proliferation during tissue injuries. They are involved in wound healing and scar formation. Fibroblasts synthesize and secrete procollagen molecules, which polymerize extracellularly to become the tropocollagen. The tropocollagen molecules (proline and lysine) assemble to form the collagen fibrils. This process involves the alignment and staggered arrangement of tropocollagen units, producing the characteristic striated appearance of collagen fibrils. Collagen fibrils aggregate to form collagen fibers, which further organize into collagen bundles. In routine histological sections stained with haematoxylin and eosin (H&E), collagen bundles appear pink due to eosin uptake. These collagen bundles provide tensile strength and structural support to various tissues and organs, including tendons and ligaments.
2. **Macrophages (Fig. 1.5; Fig. 1.6C)**
   Macrophages, also known as phagocytes, are responsible for the engulfment and digestion of dead cells, cellular debris, and pathogens. They often exhibit irregular outlines with pseudopodial extensions that aid in their phagocytic activity. In addition to phagocytosis, macrophages play a key role in the immune response by functioning as antigen-presenting cells (APCs). The cytoplasm of macrophages contains numerous lysosomes rich in hydrolytic enzymes that facilitate intracellular digestion. Their plasma membrane expresses major histocompatibility complex (MHC) class I and II molecules, as well as complement receptors such as CR3, which assist in immune recognition and phagocytosis.
3. **Plasma cells (Fig. 1.5; Fig. 1.6D)**
   They are derived from B lymphocytes following exposure to foreign antigens. They characteristically exhibit basophilic cytoplasm. On electron microscopy, the cytoplasm shows abundant, well-developed cisternae of rough endoplasmic reticulum, reflecting their active role in the synthesis of antibodies (immunoglobulin proteins).
4. **Mast cells (Fig. 1.5; Fig. 1.6E, F)**
   They are large cells containing numerous coarse basophilic granules rich in histamine. The cell surface is covered with many microvilli bearing IgE

receptors. Interaction between specific allergens and the IgE receptors results in the release of histamine, causing allergic inflammatory reactions. Histamine-containing granules in mast cells stain purple with basic dyes (such as toluidine blue) due to their high content of acid mucopolysaccharides (glycosaminoglycans). This characteristic color change is known as metachromasia.

5. **Fat cells/Adipocytes (Fig. 1.5; Fig. 1.6G)**

   The fat cells contain fat droplets and have a thin rim of cytoplasm. The nucleus is eccentrically placed at the periphery of the cell.

6. **Intercellular fibers (Fig. 1.5; Fig. 1.6A, B)**

   There are three types of intracellular fibers in the connective tissues: collagen, reticular, and elastic.

   - The collagen fibers are present in abundance in loose connective tissue and many other types of connective tissues. They provide high tensile strength and structural support.
   - The reticular fibers are synthesized by specialized fibroblasts known as reticular cells. They resemble collagen fibrils but have a higher carbohydrate content on their surface. They form the structural framework for lymphoid organs, such as the spleen.
   - The elastic fibers are branched and non-striated and are composed of elastin. They provide elasticity and resilience, allowing tissues to stretch and recoil. They are abundant in elastic cartilage and the walls of large arteries.

   Clinical Correlation: Keloids result from excessive production and deposition of collagen during wound healing.

7. **Blood capillaries**

   Blood capillaries are small blood vessels that:

   - Deliver oxygen and nutrients to connective tissue cells.
   - Remove carbon dioxide and metabolic waste products.
   - Facilitate the exchange of substances between blood and surrounding tissues, helping maintain tissue viability.

8. **Nerve fibers**

   Nerve fibers are present throughout connective tissue and provide both sensory (pain, temperature, and touch) and autonomic innervation. Autonomic nerve fibers innervate the sweat glands, smooth muscles in the vascular walls and the arrector pili muscles associated with the hair follicle. They regulate vasoconstriction and vasodilation of blood vessels (vasomotor), sweat secretion by sweat glands (sudomotor) and contraction of the arrector pili muscles (pilomotor), causing the hair to stand erect (goosebumps).

B. Dense Regular Connective Tissue

It is composed of abundant, densely packed collagen fibres arranged in parallel bundles. Between the collagen bundles are small, flattened fibrocytes, while other cell types are sparse or absent. It contains only a few capillaries. Examples include tendons, ligaments, and aponeurosis.

C. Dense Irregular Connective Tissue

It consists of thick collagen bundles arranged in an irregular and interwoven pattern. Fibroblasts are the predominant cell type, with other connective tissue cells present in smaller numbers. Examples include the fibrous capsules of joints (e.g. the shoulder joint), the capsules of organs (e.g. the spleen), and the dermis of the skin.

In both dense regular and dense irregular connective tissues, the cells and fibres are embedded in a ground substance rich in glycosaminoglycans (GAGs). This hydrated extracellular matrix provides structural support, facilitates the diffusion of nutrients and waste products, and serves as the medium through which immune cells migrate during tissue injury and infection.

MUSCULAR TISSUE

The muscle tissue is composed of muscle fibers. Each muscle fiber represent a single muscle cell. Muscle is specialized for contraction which enables movement of the body and posture maintenance. There are three types of muscle: skeletal muscle, cardiac muscle, and smooth muscle.

A. Skeletal Muscle (Fig. 1.7A; Fig. 1.8)

1. **General features:** This is named as skeletal muscle as it is attached to bones and is responsible for body movements. Contraction of skeletal muscles

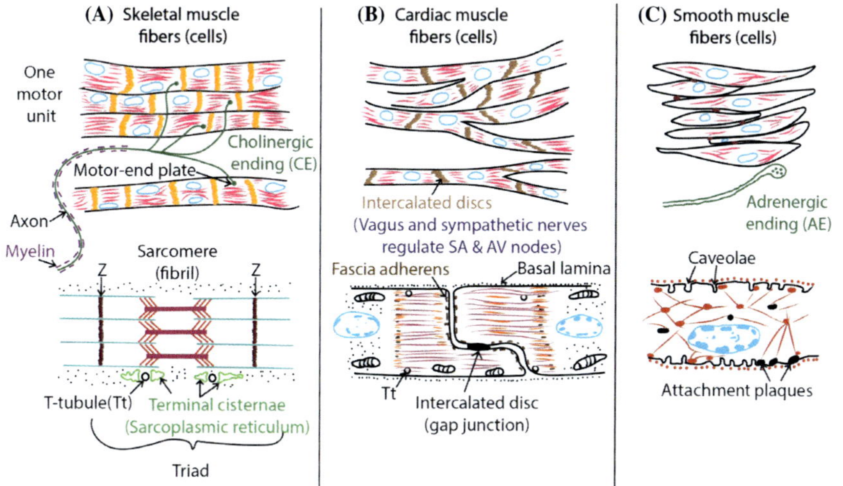

(A) Skeletal muscle fibers (cells)	(B) Cardiac muscle fibers (cells)	(C) Smooth muscle fibers (cells)
1. Contraction - Powerful - Rapid - Voluntary	1. Not under voluntary control, less forceful - Involuntary	1. Contraction - slow - sluggish - Involuntary
2. A, I bands - Striations	2. A, I bands - Striations	2. No striations
3. Myofibrils Sarcomere - Z ↔ Z lines	3. Myofibrils Sarcomeres	3. No sarcomeres
4. Triads - T tubule(Tt) - Sarcoplasmic reticulum (Calcium ions reservoir) - T tubule at A-I bands	4. Diads	4. Caveolae
5. Myoneural junction (synapse, motor-end plate)	5. Absent	5. Absent
6. Actin/myosin proteins	6. Actin/myosin proteins	6. Actin/myosin proteins
7. Multinucleated (peripheral nuclei)	7. Central nucleus (single)	7. Single nucleus
8. Glycogen +++	8. Glycogen +++	8. Glycogen +

Figure 1.7. Muscle tissue. There are three types of muscle tissues: **(A)** Skeletal muscle fibers (cells), **(B)** Cardiac muscle fibers (cells), and **(C)** Smooth muscle fibers (cells). Note that a "muscle fiber" is a "muscle cell" containing the contractile elements — actin and myosin myofilaments. The skeletal muscle cells are under voluntary control via the motor endplates, whereas the cardiac and smooth muscle cells are under involuntary control. Differences between the three types of muscle cells (fibers) in terms of structures are tabulated for comparison. Refer to the text for a detailed description of each muscle tissue.

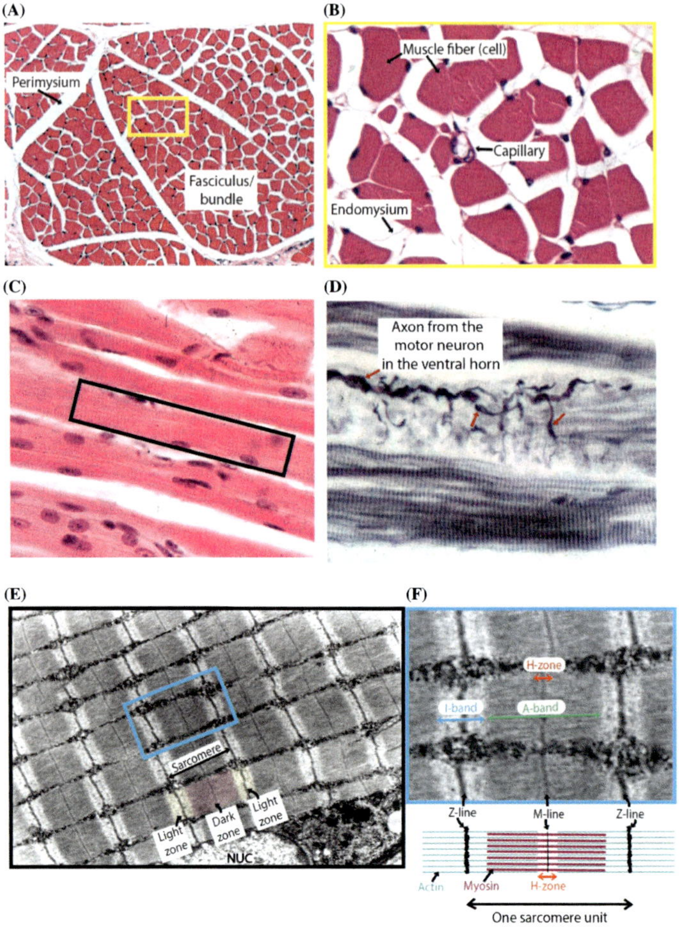

Figure 1.8. Skeletal muscle tissue. (A) Skeletal muscle fibers in a transverse section. The muscle fibers are grouped into bundles or fasciculi. Each fasciculus is surrounded by a layer of connective tissue, the perimysium. Note that a skeletal muscle fiber is a multinucleated cell whose nuclei are at the periphery. (H&E stain.) **(B)** An enlarged view of skeletal muscle fibers (cells) in a transverse section. Individual muscle fiber is surrounded by a thin layer of endomysium. A blood capillary (arrow) lies in the endomysium. (H&E stain.) **(C)** Skeletal muscle fibers in a longitudinal section. The boxed area represents a segment of a muscle fiber (cell). Note that the nuclei are located at the periphery. Faintly stained cross striations may be identified in the fiber. (H&E stain.) **(D)** Innervation of skeletal muscle fibers. A darkly stained axon, which originates from the ventral horn motor neuron, terminates as axonal swellings (arrows), forming the myoneural junctions (motor endplates) on the surface of muscle fiber. Arrival of an action potential along the axon causes depolarization and contraction of the muscle cell. (Bodian's stain.) **(E and F)** Electron micrograph. A portion of a skeletal muscle fiber (cell). The nucleus (NUC) is at the lower part of the image. The cytoplasm (sarcoplasm) contains dense glycogen masses. Parallel arrays of myofibrils (outlined in blue) show light and dark bands. The white band is bisected by the Z-line. The segment of the myofibril extending from one Z-line to another is a "sarcomere" composed of a staggering arrangement of myofilaments (actin and myosin).

moves bones at the joints enabling various voluntary activities. Skeletal muscle contraction is rapid and powerful and is under voluntary control.

The skeletal muscle is invested by layers of connective tissue, epimysium, perimysium and endomysium. At the microscopic level, the muscle is organized into many bundles or fasciculi (singular: fasciculus) **(Fig. 1.8A, B)**. Each fasciculus is surrounded by the perimysium. An individual muscle fiber (muscle cell) is surrounded by the endomysium. The epimysium, which is a dense connective tissue sheath, covers the entire muscle (eg., the biceps brachii). Blood vessels and nerve fibers travel within in the connective tissue coverings to supply and innervate the muscle fibers **(Fig. 1.8B)**.

2. **Contractile elements (Fig. 1.8C, E, F):** A skeletal muscle fiber is a long, multinucleated muscle cell with its nuclei located at the periphery beneath the plasma membrane, known as sarcolemma. The cytoplasm or sarcoplasm is densely packed with parallel arrays of myofibrils which are composed of the contractile elements: actin and myosin filaments. On microscopic examination, the parallel arrangement of actin and myosin filaments gives skeletal muscle its characteristic striated appearance, with alternating dark bands (A-bands) and light bands (I-bands). Each I-band is bisected by a Z-line (Z-disc), and the segment of myofibril between two adjacent Z-lines is called a sarcomere, the structural and functional unit of muscle contraction. The actin filaments are anchored to the "Z" line, while the myosin filaments lie between them with partial overlapping. The actin filament is composed of G-actin, tropomyosin, and the troponin complex, whereas each myosin molecule consists of a long tail and globular heads that possess ATPase activity. During muscle contraction, calcium ions (Ca^{2+}) released from the sarcoplasmic reticulum, a specialised form of smooth endoplasmic reticulum. Interaction between the two contractile filaments, with the availability of calcium ions, causes a "sliding filament mechanism" between them. This shortens the sarcomeres, resulting in the contraction of the entire muscle fiber.
3. **Innervation and contraction of muscle fiber:** The muscle fibers are innervated by the motor neurons whose cell bodies are located in the ventral horn of the spinal cord or in the motor nuclei of cranial nerves, such as the facial nerve. The axon of a motor neuron extends to the skeletal muscle fiber and the axon terminal contacts the sarcolemma of the skeletal muscle, to establish a neuromuscular junction, also known as the "motor end plate" **(Fig. 1.8D)**. When an action potential reaches the axon terminal,

the neurotransmitter acetylcholine (ACh) is released into the synaptic cleft. Acetylcholine binds to nicotinic acetylcholine receptors on the sarcolemma, causing depolarisation of the muscle fiber membrane. The action potential then travels along the sarcolemma and into the transverse (T) tubules (invaginations of the sarcolemma), where it triggers the sarcoplasmic reticulum to release calcium ions (Ca^{2+}). The close association of a T-tubule with two terminal cisternae of the sarcoplasmic reticulum forms a structure known as the "triad". The released calcium initiates the sliding filament mechanism which shortens the sarcomeres and ultimately produces contraction of the skeletal muscle fiber.

4. **Muscle spindles (neuromuscular spindles):** They are specialised sensory receptors (stretch) embedded within the skeletal muscle, near the myotendinous junction. They detect changes in muscle length and the rate of muscle stretch. Each muscle spindle contains specialised intrafusal muscle fibres, which are of two types: nuclear bag fibres and nuclear chain fibres. These fibres are innervated by sensory nerve fibers, namely annulospiral (primary) and flower-spray (secondary) fibers. When a muscle is stretched, the intrafusal fibres are also stretched, stimulating these sensory fibers. The resulting nerve impulses travel along afferent (sensory) fibres to the spinal cord, where they synapse directly with α-motor neurons. These motor neurons then stimulate the surrounding extrafusal muscle fibres to contract, opposing the stretch and restoring the muscle to its original length. This reflex response is known as the stretch reflex and is demonstrated clinically by the biceps tendon reflex. Thus, muscle spindles play an essential role in regulating muscle length, maintaining muscle tone, and coordinating posture and movement.

B. Cardiac Muscle (Fig. 1.7B; Fig. 1.9A, B)

The cardiac muscle is found exclusively in the heart wall and consists of three layers: the endocardium (inner layer), the myocardium (middle layer), and the epicardium (inner layer). The cardiac muscle forms the bulk of the myocardium, and contracts rhythmically and forcefully during ventricular systole to pump blood throughout the body. Unlike skeletal muscle, cardiac muscle contraction is involuntary and is regulated by the heart's intrinsic conducting system.

The cardiac muscle fibers are branched (or syncytial) and are uninucleated, with a centrally located nucleus. Adjacent cardiac muscle cells are connected by specialized cell junctions, the intercalated discs which provide both strong

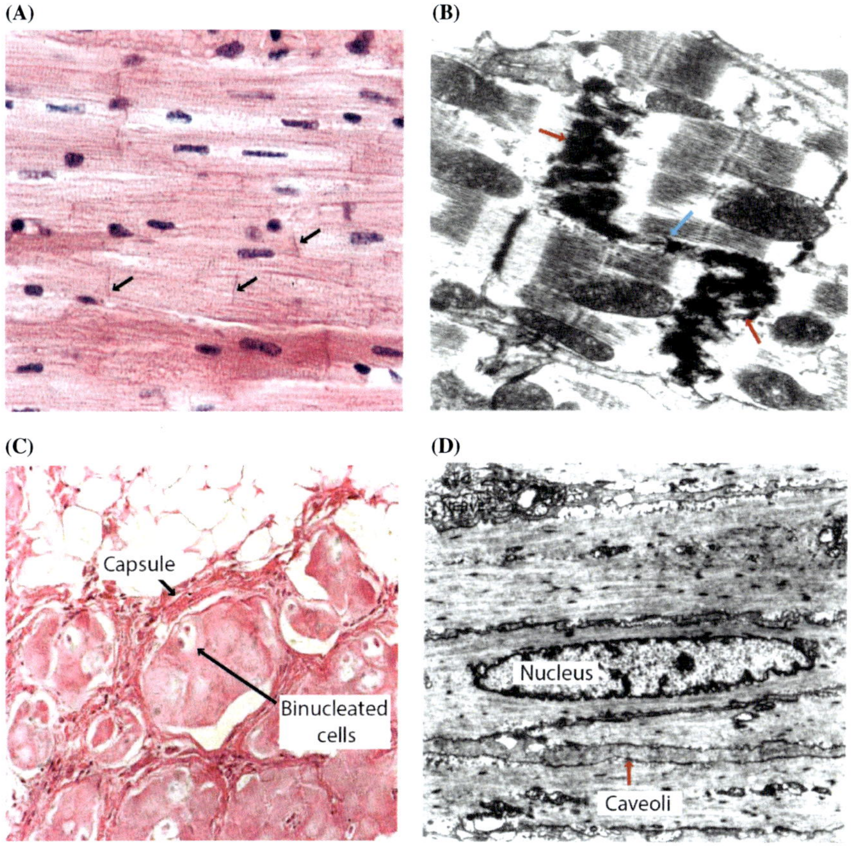

Figure 1.9. **(A)** Cardiac muscle fibers (tissue) in a longitudinal section. Arrows (red) indicate intercalated discs, which represent specialized junctions between cells. The nucleus is centrally located. (H&E stain.) **(B)** Electron micrograph of an intercalated disc. It is made up of two parts: transverse part (desmosomes or fascia adherens, red arrow) and the horizontal part (gap junction, blue arrow). Note the dark and light bands in the cell. **(C)** Purkinje fibers in a transverse section. They are in bundles enclosed by a layer of capsule (connective tissue) localized in the subendocardial region. Purkinje fibers are modified cardiac muscle fibers. They are binucleated cells (arrows). Intercalated discs are absent. Note that gap junctions are present between cells. The junctions facilitate the conduction of nerve impulses between cells. (H&E stain.) **(D)** Electron micrograph of smooth muscle fibers (cells) in a longitudinal section. Note that the cells are spindle-shaped or fusiform. The nucleus is centrally located. The plasma membrane (sarcolemma) shows many caveoli (invaginations) for the internalization of calcium ions from the exterior. Dense patches (circles) equivalent to Z-lines are widely distributed. Actin and myosin filaments are present. Note the lack of sarcomeres.

mechanical attachment and electrical continuity between cells. The intercalated discs not only hold the cells together but they also provide direct communications (gap junctions) for the transport of ions across the cells, such as Na^+, during cardiac muscle cell depolarization.

Microscopically, the cardiac muscle is striated with A- and I-bands on individual myofibrils and sarcomeres.

A unique feature of the cardiac muscles is the presence of intercalated discs, which represent specialized cell junctions as mentioned above. Cardiac muscle does not possess neuromuscular junctions (motor end plates). Instead, cardiac muscle cell contraction is initiated by the conducting system of the heart, beginning at the sinoatrial (SA) node (pacemaker). The electrical impulse then travels to the atrioventricular (AV) node, continues through the bundle of His and is distributed by the Purkinje fibers **(Fig. 1.9C)**, which are modified cardiac muscle fibers responsible for rapid electrical conduction. This coordinated conduction ensures the rhythmic contraction of the atria and ventricles.

The cardiac muscle contraction is is regulated by the autonomic nervous system (involuntary control). Both parasympathetic fibers, carried by the vagus nerve (cranial nerve X), and sympathetic nerve fibers which form the cardiac nerve plexus, innervate the SA and AV nodes to regulate the heart rate. Parasympathetic fibres decrease the heart rate, whereas sympathetic nerve fibres increase both the heart rate and the force of contraction.

Cardiac muscle cells have very limited regenerative capacity and do not proliferate significantly. Consequently, following injury, such as a myocardial infarction (heart attack), damaged cardiac muscle cells cannot be replenished by cell proliferation and are replaced by fibrous scar tissue, which may impair the pumping function of the heart.

C. Smooth Muscle (Fig. 1.7C; Fig. 1.9D)

The smooth muscle cells are spindle-shaped (fusiform), and uninucleated cells with a centrally located nucleus. Unlike skeletal and cardiac muscle, smooth muscle is non-striated because its contractile proteins are not arranged into sarcomeres. Consequently, A-bands, I-bands and sarcomeres are absent.

Although smooth muscle contains actin and myosin filaments, these filaments are arranged in an irregular network and are anchored to dense bodies within the cytoplasm and attachment plaques (dense plaques) on the sarcolemma, allowing the cell to contract efficiently. Unlike skeletal and cardiac muscle, smooth muscle lacks transverse (T) tubules. Instead, the sarcolemma contains numerous small flask-shaped invaginations called caveolae, which facilitate the entry of calcium ions (Ca^{2+}) required for muscle contraction.

The contractile elements and actin and myosin filaments are anchored to the dense bodies within the cytoplasm and attachment plaques (dense plaques) on the sarcolemma, allowing the cell to contract efficiently. Unlike skeletal and cardiac muscle, smooth muscle lacks transverse (T) tubules. Instead, the sarcolemma contains numerous small flask-shaped invaginations called caveolae, which facilitate the entry of calcium ions (Ca^{2+}) required for muscle contraction.

Smooth muscle is widely distributed throughout the body and is found in the muscularis externa in the gastrointestinal tract, tunica media of blood vessels, ureters, urinary bladdet, uterus, bronchus and ciliary body of the eye, arrector pili muscle associated with the hair follicle in the skin, and myoepithelial cells of mammary glands. Smooth muscle is involuntarily controlled and is innervated by autonomic nerve fibers (postganglionic sympathetic and postganglionic parasympathetic nerve fibers). Unlike skeletal muscle, smooth muscle does not possess specialised neuromuscular junctions.

Instead, autonomic nerve terminals release neurotransmitters, such as acetylcholine and noradrenaline (norepinephrine), from varicosities near the muscle cells, allowing the neurotransmitters to diffuse to their receptors. Electrical impulses may also spread from one smooth muscle cell to another cell via gap junctions, enabling coordinated contraction, particularly in single-unit (visceral) smooth muscle.

Smooth muscle contracts slowly, rhythmically, and in a sustained manner, making it well suited for functions such as peristalsis in the gastrointestinal tract, regulation of blood vessel diameter, and movement of urine through the ureters.

NERVOUS TISSUE

Classification

The nervous tissue is the main component of the nervous system which can be classified anatomically into:

1. **Central nervous system (CNS):** This comprises the brain and spinal cord.
2. **Peripheral nervous system (PNS):** It consists of cranial and spinal nerves and associated peripheral ganglia and sensory receptors.

Functionally, the nervous system is divided into:

1. **Somatic nervous system:** It is responsible for the innervation of structures derived from the embryonic somites, particularly skeletal muscles, enabling voluntary movement.
2. **Autonomic nervous system:** It is responsible for the innervation of smooth muscle, cardiac muscle, and glands, regulating involuntary body functions such as heart rate, digestion, and glandular secretion.

General Arrangement of Nervous Tissue

Histologically, the nervous tissue is composed of three main structural components (**Fig. 1.10**):

1. Neurons
2. Neuroglial cells
3. Blood vessels and the associated connective tissue elements

In this textbook, a segment of the spinal cord has been used as a model to illustrate the general arrangement of nervous tissue and cell types present in the CNS.

The brain and spinal cord are generally organized into two distinct regions: (A) gray matter and (B) white matter.

A. **Gray matter:** It consists of neuronal cell bodies, dendrites, synapses, and supporting neuroglial cells including astrocytes, oligodendrocytes and microglia. In the spinal cord, it is located around the central canal and appears as a butterfly-shaped area, where it is divided into different zones, namely, anterior (ventral), posterior (dorsal), and lateral horns.
B. **White matter:** It mainly consists of neuronal processes (mainly of myelinated axons), neuroglial cells and blood vessels. Nerve cell bodies are absent.

Classification of Neurons

Neurons are classified based on their functions as follows:

A. **Sensory (Afferent) neurons:** These neurons are located primarily in the dorsal root ganglion (sensory), attached to the spinal cord or in the cranial

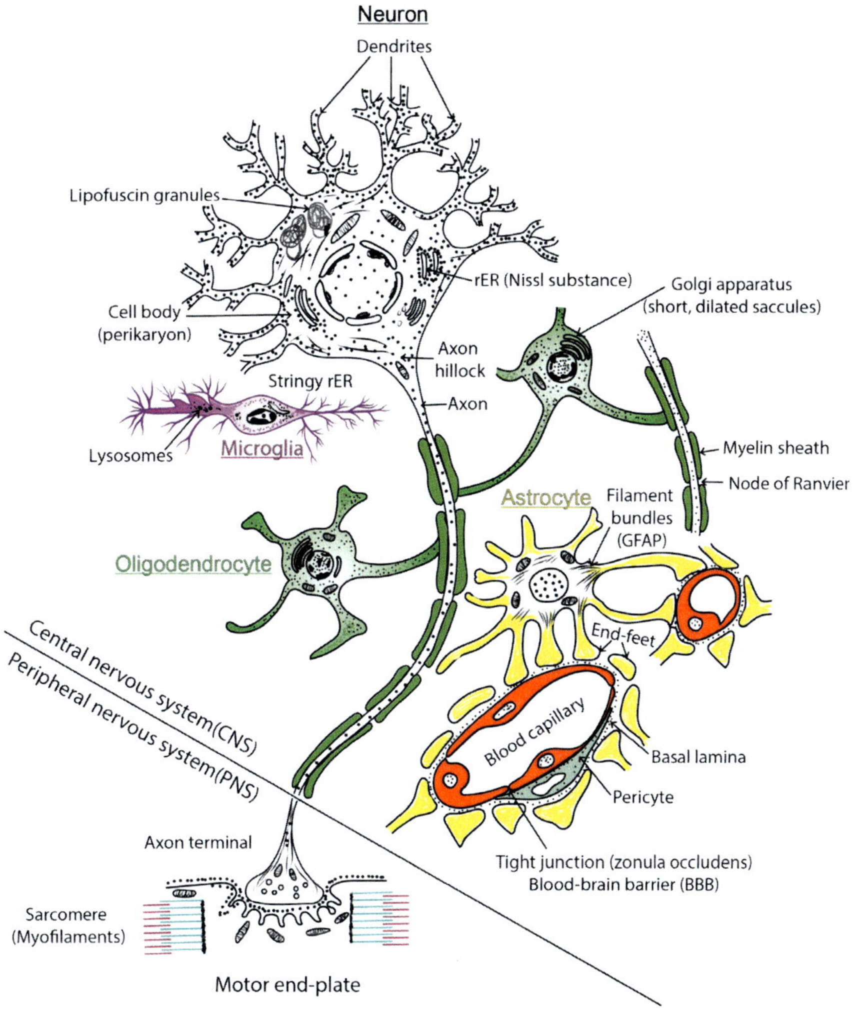

Figure 1.10. Nervous tissue. Showing the cellular components (neurons and neuroglia) of the nervous tissue in the central nervous system (CNS). The oblique line across the figure below marks the junction between the CNS and the peripheral nervous system (PNS). Note the motor neuron in the CNS innervates the muscle fiber (cell) at the motor endplate. The neuron has long branching dendrites and a long extending axon, which is insulated by a layer of myelin sheath formed by the oligodendrocytes. The astrocytes show radiating processes; some of them impinge on the outer walls of the blood capillary. Microglia are immune cells in the CNS.

ganglia associated with some cranial nerves, such as the trigeminal nerve. Their function is to receive sensory information from receptors and transmit it to the central nervous system (CNS).

B. **Motor (Efferent) neurons:** These neurons are distributed in the gray matter in the ventral or anterior horn of the spinal cord. They transmit impulses from the CNS to skeletal muscles, producing muscle contraction, or to glands, stimulating secretion.

C. **Interneurons:** They are located entirely within the CNS and form connections between sensory and motor neurons, as well as with other interneurons. They play an essential role in processing, integrating, and coordinating neural information and are generally smaller than motor neurons.

D. **Projection neurons:** These neurons have long axons that extend to distant regions of the CNS, allowing communication between different parts of the brain and spinal cord. In the spinal cord, many projection neurons are found in the dorsal horn.

Neurons are also classified according to the branching pattern of their processes: axons and dendrites. In general, each neuron has a single axon, which conducts nerve impulses away from the cell body (soma, perikaryon). The dendrites, which are variable in numbers, conduct impulse toward the cell body.

A. Unipolar and pseudounipolar neurons

1. **Unipolar neurons:** These neurons possess a single process extending from the cell body and are mainly found in the developing nervous tissue.
2. **Pseudounipolar neurons:** These are found primarily in the sensory ganglia of the peripheral nervous system such as the dorsal root (spinal) ganglion and the sensory ganglia of certain cranial nerves. They are sensory neurons. A single process arises from the cell body and bifurcates into two branches. The peripheral process functions like a dendrite, while the central process functions as an axon.

B. **Bipolar neurons:** These neurons possess one axon and one dendrite, arising from opposite poles of the cell body. They are found in the olfactory epithelium and the retina of the eye, where they transmit sensory information related to smell and vision respectively.

C. **Multipolar neurons:** These are the most common type of neurons and are found throughout the CNS. They possess one axon and multiple dendrites that radiate from the cell body, allowing them to receive input from many neurons. Typical examples include motor neurons in the ventral horn of the spinal cord, pyramidal neurons in the cerebral cortex, and Purkinje neurons in the cerebellar cortex.

Neurons in the brain may also be classified into Golgi Type I and Golgi Type II neurons, based on the length of their axons, as demonstrated by the Golgi silver staining method under the light microscope.

A. **Golgi Type I neurons:** They have long axons, multiple dendrites, and large cell bodies. Typical examples include pyramidal neurons in the cerebral cortex and motor neurons in the ventral horn of the spinal cord.
B. **Golgi Type II neurons:** They have short axons and many branching dendrites radiating from a stellate-shaped cell body. Examples include stellate interneurons of the cerebral cortex and granule cells of the cerebellar cortex.

A Typical Neuron (Fig. 1.10; Fig. 1.11A, B)

Structural Parts

A typical neuron of the central nervous system (e.g., a motor neuron) consists of three structural parts:

1. Perikaryon (soma or cell body)
2. Dendrites
3. Axon

A. **Perikaryon (soma):** The perikaryon or cell body contains a large round nucleus with a prominent nucleolus and predominantly euchromatin, reflecting its high level of transcriptional activity. The cytoplasm contains patchy basophilic structures known as the Nissl substance (Nissl bodies), which correspond to aggregates of free ribosomes and rough endoplasmic reticulum seen under the electron microscope. Following axonal injury, the neuron undergoes chromatolysis or axonal reaction, during which the Nissl substance disperses, and the cytoplasm darkens. Under the electron microscope, the cytoplasm shows the presence of microtubules,

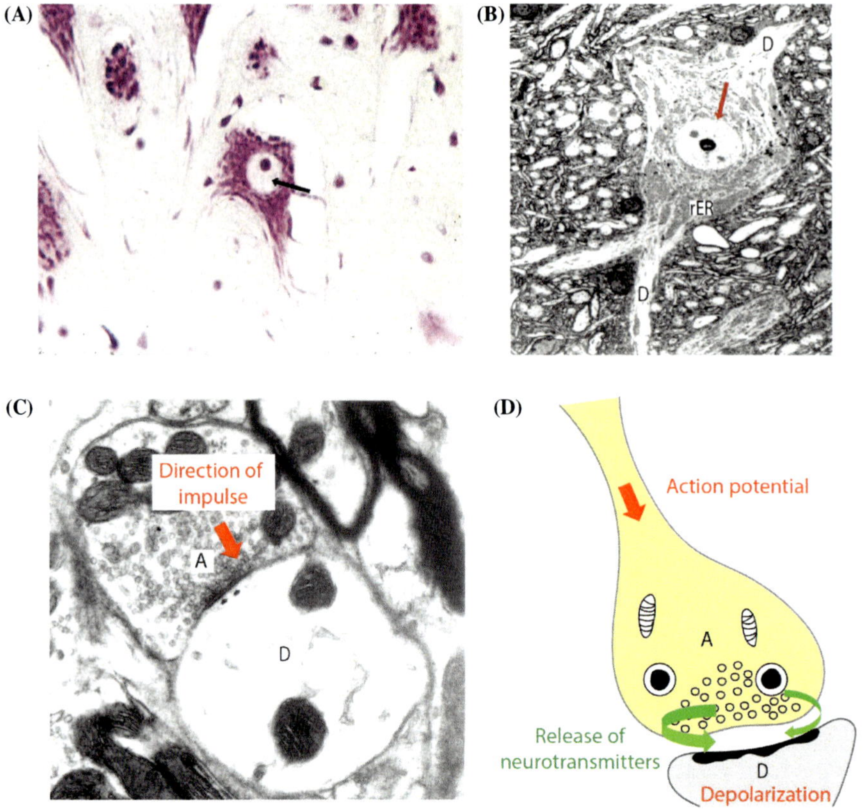

Figure 1.11. Nervous tissue — CNS. (A) A motor neuron in the cerebral cortex stained with cresyl fast violet. (Nissl stain.) The pale nucleus (arrow) shows a conspicuous nucleolus. The cytoplasm is rich in Nissl substance. **(B)** Electron micrograph of a motor neuron in the spinal cord. The pyramidal-shaped cell body shows a projection of dendrites. The nucleus (arrow) contains mainly euchromatin and a distinct nucleolus. ***Quiz:*** *What is the function of the nucleolus?* The cytoplasm has abundant cisternae of rough endoplasmic reticulum (Nissl substance) responsible for protein synthesis. **(C)** Electron micrograph showing a typical axo-dendritic synapse between an axon (A) and a dendrite (D). The axon terminal contains many presynaptic vesicles bearing neurotransmitters, e.g., acetylcholine. Both the pre- and postsynaptic membranes are thickened (double arrowheads). Red arrow indicates the direction of the impulse. **(D)** The arrival of axon potential (red arrow) at the axon terminal (A) triggers the release of a neurotransmitter (curved green arrows) into the synaptic cleft. The neurotransmitter either excitatory or inhibitory initiates the depolarization of dendrite (D).

neurofilaments, microfilaments, smooth endoplasmic reticulum, Golgi apparatus, lipofuscin granules, and mitochondria.

B. **Dendrites:** They are highly branched neuronal processes that receive synaptic inputs from other neurons and transmit these signals toward the cell body (soma). Structurally, dendrites resemble the perikaryon because they contain cytoplasm with organelles involved in protein synthesis. The proximal portions of dendrites contain cisternae of rough endoplasmic reticulum, neurofilament bundles, microtubules, free ribosomes, mitochondria, and smooth endoplasmic reticulum. The rough endoplasmic reticulum gradually becomes less abundant in the distal branches. The Golgi apparatus is generally confined to the cell body and may occasionally extend into the proximal dendrite.

Most dendrites possess numerous irregular projections called dendritic spines, which increase the surface area available for synaptic contacts and play an important role in synaptic plasticity, including learning and memory. The dendritic spines generally lack microtubules but contain actin filaments along with occasional ribosomes. Under the electron microscope, the dendritic spine head is characterized by an electron-dense postsynaptic density and actin-rich cytoskeleton.

C. **Axon:** A neuron typically has a single axon that originates from the axon hillock, followed by the axon initial segment and the axon proper. The axon gives rise to terminal branches that end as synaptic boutons (terminal boutons or end bulbs), which form synapses with target cells.

The axon hillock is a funnel-shaped region that serves as the transition between the soma and the axon. The axon initial segment is the site where action potentials are initiated because it contains a high density of voltage-gated sodium channels. Ultrastructurally, the initial segment is characterized by bundles of microtubules and neurofilaments, very few ribosomes, and a specialized submembranous dense undercoat (membrane-associated cytoskeleton).

The axon proper contains microtubules, neurofilaments, smooth endoplasmic reticulum, mitochondria and numerous transport vesicles. These structures support axonal transport between the cell body and the axon terminals. In contrast to the soma and proximal dendrites, the axon lacks free ribosomes, rough endoplasmic reticulum, and the Golgi apparatus.

Axons may be myelinated or unmyelinated. In the CNS, myelin around the axon is produced by oligodendrocytes, whereas in the PNS, myelin is produced by Schwann cells. A single oligodendrocyte can myelinate multiple axons, whereas each Schwann cell myelinates a single segment of one axon.

Axonal Transport

Although the axon contains most of the organelles, it lacks rough endoplasmic reticulum and the Golgi apparatus. Therefore, most proteins and membrane components required by the axons and its terminals are synthesized in the cell body (soma) and transported along the axon. Axonal transport is classified into two major types:

a. *Slow axonal transport* (1 mm/day): This transport primarily carries tubulin and neurofilament proteins as well as other soluble proteins required for the growth and maintenance of the axon.
b. *Fast axonal transport* (10 to 1000 mm/day): Fast axonal transport occurs not only in an anterograde direction (from the cell body to the axon) but also in a retrograde direction or reverse manner (axon to cell body). Fast anterograde transport carries membrane-bound organelles, synaptic vesicles, mitochondria, membrane proteins, enzymes and neurotransmitter precursors to the axon terminals. Fast retrograde transport returns endocytic vesicles, worn-out organelles, and neurotrophic factors from the axon terminals to the cell body for recycling.

Horseradish peroxidase (HRP), the neuronal protein tracer, has been widely used to identify and trace the origin of neuronal pathway in experimental neuroanatomy. In such experiments, the HRP is taken up at axon terminals or injured axons and transported retrogradely to the cell body (soma).

Synapse

a. *General features and classification*

A synapse is a specialized cell junction through which a neuron communicates with another neuron or an effector cell (such as a muscle cell). Most synapses occur between the axon terminal of one neuron and another neuron. When the contact is between an axonal terminal and a skeletal muscle cell, it is called a neuromuscular (myoneural) junction. The primary function of a synapse is to transmit nerve impulses from one cell to another.

This section focuses on synapses in the CNS. Based on the synaptic configurations, synapses are classified as follows:

i) *Axodendritic synapse:* The most common type, in which an axon terminal forms a synapse with a dendritic process, most frequently on a dendritic spine.
ii) *Axoaxonic synapse:* A synapse between the axon terminal of a neuron and the axon or axon terminal of another neuron.
iii) *Axosomatic synapse:* A synapse between the axon terminal and the soma of another neuron.

The most common type of synapse is the axodendritic and axosomatic. There are rare synapse types which include dendro-dendritic synapse which occurs between the dendrites of two neurons and somatosomatic synapse which occurs between the cell bodies (somata) of two neurons.

The synapse are further classified into two main categories based on their structures and mechanism of signal transmission.

i) *Chemical synapse:* This is the most common type of synapse. Transmission occurs through the release of neurotransmitters across a synaptic cleft and is unidirectional.
ii) *Electrical synapse:* This is formed by a gap junction (nexus), which allows rapid conduction and is often bidirectional.

(b) *Ultrastructure of a synapse* (**Fig. 1.11C, D**):
Under the electron microscope, a typical synapse consists of three main components:

i) Presynaptic terminal: Presynaptic membrane of an axon terminal (end bulb, or bouton terminal) containing numerous synaptic vesicles.
ii) Synaptic cleft: A narrow extracellular space that separates the pre and postsynaptic membranes.

iii) Postsynaptic membrane: The specialized membrane of the receiving neuron, located on a dendrite, dendritic spine and soma. It contains an electron-dense postsynaptic density (PSD).

Both the presynaptic and postsynaptic membranes are electron-dense specializations. The postsynaptic membrane is thicker due to the presence of the postsynaptic density (PSD), previously referred to as the subsynaptic web. The PSD is a protein-rich specialization containing neurotransmitter receptors and intracellular signaling molecules. The synaptic cleft is approximately 200–300Å (20–30 nm) wide and contains extracellular matrix proteins and cell adhesion molecules, which maintain close apposition between the pre- and postsynaptic membranes and facilitate efficient synaptic transmission. The cytoplasm of the presynaptic axon terminal contains numerous synaptic vesicles, mitochondria and cytoskeletal elements. Synaptic vesicles measure approximately 400 and 600Å (40–60 nm) in diameter. They store neurotransmitters and release them into the synaptic cleft by exocytosis. Two principal types of synaptic vesicles are recognized: a) small clear (agranular) vesicles and b) dense-core vesicles, which are generally larger than small clear vesicles.

Historically, cholinergic synapses were described as containing predominantly small clear vesicles, whereas adrenergic and noradrenergic synapses were characterized by the presence of dense-core vesicles. However, it is now recognized that vesicle morphology alone is not sufficient to identify the neurotransmitter present, as many neurons contain multiple synaptic vesicle populations.

Some neurons may release more than one neurotransmitter, a phenomenon known as co-transmission. In addition to classical neurotransmitters such as glutamate, gamma-aminobutyric acid (GABA), serotonin, and dopamine, many neurons also release neuropeptides, including substance P, calcitonin gene-related peptide (CGRP), and neuropeptide Y (NPY). These neuropeptides function primarily as neuromodulators. Neurotransmitters are functionally classified as excitatory or inhibitory. In the CNS, glutamate is the principal excitatory neurotransmitter, whereas GABA is the major inhibitory neurotransmitter. Inhibitory synapses commonly contain flattened small synaptic vesicles, while excitatory synapses are associated with round clear synaptic vesicles.

Neuroglial Cells (Glia) (Fig. 1.10)

Neuroglial cells, or glia, are non-neuronal supporting cells of the nervous system. They are present in both the gray and white matter of the CNS. Unlike mature neurons, which are generally postmitotic, most neuroglial cells retain the capacity to proliferate, although the extent of proliferation varies among different glial cell types. Developmentally, astrocytes, oligodendrocytes and ependymal cells are derived from the neuroectoderm, whereas microglial cells are believed to originate from primitive yolk sac erythromyeloid progenitors that migrate into the developing CNS during early embryogenesis.

Because of their proliferative capacity, neuroglial cells can give rise to brain tumors, collectively known as gliomas. These include astrocytomas, oligodendrogliomas and glioblastoma (GBM), which is thought to arise predominantly from astrocytic lineage cells or neural progenitor cells.

Neuroglial cells are classified into four major types based on their structure and functions **(Fig. 1.10)**.

1. Oligodendrocytes
2. Astrocytes
3. Microglia
4. Ependymal cells

A. Oligodendrocytes

These cells are the predominant form of neuroglial cells in the CNS, dominating the white matter and heavily populating the grey matter. They are generally regarded as the most abundant glial cell type in the adult CNS, although the exact proportion varies among different brain regions and methods of quantification. They possess relatively fewer cytoplasmic processes compared with astrocytes, hence the prefix oligo, which stands for "few". Based on ultrastructural characteristics observed under the electron microscope, oligodendrocytes have traditionally been classified into:

i) Light oligodendrocytes
ii) Medium oligodendrocytes
iii) Dense (dark) oligodendrocytes

The light oligodendrocytes are considered immature cells, that differentiate into medium and subsequently dark (dense) oligodendrocytes. The dark oligodendrocytes represent the predominant mature form in the adult CNS.

The main function of oligodendrocytes is to form the myelin sheath around axons in the CNS. A single oligodendrocyte can myelinate segments of multiple axons. In addition to myelination, oligodendrocytes provide metabolic and trophic support to axons, helping to maintain their survival and normal function. Recent studies also suggests that oligodendrocytes contribute to learning and memory by modifying myelin in response to neuronal activity, a process known as adaptive myelination.

B. Astrocytes

Astrocytes constitute approximately 20–40% of the total glial cells, depending on the different regions in the CNS. They are star-shaped cells with numerous radiating long processes that terminate as enlarged "end-feet" which closely surround cerebral blood vessels. Astrocytic end-feet invest nearly the entire surface of CNS capillaries and extend to the brain surface beneath the pia mater to form the glia limitans.

Astrocytes play an essential role in maintaining CNS homeostasis. They provide metabolic support to neurons, and help maintain the integrity of the blood-brain barrier by supporting endothelial cells and pericytes. Astrocytes express glial fibrillary acidic protein (GFAP), an intermediate filament protein commonly used as an astrocytic marker. During CNS injury, astrocytes become reactive, showing increased GFAP expression and producing numerous cytokines and growth factors, including vascular endothelial growth factor (VEGF).

Ultrastructurally, astrocytes exhibit an oval nucleus with finely dispersed chromatin. Their pale cytoplasm contains bundles of intermediate filaments, and glycogen granules. Glycogen is particularly abundant within the astrocytic end-feet.

Astrocytes provide structural support and participate in tissue repair. Following CNS injury, they proliferate and undergo hypertrophy, producing a glial scar (reactive astrogliosis) that helps limit tissue damage. Reactive astrocytes secrete neurotrophic factors, including brain-derived neurotrophic factor (BDNF), neurotrophin-3 (NT-3), and insulin-like growth factor-1 (IGF-1), which support neuronal survival and repair.

C. Microglial cells

Microglia constitute 5–15% of the glial cells in the CNS, with regional variation. As the name implies, they are small and elongated cells that serve as the resident immunocompetent cells of the CNS, including the brain, spinal cord, and retina. They are derived from yolk sac erythromyeloid progenitors that migrate into the developing brain during embryogenesis and are distinct from neuroectoderm-derived macroglia (astrocytes and oligodendrocytes).

In the healthy CNS, microglia exhibit a ramified morphology and continuously survey the surrounding environment with their highly motile processes. Following injury, infection, or neurodegeneration, they become activated, proliferate, migrate to sites of injury, phagocytose cellular debris, and release inflammatory mediators, including tumour necrosis factor-α (TNF-α), interleukin-1β (IL-1β), reactive oxygen species, and nitric oxide (NO). Activated microglia also produce anti-inflammatory cytokines and neurotrophic factors that contribute to tissue repair.

Microglia can be identified using immunohistochemical markers including Iba1, CD11b (OX-42 in rodents), CD68, TMEM119 and isolectin B4 (commonly used in experimental studies). Amoeboid microglia represent the predominant developmental phenotype and gradually differentiate into highly ramified microglia in the mature CNS.

Microglia play important roles in both normal CNS physiology and disease. In addition to immune surveillance and synaptic pruning during development, chronically activated microglia are implicated in numerous neurological disorders, including traumatic brain injury, ischemic stroke, Alzheimer's disease, Parkinson's disease, multiple sclerosis, and chronic pain.

D. Ependymal cells

Ependymal cells are specialized neuroglial cells that line the ventricles of the brain and the central canal of the spinal cord. They range from cuboidal to low columnar in shape and possess numerous microvilli and motile cilia on their apical surface. The coordinated beating of the cilia facilitates the circulation of cerebrospinal fluid (CSF), while the microvilli participate in the absorption and exchange of substances between the CSF and ependymal cells.

Specialized ependymal cells lining the floor and walls of the third ventricle are known as tanycytes. These cells exhibit long processes that extend into the hypothalamus and participate in the transport of molecules between the CSF and hypothalamic neurons, thereby contributing to neuroendocrine regulation.

E. Choroid plexus

The choroid plexus is a specialized vascular structure located within the ventricles of the brain. It consists of a highly vascular core of vascular pia mater (connective tissue) containing fenestrated capillaries, covered by a layer of simple cuboidal epithelial cells, which are modified ependymal cells. The choroid plexus is responsible for the production of cerebrospinal fluid (CSF).

PERIPHERAL NERVOUS SYSTEM

Spinal Nerves and Cranial Nerves

There are 12 pairs of cranial nerves that arise from the brain stem, and 31 pairs of spinal nerves from different segments of the spinal cord. The spinal nerves comprise 8 cervical, 12 thoracic, 5 lumbar, 5 sacral, and one coccygeal pair of nerves.

The various spinal nerves and associated ganglia form several nerve plexuses (e.g., brachial plexus), which distribute the major nerves to the different body parts (e.g., brachial plexus supplying the upper limbs and lumbosacral plexus supplying the lower limbs). For the convenience of description, we shall take a segment of the median nerve to examine the histology of the PNS **(Fig. 1.12)**.

In a transverse section, peripheral nerve (median nerve is shown in histology illustration **Fig 1.12**) consist of numerous nerve fibres (both sensory and motor) arranged into bundles or fasciculi. Each fascicle is enclosed by the **perineurium**, which forms the blood-nerve barrier. Each individual nerve fibre is surrounded by delicate connective tissue called the **endoneurium**. The entire group of nerve bundles are surrounded by dense connective tissue called the **epineurium**, which contains larger blood vessels and provides mechanical support to the nerve.

Schwann cells ensheath all peripheral axons. A single myelinating Schwann cell forms one internodal myelin segment around a single axon, In contrast, a single non-myelinating Schwann cell may envelop multiple small unmyelinated axons, without forming myelin.

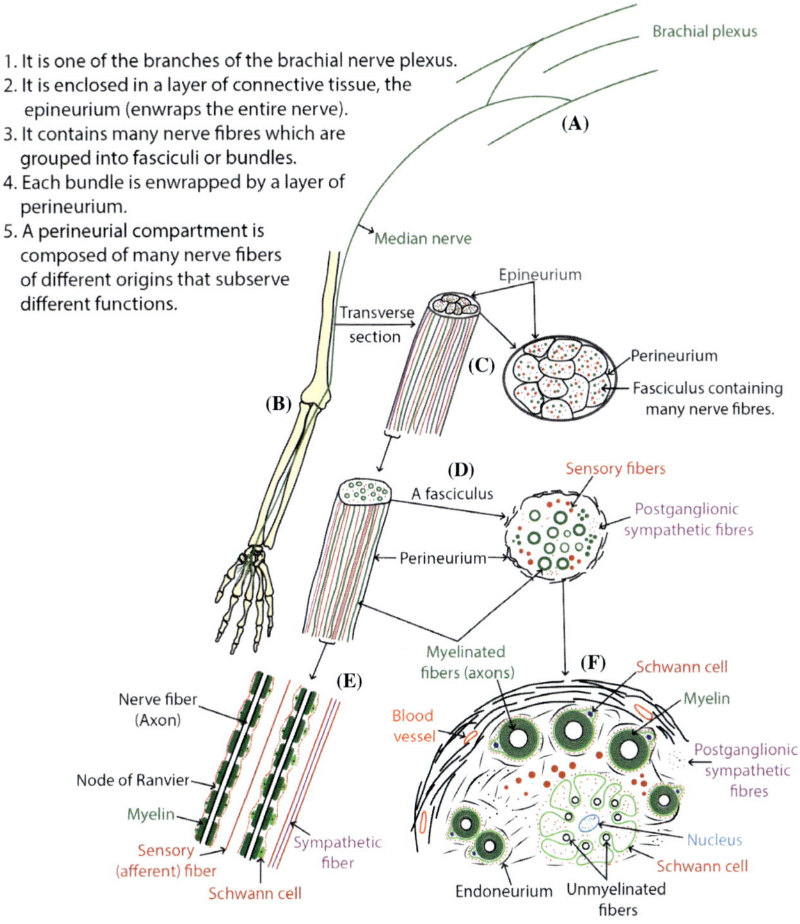

Nerve fibers:

1. Sensory fibers are also called the afferent fibers (they represent the peripheral process of the dorsal root ganglion cells).
2. Axons (motor fibers, efferent fibers)- they arise from the ventral horn motor neurons. They are myelinated; hence, myelinated axons (fibers).
3. Sympathetic fibers (Postganglionic fibers) supplying the sweat glands, arrector pili muscle, and smooth muscles in vascular walls.

Figure 1.12. Peripheral nervous system. (A, B) Showing the organization of a peripheral nerve, e.g., the median nerve that originates from the brachial nerve plexus in the upper limb. **(C)** In a longitudinal or transverse section, the entire nerve is invested by a layer of connective tissue, the epineurium. **(D)** The nerve contains many nerve fibers, which are grouped into many bundles or fasciculi (sing. fasciculus), each enclosed by a layer of connective tissue, the perineurium. **(E)** In an enlarged view, some of the nerve fibers are covered with a myelin sheath formed by the Schwann cells. Nodes of Ranvier are regular interrupted gaps along the myelin sheath; they facilitate saltatory conduction. **(F)** Individual nerve fibers in the nerve fibers are surrounded by small amounts of connective tissue, the endoneurium. Accompanying the myelinated axons (fibers) are some unmyelinated nerve fibers. Some of them represent the postganglionic sympathetic fibers.

Dorsal Root Ganglion (Fig. 1.13A to C)

The dorsal root or sensory ganglion is associated with the dorsal root of the spinal nerve. It contains the cell bodies of pseudounipolar sensory neurons, each of which is surrounded by satellite glial cells that provide structural, metabolic, and homeostatic support to the neuron.

Each pseudounipolar neuron possesses a single process (common stem or neurite) that bifurcates into a peripheral process and a central process. The peripheral process functions as a dendrite and terminates in various sensory receptors within the skin, joint capsules, ligaments, and muscles or as free nerve endings in the epidermis. These peripheral processes are afferent fibers because they transmit sensory impulses from the receptors towards the CNS. The sensory impulse is conducted through the central process, which functions as an axon, to synapse with second-order neurons in the spinal cord. Although the peripheral process is functionally equivalent to a dendrite, both peripheral and central processes are structurally axons.

The spinal nerve is a mixed nerve because it contains sensory fibers (peripheral processes of sensory neurons), motor fibers (axons of somatic motor neurons) and autonomic fibers **(Fig. 1.12A to F; Fig. 1.13A)**. The axons of somatic motor neurons arise from the neuronal cell bodies located in the ventral (anterior) horn of the spinal cord and terminate at the motor endplates (neuromuscular junctions) on extrafusal skeletal muscle fibres. Branches of some motor axons also innervate intrafusal muscle fibres of the muscle spindle **(Fig. 1.13A)**. The autonomic fibres within spinal nerves consist primarily of postganglionic sympathetic fibres originating from the sympathetic chain ganglia. These fibres innervate sweat glands, vascular smooth muscle, and arrector pili muscles.

The axons of myelinated peripheral nerve fibres are ensheathed by a myelin sheath which is produced by Schwann cells **(Fig. 1.12E, F)**. Each myelinating Schwann cell forms a single internodal myelin segment around one axon. In addition to forming myelin, Schwann cells provide structural and metabolic support to axons and play a crucial role in peripheral nerve regeneration following injury by promoting axonal remyelination.

Clinical Considerations

Because a spinal nerve contains sensory, motor, and autonomic nerve fibers, injury to the nerve results in motor weakness (or paralysis of the muscles it

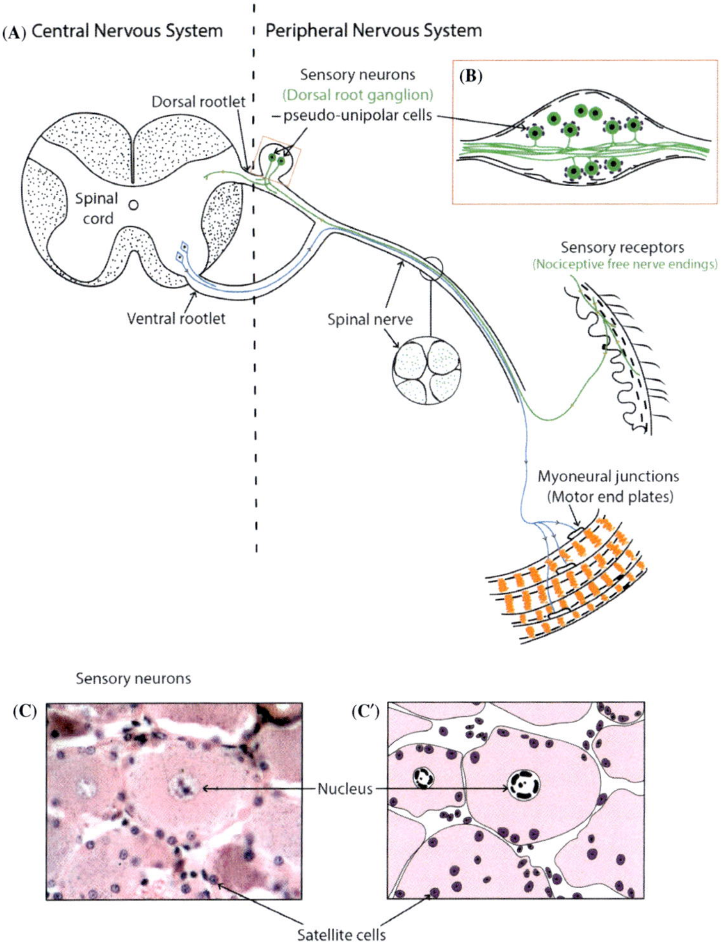

Figure 1.13. Peripheral nervous system (PNS). (A) The PNS is composed of dorsal and ventral rootlets attached to the spinal cord, spinal nerve, and sensory receptors. Both rootlets join to give rise to the spinal nerve (dorsal ramus is omitted). The dorsal root ganglion (sensory ganglion) is associated with the dorsal rootlet. It contains the dorsal root (or sensory) neurons, which are pseudounipolar neurons (red) bearing a peripheral or sensory process (fiber) and a central process. The peripheral process terminates in the sensory receptors (e.g., Pacinian corpuscle, free nerve endings). The central process (red) of the neuron projects into the dorsal horn of the spinal cord. The ventral rootlet carries the axons (blue) of the motoneurons (ventral horn neurons), which innervate the muscle fibers at the myoneural junction (motor endplates). The spinal nerve contains both sensory and motor fibers; hence, it is a mixed nerve. **(B)** Dorsal sensory ganglion contains pseudounipolar neurons, each bearing a peripheral or sensory process and a central process, which projects into the spinal cord. The peripheral processes are also called the afferent fibers because they transmit impulses from the peripheral receptors to the spinal cord interneurons (relay neurons). The boxed area is enlarged. **(C & C')** Dorsal root or sensory ganglion cells or sensory neurons. The cell body is surrounded by satellite cells, which provide nutritional support to the sensory neurons. (H&E stain.)

supplies) and sensory loss within the corresponding dermatome. In addition, interruption of autonomic nerve fibers produces autonomic dysfunction, including reduced sweating (anhidrosis), vasodilation resulting in warm, dry skin, and loss of pilomotor activity (piloerection/ goosebumps).

Sensory Receptors

The peripheral processes of primary sensory neurons whose cell bodies are located in the dorsal root ganglion, terminate either as free nerve endings or within specialized encapsulated or non-encapsulated sensory receptors in the skin, muscles, tendons, and joints. Major sensory receptors include:

1. **Meissner's corpuscle** — located in the dermal papilla of skin; function as receptors for light touch (low-frequency vibration).
2. **Pacinian corpuscle** — located in the deep dermis or subcutaneous tissue; function as receptors for deep pressure (high-frequency vibration).
3. **Merkel disc** — located in the basal layer of the epidermis; function as receptors for fine touch.
4. **Muscle spindles** — located within skeletal muscles; function as stretch receptors (proprioceptors) that detect changes in muscle length and contribute to the maintenance of muscle tone.

The cell bodies of all primary sensory neurons associated with these receptors are located within the dorsal root (spinal sensory) ganglia, except for sensory receptors of the head and face, whose primary sensory neuron cell bodies are located in the sensory ganglia of certain cranial nerves (e.g., the trigeminal ganglion).

CARTILAGE AND BONE TISSUE

Both cartilage and bone are specialized supporting connective tissues and therefore share several common histological features. They consist of two main structural components: cells and an extracellular matrix, composed of collagen fibers and ground substance. The extracellular matrix provides the strength and resilience that enable cartilage and bone to support the body and maintain its structural integrity. Cartilage forms the articular surfaces of synovial joints (e.g., the shoulder joint), where its smooth, resilient surface reduces friction and distributes mechanical loads during movement.

Cartilage

Types of cartilage (Fig. 1.14; Fig. 1.15)

There are three types of cartilage. The principal cellular components are chondrocytes, the mature cartilage cells, and chondroblasts, their less mature precursors. The cells are embedded within an abundant extracellular matrix composed of collagen fibers and a highly hydrated ground substance rich in glycosaminoglycans (GAGs) and proteoglycans. The classification of cartilage is based primarily on the type and relative abundance of the fibers present within the extracellular matrix. The ground substance occupies the spaces between the cells and fibers and contributes to the resilience and compressive strength of cartilage.

1. ***Hyaline cartilage*** **(Fig. 1.15A):** This is the most common type of cartilage. Its principal cells are chondrocytes, which are often arranged in small clusters (typically 2–4 cells). Each chondrocyte occupies a lacuna, an empty-appearing space in histological sections that results from tissue shrinkage during tissue processing. The extracellular matrix consists of a highly hydrated ground substance, together with abundant type II collagen fibrils. These collagen fibrils are too fine to be distinguished in routine H&E-stained sections, giving the matrix its characteristic glassy (hyaline) appearance. Hyaline cartilage is found on the articular surfaces of synovial joints, such as the shoulder joint (between the head of the humerus and the glenoid cavity of the scapula) and the knee joint (between the femur and tibia). It provides a smooth, low-friction surface that facilitates joint movement and distributes mechanical loads during weight-bearing and motion. Degeneration and progressive loss of articular cartilage are characteristic features of osteoarthritis. Because cartilage is avascular, its capacity for repair and regeneration is limited.

   Other common. examples of hyaline cartilage include the C-shaped tracheal rings, the cartilage plates of the bronchi, and most laryngeal cartilages (except the epiglottis). During embryonic development, hyaline cartilage forms the preexisting "cartilage model" that is subsequently replaced by bone during endochondral ossification.

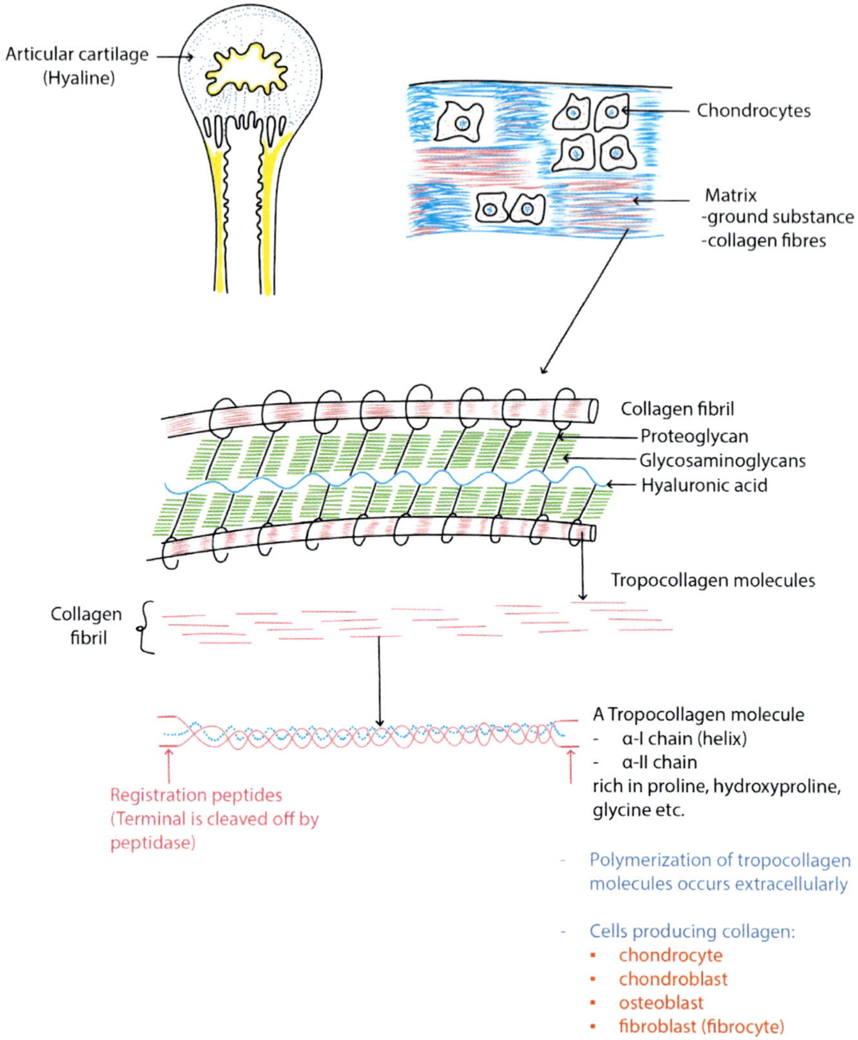

Figure 1.14. Cartilage tissue. The epiphysis of a long bone, e.g., humerus or femur, is lined by a layer of cartilage- articular cartilage. It is made up of cartilage cells (chondrocytes) and the matrix is composed of fine collagen fibrils and ground substance. Note that the collagen fibrils are linked to proteoglycans, hyaluronic acid, and glycosaminoglycans.

Most hyaline cartilage is covered on its surface by a layer of dense connective tissue called the perichondrium, which consists of an outer fibrous layer rich in collagen fibers and an inner chondrogenic layer containing chondroblasts. Articular cartilage is an important exception and lacks a

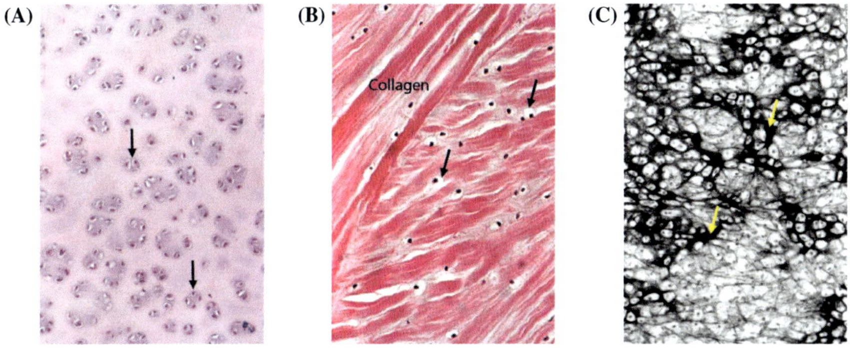

Figure 1.15. Cartilage tissue. (A) Hyaline cartilage shows clusters of chondrocytes in lacunae (black arrows) (e.g., costal cartilage, trachea). Note its "glassy" matrix whose collagen fibrils are not visible. **(B)** Fibrocartilage shows large bundles of collagen fibers (e.g., articular disc). Chondrocytes (arrows) in lacunae are widely distributed. **(C)** Elastic cartilage stained with Verhoeff staining (e.g., epiglottis]). Elastic fibers stained in black course between the chondrocytes (yellow arrow). A, B: H&E stain. C: Verhoeff stain.

perichondrium. Because cartilage contains no blood vessels, chondrocytes receive nutrients by diffusion through the extracellular matrix from blood vessels in the perichondrium or, in the case of articular cartilage, from the synovial fluid.

Cartilage grows by appositional growth, in which chondroblasts in the inner layer of the perichondrium differentiate and secrete new extracellular matrix onto the cartilage surface, and by interstitial growth, in which chondrocytes divide within the matrix and produce additional extracellular matrix from within the cartilage. Both chondroblasts and chondrocytes synthesize the collagen fibrils and ground substance of the cartilage matrix.

2. ***Elastic cartilage* (Fig. 1.15C):** Elastic cartilage consists primarily of chondrocytes and chondroblasts embedded within an extracellular matrix. Its distinguishing feature is the presence of an abundant network of branched elastic fibers, composed of elastin and fibrillin-containing microfibrils, in addition to type II collagen fibrils. These elastic fibers impart flexibility and resilience, enabling the cartilage to withstand repeated bending and deformation while maintaining its original shape. Elastic cartilage is found in structures that require both support and flexibility, including the auricle (pinna) of the external ear, the epiglottis, the external acoustic meatus, and the auditory (Eustachian) tube. Elastic cartilage is surrounded by a layer of

perichondrium, which provides nourishment and contributes to appositional growth. The elastin in elastic cartilage is synthesized by chondrocytes. In contrast, elastin in the wall of elastic arteries, such as the aorta, is produced mainly by vascular smooth muscle cells. The abundant elastic lamellae within the aortic wall allow the vessel to expand during systole and recoil during diastole, helping to maintain continuous blood flow.

3. ***Fibrocartilage* (Fig. 1.15B):** This cartilage contains relatively few chondrocytes, which are often arranged in rows between thick bundles of collagen fibers. In some regions, chondrocytes are interspersed with fibroblasts and fibrocytes. A prominent feature of the fibrocartilage is the abundance of type I collagen fibers, which provide the tissue with high tensile strength while also resisting compressive forces. Fibrocartilage is found in structures subjected to considerable mechanical stress, including the intervertebral discs, the menisci (semilunar cartilages) of the knee, and the articular discs of joints, such as the temporomandibular joint. In these locations, fibrocartilage helps absorb shock, improve joint congruity, and, in certain joints, deepen the articular surfaces to enhance joint stability and movement. Unlike hyaline and elastic cartilage, fibrocartilage lacks a perichondrium.

Bone and Its Tissue

Bones form the skeletal framework of our body, providing structural support, protection for vital organs and attachment sites for muscles that enable locomotion. Bone tissue is therefore structurally adapted to perform these diverse functions.

1. **Gross features (Fig. 1.16A to D):** When a typical long bone, such as the humerus, is sectioned longitudinally, its outer surface is covered by a dense connective tissue membrane called the periosteum. The inner layer of the periosteum contains osteoprogenitor (osteogenic) cells, which differentiate into osteoblasts during bone growth and repair following a fracture. The wall of the shaft (diaphysis) of a long bone consists of compact (cortical) bone, a dense tissue composed of bone cells embedded in a mineralized extracellular matrix containing ground substance, collagen fibers and inorganic mineral salts. Mature bone cells, known as osteocytes, reside within small spaces

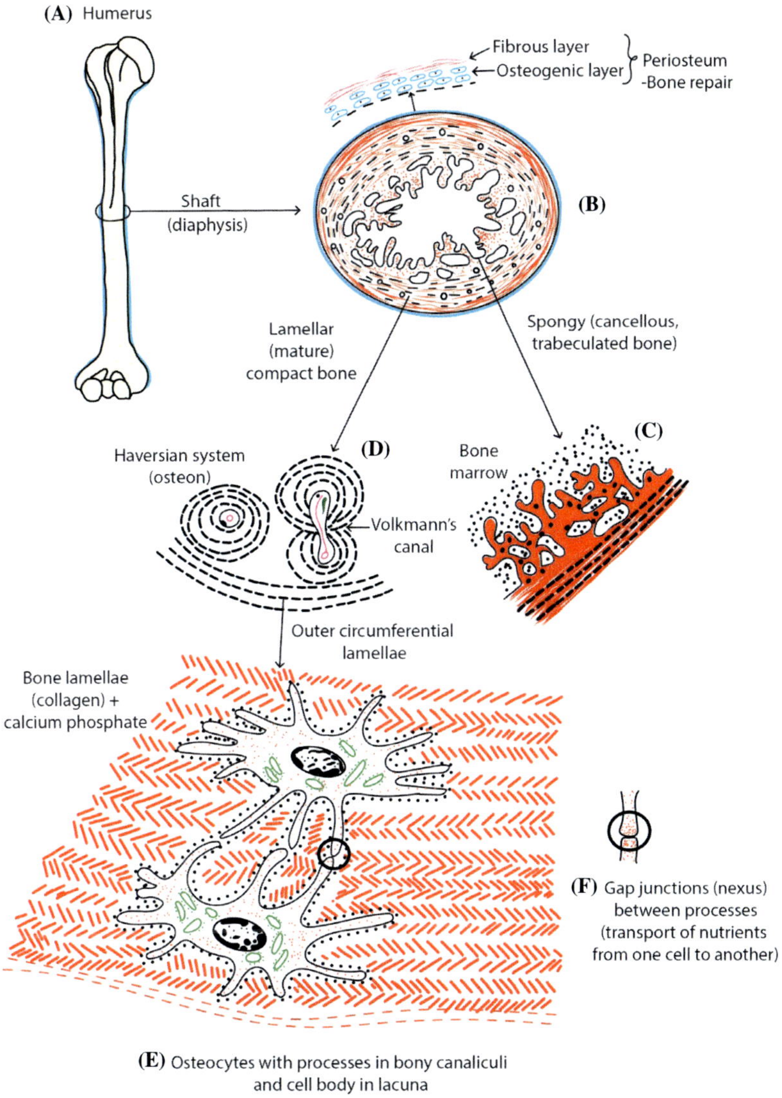

Figure 1.16. Bone tissue. **(A)** Showing the shaft (diaphysis) of the humerus. **(B)** In a transverse section of the shaft, the surface of the bone is covered with a layer of periosteum containing some osteogenic cells. **(C)** Facing the marrow cavity is the spongy (cancellous) bone filled with marrow cells in between. **(D)** The solid part of the bone is made up of cylindrical Harversian systems (osteons). **(E)** An enlarged view of osteocytes housed in a bony lacuna. Between the osteocytes are bony lamellae composed of bundles of collagen fibers impregnated by calcium phosphate. The osteocyte has long, extending processes lying in the body canaliculi. **(F)** The processes from the osteocyte make contact with those of the adjacent cells via the gap junction.

called lacunae. The compact bone of the diaphysis surrounds the medullary (marrow) cavity, which is lined by the endosteum. Cancellous (spongy or trabecular) bone, consisting of an interconnected network of bony trabeculae enclosing marrow spaces, is found predominantly in the epiphyses of long bones. In these regions, the marrow spaces of the cancellous bone are continuous with the medullary cavity.

2. **Microscopic features:** In a ground section of compact bone, the mature bone cells (osteocytes) are housed within lacunae. Each osteocyte extends numerous slender cytoplasmic processes through tiny canals known as canaliculi, where they establish contact with the processes of adjacent osteocytes through gap junctions. This interconnected network facilitates cell-to-cell communication and the exchange of nutrients and metabolites **(Fig. 1.16E, F)**. The osteocytes are arranged in concentric layers (lamellae) surrounding the central Haversian canal, which contains neurovascular structures **(Fig. 1.17A; Fig. 1.18A)**. Adjacent Haversian canals are interconnected by Volkmann's canals, which transmit blood vessels and nerves between neighbouring osteons and the periosteal and endosteal surfaces. The extracellular matrix between adjacent lamellae consists predominantly of type I collagen fibers that are mineralized with hydroxyapatite crystals, providing the bone with both tensile strength and compressive resistance. A Haversian canal surrounded by concentric lamellae containing osteocytes forms a Haversian system, or osteon, the fundamental structural and functional unit of compact bone. The shaft (diaphysis) of a long bone is composed of numerous osteons that are aligned parallel to the long axis of the bone **(Fig. 1.17A)**. This highly organized arrangement provides an efficient vascular supply to the bone while imparting strong mechanical support to resist bending.
3. **Bone formation and deposition (Fig. 1.17B; Fig. 1.18B):** Bone is formed by osteoblasts, which are cuboidal to columnar, bone-forming cells with basophilic cytoplasm. Osteoblasts are polarized cells that synthesize and secrete osteoid, the unmineralized organic bone matrix, onto the bone surface. Osteoid consists of type 1 collagen fibers, together with ground substance containing proteoglycans and non-collagenous proteins. As osteoid is deposited, the osteoprogenitor cells continue to proliferate and differentiate into new osteoblasts to maintain the osteoblast population.

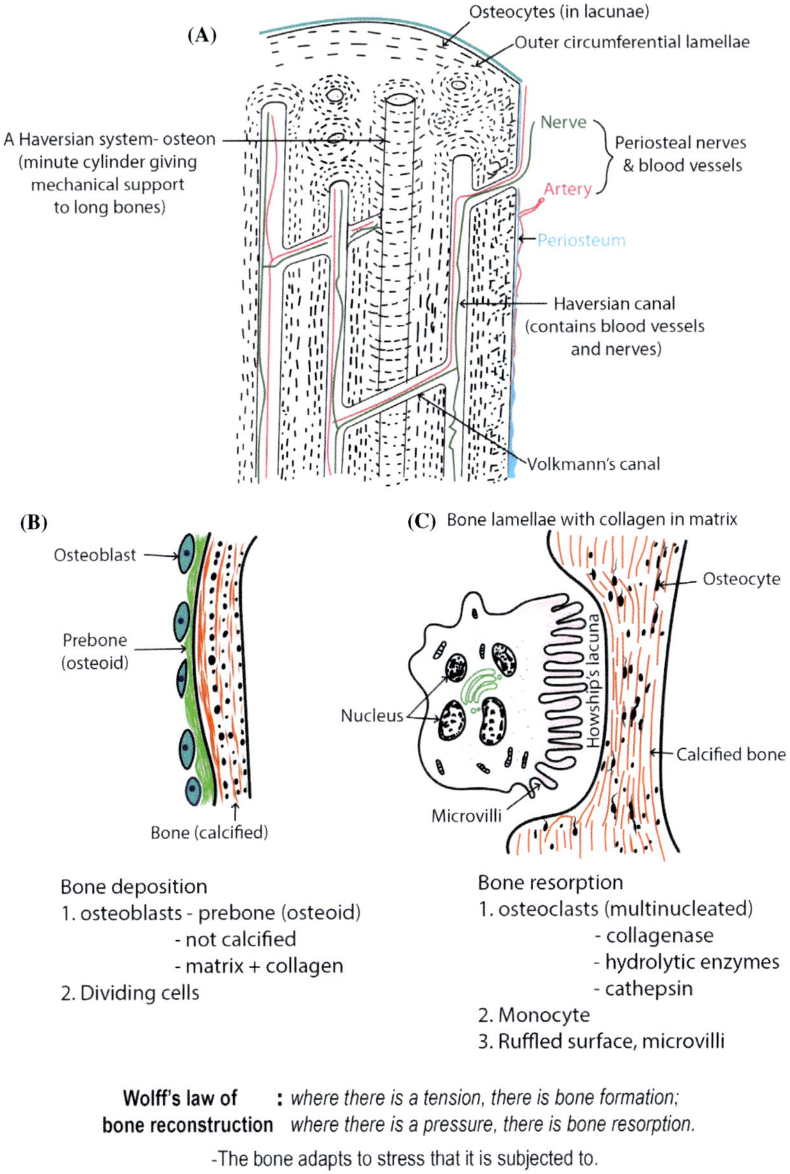

Figure 1.17. Bone tissue. (A) Longitudinal section of the shaft of a long bone showing multicylinders of the Haversian system (osteon) that provide mechanical support to the bone. The Haversian canal conveys blood vessels and nerves derived from the periosteal surface. Interconnecting the Harversian canals is Volkman's canal. **(B)** Osteoblasts deposit bone first as the prebone (osteoid), which is then calcified distally. **(C)** A multinucleated osteoclast in the Howship's lacuna is indicative of active bone resorption. Note that the secretory surface of the cell is "ruffled," showing many microvilli.

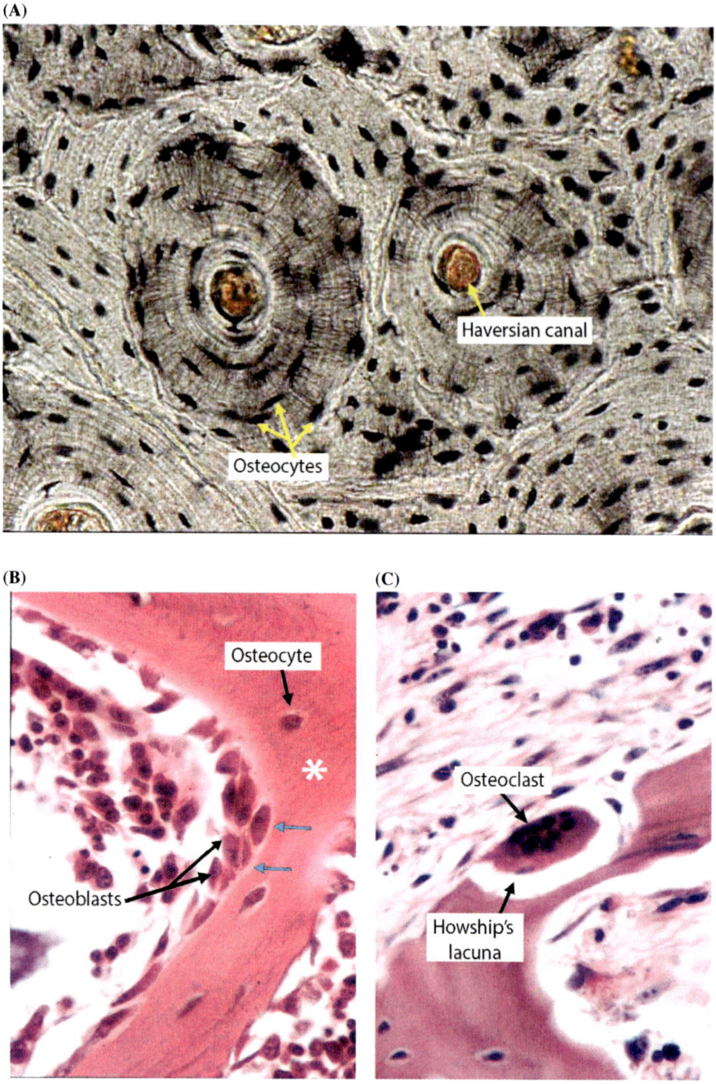

Figure 1.18. Bone tissue. (A) Haversian systems (osteons) in a long bone. Each osteon is composed of the centrally located Haversian canal containing blood vessels and nerves. The canal is surrounded by concentric layers of bony lamellae. Between the bony lamellae are the osteocytes; each is housed in a lacuna. The radiating processes from the osteocytes lie in the bony caliculi. Prepared from a ground bone section without staining. **(B) Bone formation**. During the process, prebone (osteoid, not calcified) (note the light zone indicated by blue arrows) is first deposited by a cluster or layer of osteoblasts. The newly formed bone is then calcified (white asterisk), which shows embedded osteocytes (black arrow). **(C) Bone resorption** is by osteoclasts (a cell is labeled). The bone surface is "excavated" or "remodeled" by osteoclasts, which release different hydrolytic enzymes, including collagenase. Osteoclastic actions result in the formation of Howship's lacuna (black arrow) on the surface of the bony spicules. (H&E stain.)

Some active osteoblasts remain on the bone surface or become flattened bone-lining cells, whereas others become embedded within the newly formed matrix and differentiate into osteocytes, which reside in lacunae. Osteocytes are terminally differentiated cells and normally do not undergo mitosis. Following osteoid deposition, the matrix undergoes mineralization through the deposition of hydroxyapatite crystals, resulting in the formation of mature lamellar bone. Repeated cycles of osteoid deposition and mineralization produce successive layers (lamellae) of bone, contributing to bone growth, remodeling, and repair.

4. **Bone resorption (Fig. 1.17C; Fig. 1.18C):** Following bone formation, some bony surface areas are removed and replaced through the process of bone remodeling. During growth, remodeling allows bones to change their shape and accommodate the expansion of adjacent organs, such as the growing brain. Bone remodeling continues throughout life and is essential for maintaining bone strength and repairing microscopic damage. Osteoclasts are responsible for bone resorption. They are large, multinucleated cells derived from hematopoietic stem cells of the monocyte–macrophage lineage. The bone-facing surface of an active osteoclast forms a specialized ruffled border, which greatly increases the surface area available for bone resorption. Osteoclasts first acidify the resorption lacuna to dissolve the inorganic mineral component of bone and then secrete lysosomal enzymes, including cathepsin K and matrix metalloproteinases, to degrade the organic matrix, particularly type I collagen in the bone. Bone resorption by osteoclasts results in the formation of shallow depressions on the bone surface known as Howship's lacunae, which are characteristic sites of active osteoclastic activity (bone resorption).
5. **Hormones and bone:** Bone remodeling is regulated by several hormones, including parathyroid hormone (PTH), calcitonin, growth hormone, thyroid hormones, and the sex hormones. Estrogen plays a crucial role in maintaining bone mass by inhibiting osteoclast formation and activity while promoting osteoblast survival. The decline in estrogen levels after menopause in women accelerates osteoclast-mediated bone resorption, resulting in reduced bone mass and an increased risk of osteoporosis.
6. **Bone ossification:** Bones are formed by two distinct modes of ossification: endochondral ossification and intramembranous ossification. Most long bones, such as the humerus and femur develop by endochondral ossification,

whereas many flat bones of the skull bones (frontal, parietal, and occipital) develop by intramembranous ossification.

a. *Endochondral ossification* **(Fig. 1.19; Fig. 1.20):** This is a relatively slower process than intramembranous ossification, and is exemplified by the development of the humerus. It begins with the formation of a pre-existing hyaline cartilage model. As the cartilage model enlarges during fetal development, chondrocytes (cartilage cells) in its central region undergo hypertrophy, the surrounding cartilage matrix becomes calcified, and the chondrocytes subsequently degenerate, leaving cavities within the calcified cartilage. Osteoprogenitor cells from the surface invade these cavities to form the primary ossification centre in the diaphysis. Osteoprogenitor cells differentiate into osteoblasts, which lay the first bone tissue at the primary ossification center. After birth, secondary ossification centers develop in both ends of the cartilage model (epiphysis). As bone growth continues, a plate of hyaline cartilage, the epiphyseal (growth) plate, persists between the epiphysis and the diaphysis (shaft) until skeletal maturity. The epiphyseal plate consists of distinct zones of chondrocyte activity: the resting (reserve) zone, proliferative zone, hypertrophic zone, calcification zone, and ossification (resorption) zone. These sequential zones are responsible for the longitudinal growth of long bones. Growth of the epiphyseal plate in a long bone is regulated by growth hormone (somatotropin), insulin-like growth factor-1 (IGF-1), thyroid hormones, and sex hormones, particularly estrogen.

   Bone growth in diameter (appositional growth) occurs by the addition of new bone to the outer surface of the shaft by osteoblasts derived from osteoprogenitor cells in the periosteum. At the same time, osteoclasts resorb bone from the inner (endosteal) surface, enlarging the medullary cavity. The coordinated actions of osteoblasts and osteoclasts allow the long bone to increase in diameter while maintaining its shape and strength. Bone remodeling also contributes to the development of the funnel-shaped metaphysis.

b. *Intramembranous ossification* **(Fig. 1.21; Fig. 1.22):** There is no preexisting cartilage model in intramembranous ossification. Ossification begins in

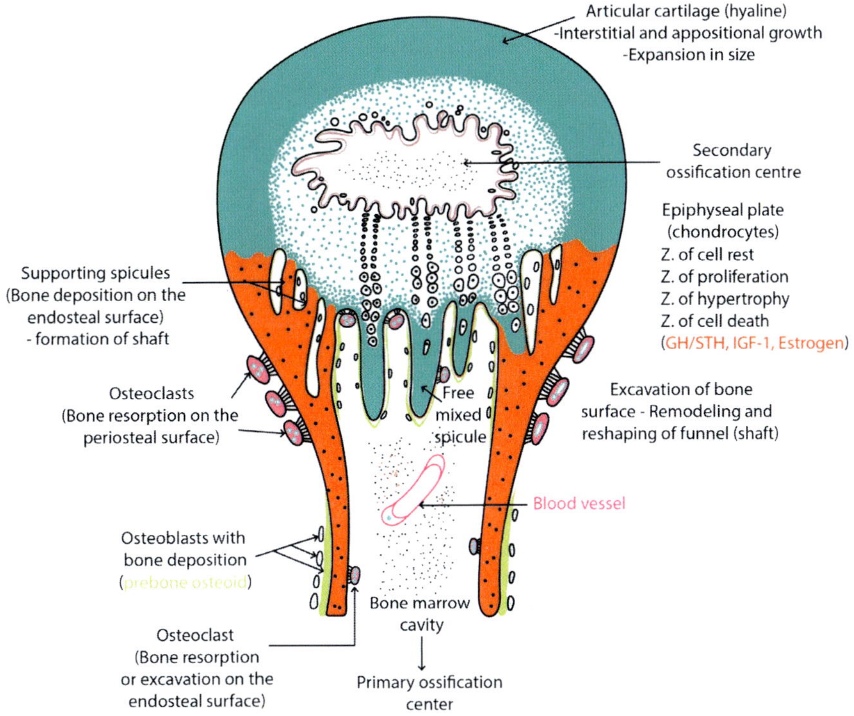

1. How does a long bone e.g. humerus grow in length?
   A. *Proliferation of chondrocytes in the epiphyseal plate.*
   B. *Somatotropin or growth hormone stimulates the growth of the plate through Insulin-like growth factor (IGF-1) from the liver. Both hormones together with estrogen act on chondrocyte and osteoblast growth - cell proliferation.*
   C. *Gigantism and Dwarfism - Excess or Deficiency of STH.*

2. At 21 years of age, the epiphyseal plate is disrupted. There is then a direct communication between the epiphyseal cavity and diaphyseal cavity - Fusion (the person can no longer grow taller after this).

3. How does the shaft (diaphysis) grow or increase in diameter?
   Opposing activity of osteoblats and osteoclasts on the periosteal and endosteal surface, respectively.

Figure 1.19. Endochondral ossification. Showing the proximal end (epiphysis) of a long bone, e.g., the humerus, which is formed by endochondral ossification. It is covered by a layer of articular cartilage (hyaline). Below it is the epiphyseal plate composed of columns of chondrocytes at different stages of maturation. The epiphyseal plate accounts for the growth of the long bone, both in length and size. (For a detailed description, please refer to the text).

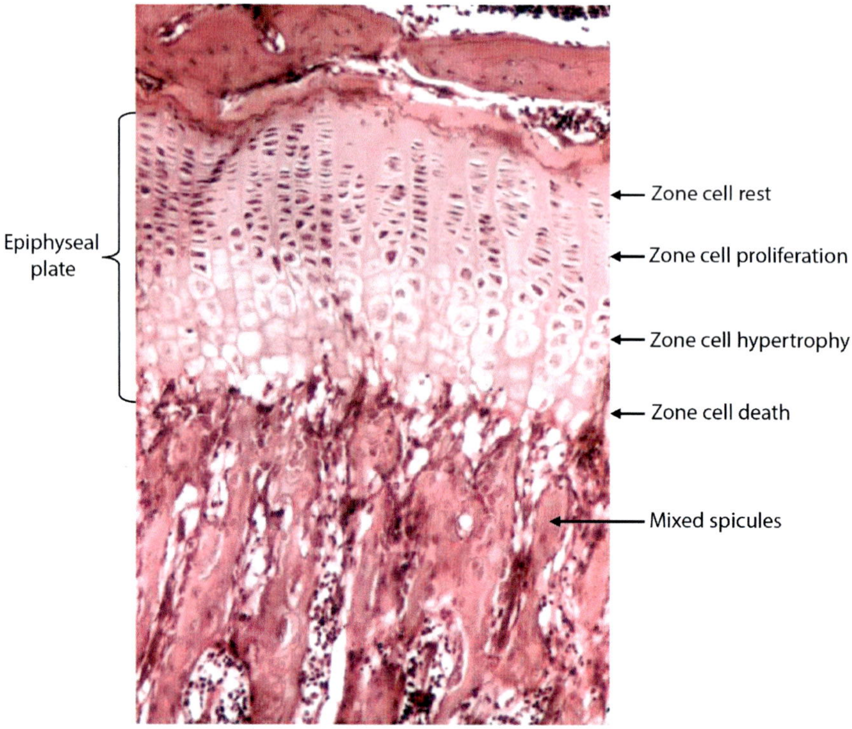

Figure 1.20. Endochondral ossification of a long bone, e.g., humerus, tibia. Showing the epiphyseal or growth plate (hyaline cartilage). It is made up of many layers and columns of chondrocytes at different stages of activity (zone of cell rest, zone of cell proliferation, zone of cell hypertrophy, and zone of cell death). The epiphyseal plate is under the influence of the growth hormone (somatotrophin), insulin-like growth factor, and estrogen. The mixed spicules project into the bone marrow (lower part of the figure). (H&E stain.)

an embryonic connective tissue (mesenchyme) membrane. Mesenchymal cells differentiate into osteoprogenitor cells and subsequently into osteoblasts, which secrete osteoid that later mineralizes to form bone. The earliest bone formed consists of bony spicules, containing osteocytes enclosed within bony lacunae. As ossification progresses, these spicules enlarge and fuse to form interconnected bony trabeculae, producing spongy or trabeculated bone. The spaces between the trabeculae become occupied by bone marrow and blood vessels, forming the diploë of flat bones. Subsequently, osteoblasts deposit additional bone on both the outer and inner surfaces of the trabecular bone, forming the outer and inner compact (cortical) bone layers, as seen in adult skull bones,

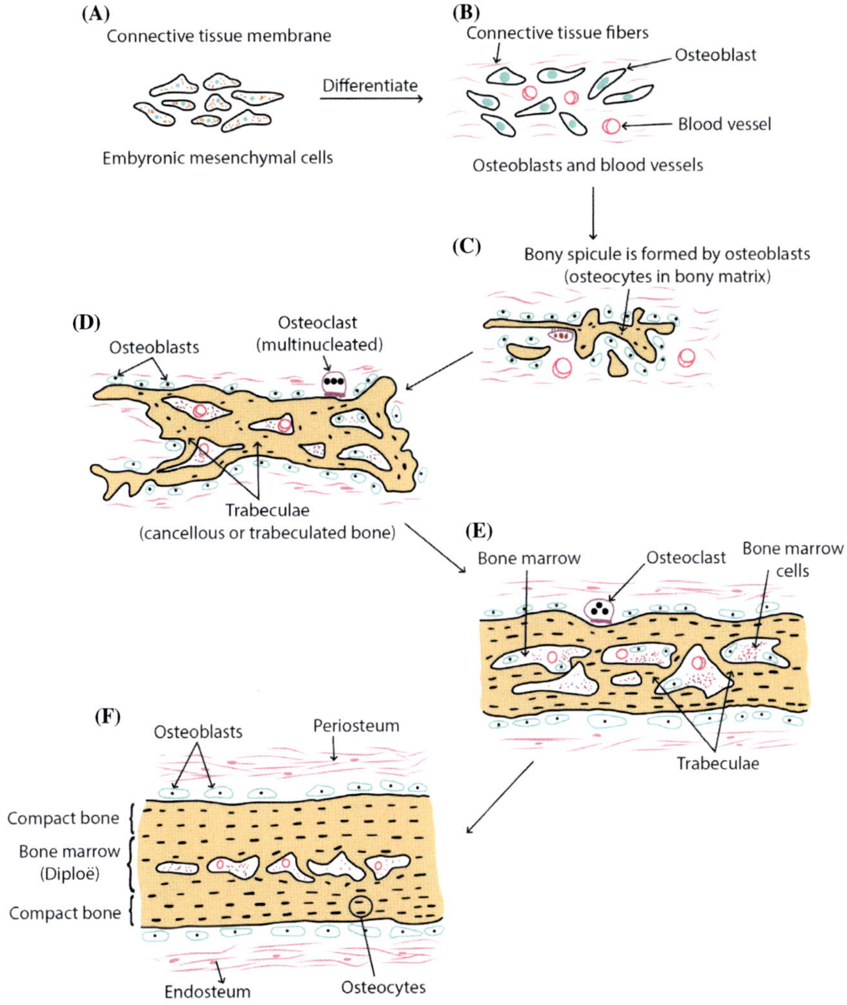

Figure 1.21. Intramembranous ossification. **(A)** Embryonic mesenchymal cells in a connective tissue membrane differentiate to become osteogenic cells and cells that differentiate to form the blood vessels. **(B)** The osteogenic cells further differentiate to become the osteoblasts. **(C)** Osteoblasts lay down bone material to form bony spicules. **(D)** Fusion of bony spicules forms the larger bony trabeculae. Some areas of the bony trabeculae are "trimmed" off by active osteoclasts through bone resorption. **(E)** More bone is deposited on the surface, but the central areas remain "spongy" with future marrow cavities. **(F)** More bone is added on the surfaces to form the compact bone with layers of bony lamellae.

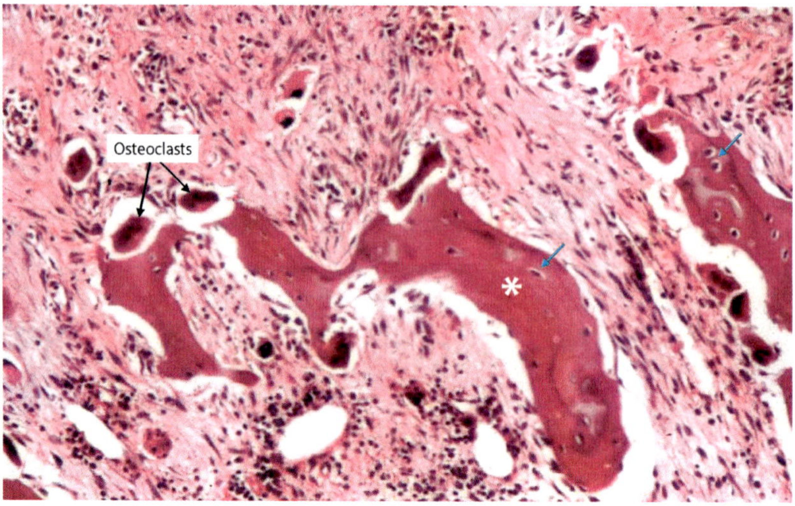

Figure 1.22. Intramembranous ossification (e.g., frontal, parietal bones, etc). Ossification begins with the formation of bone spicules (white asterisk). Embedded in the bony spicules are osteocytes (blue arrows). Multinucleated osteoclasts involved in bone resorption are on the surface of the bony spicules (black arrows). Between the bony spicules are mesenchymal cells; some have differentiated into osteoblasts. (H&E stain.)

including the frontal, parietal, and occipital bones. Throughout life, osteoblasts and osteoclasts work in concert to maintain bone formation and remodeling.

Quizzes and some points for consideration

1. How does a long bone (e.g., femur) grow in length?
   a. Growth in length occurs through the proliferation and hypertrophy of chondrocytes in the epiphyseal (growth) plate, followed by replacement of cartilage with bone (endochondral ossification).
   b. Growth hormone (GH), also known as somatotropic hormone (STH) stimulates the growth of the epiphyseal plate by promoting the production of insulin-like growth factor (IGF-1) in the liver. Both hormones, together with estrogen and other sex hormones, stimulate the proliferation and activity of chondrocytes and osteoblasts, resulting in bone growth.
   c. Gigantism and dwarfism result from excessive and deficient secretion of GH during childhood, respectively.

2. What is meant by "fusion" of the epiphysis and diaphysis? Why does a person stop growing taller after skeletal maturity (approximately 18–21 years of age)?
3. How does the shaft (diaphysis) of a long bone increase in diameter?

   The diameter of the shaft increases by appositional growth. Osteoblasts in the periosteum deposit new bone on the outer surface of the shaft, while osteoclasts resorb bone from the inner (endosteal) surface facing the medullary cavity. The coordinated activities of osteoblasts and osteoclasts increase both the diameter of the shaft and the size of the medullary cavity while maintaining bone strength.
4. What are the functions of periosteum? What role does it play in the repair of a bone fracture?

SKIN

The skin is the largest organ of the body, covering its entire external surface. Together with its appendages (hair, nails, sweat glands, and sebaceous glands), it forms the integumentary system.

The skin provides protection against invasion of pathogens, mechanical injury, harmful chemicals, ultraviolet (UV) radiation, and dehydration. It plays a vital role in thermoregulation through sweat production and regulation of cutaneous blood flow. Because of the abundance of sensory nerve endings in its superficial layers, the skin also functions as a sensory organ, detecting touch, pressure, pain, and temperature. In addition, it contributes to the excretion of metabolic wastes through sweat.

Histologically, the skin consists of three main layers: epidermis, dermis, and hypodermis (subcutaneous layer or superficial fascia in gross anatomy). The hypodermis contains variable amounts of adipose tissue (subcutaneous fat) and anchors the skin to the underlying structures. In this chapter, the focus will be on the epidermis and dermis.

Histology of skin

There are two main types of skin: thin skin and thick skin **(Fig. 1.23A, B)**. The major difference between them is the thickness of the stratum corneum, the outermost layer of the epidermis composed of layers of dead, keratinized epithelial cells that are continuously shed from the surface. **Thin skin** has a

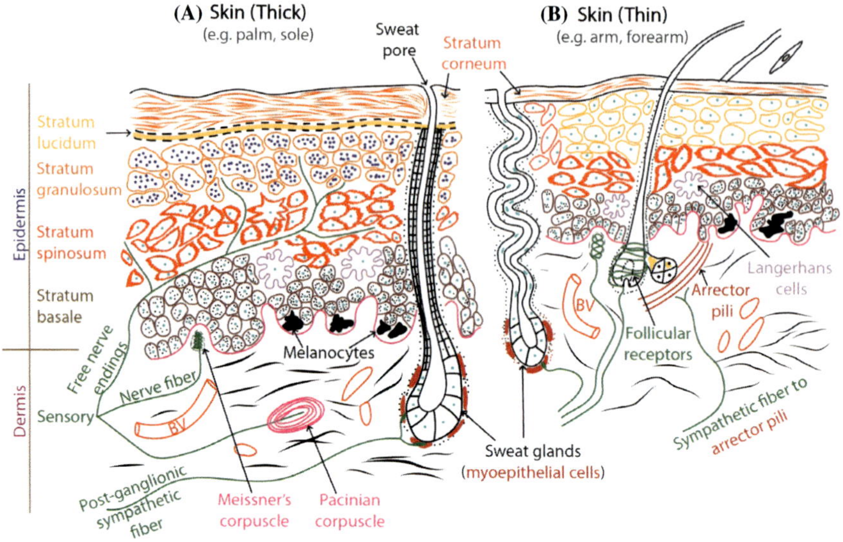

1. Nerve endings - Free nerve endings (nociceptors)
   (sensory) - Meissner's corpuscle (simple touch)
   - Pacinian corpuscle (deep pressure)
   - Follicular nerve plexus (mechanoreceptors)

2. Melanocytes - Production of melanin
   Langerhans cells - immune cells in epidermis, antigen presentation; circulate to lymph
   (dendritic cells) node - monocyte origin (bone marrow)

3. Sympathetic nerve supply: A. Arrector pili
   B. Sweat glands, myoepithelial cells
   C. Blood vessels

4. Differences:

Thick skin	Thin skin
-No arrector pili	-Arrector pili
-No hair follicle	-Hair follicle
-No sebaceous glands	-Sebaceous glands
-Stratum lucidum	-No stratum lucidum
-Thick layer of stratum corneum	-Thin layer of stratum corneum

Figure 1.23. (A) Thick skin. (B) Thin skin. Examples of thick skin include the palm and the sole of the foot. The rest of the body surface is covered by thin skin. In the thick skin **(A)**, the epidermis has a thick layer of stratum corneum. Below it is the stratum lucidum, stratum granulosum, stratum spinosum, and stratum basale (germinativum). The same layers are present in the thin skin **(B)** except for the stratum lucidum. Both types of skin are richly innervated by sensory nerves (pain, temperature, and touch). Note that the nerve endings ramify freely in the epidermis. In addition, there are postganglionic sympathetic fibers supplying the sweat glands and associated myoepithelial cells, arrector pili muscle associated with the hair follicle, and blood vessels (BV). Note that the epidermis is avascular. The differences between the two types of kin are listed with the figure.

relatively thin layer of stratum corneum **(Fig. 1.24A)** and covers most of the body surface. It typically contains hair follicles, sebaceous glands, and sweat glands. Thick skin has a much thicker stratum corneum **(Fig. 1.24B)** and is found only on palms of the hands, and soles of the feet. It is adapted to withstand greater mechanical stress and friction. Thick skin lacks hair follicles and sebaceous glands but contains numerous eccrine sweat glands.

Under the microscope, both thin and thick skin consist of two main layers: the epidermis and the dermis. The epidermis is a keratinized stratified squamous epithelium, whereas the dermis is a layer of connective tissue that supports and nourishes the epidermis.

Epidermis

The epidermis is composed of keratinized stratified squamous epithelium arranged into distinct layers (strata), which represent successive stages of keratinocyte differentiation.

A. **Stratum basale (basal layer):** It is the deepest layer of the epidermis, resting directly on the basement membrane. This layer consists of a single layer of cuboidal to low columnar cells, which are highly proliferative and produce new keratinocytes that migrate toward the skin surface. The basal layer also contains melanocytes and a small number of Merkel cells.
B. **Stratum spinosum (spiny cell layer):** It is composed of several layers of polygonal keratinocytes connected by numerous desmosomes. During routine histological preparation, the cells shrink, producing the characteristic spiny appearance. Langerhans cells are commonly found in this layer.
C. **Stratum granulosum (granular layer):** It consists of three to five layers of flattened cells containing abundant keratohyalin granules in their cytoplasm. The cells also contain lamellar granules, which release lipids that contribute to the epidermal water barrier.
D. **Stratum lucidum (clear layer):** It is a translucent layer of anucleate keratinocytes and is readily visible only in thick skin under a microscope.
E. **Stratum corneum (keratinized layer):** It is the outermost layer of epidermis, containing many layers of dead and keratinized cells that form a water-resistant protective barrier. These cells are continuously shed from the surface and are replaced by new cells derived from the proliferative cells of the stratum basale.

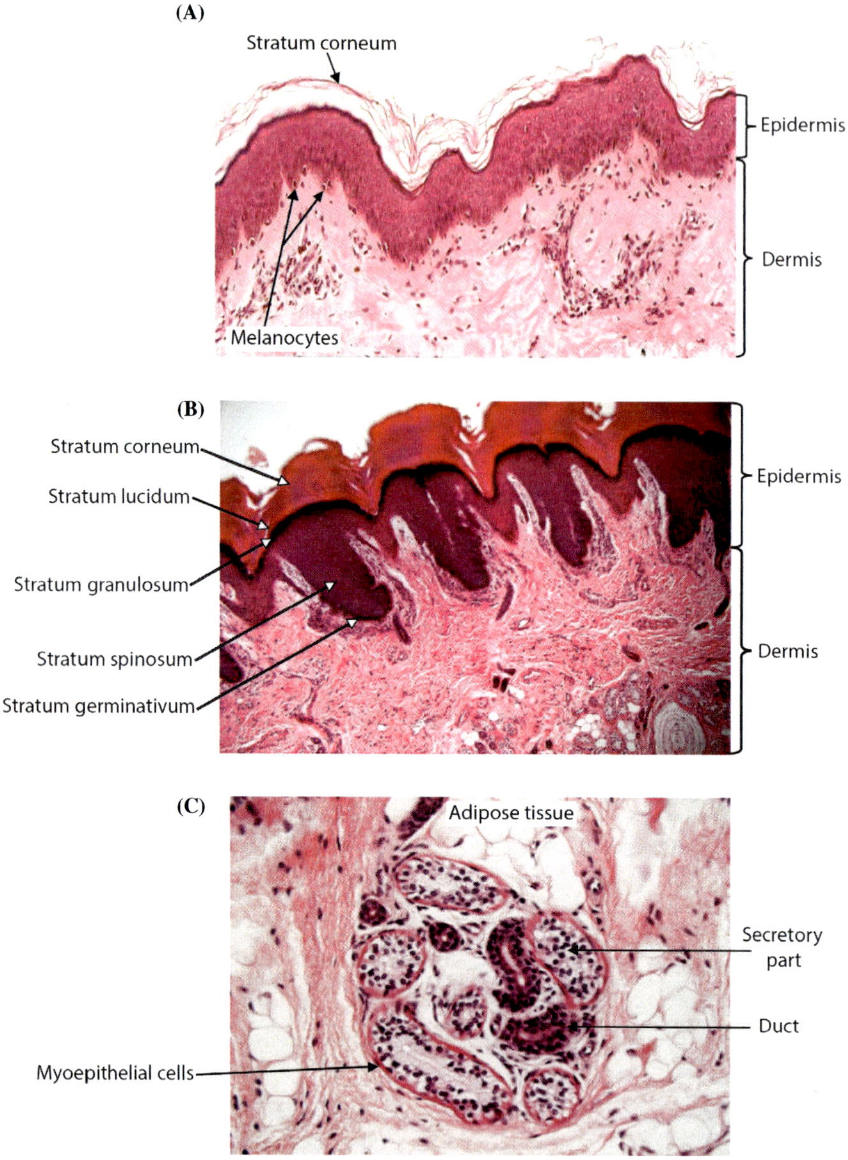

Figure 1.24. (A) Thin skin. (B) Thick skin. Note that the stratum corneum is relatively thin in the thin skin compared with the thick skin. The epidermis is composed of epithelial cells (epithelium) resting on the dermis, which is mainly connective tissue filled with massive collagen fibers (pinkly stained). The epidermis is subdivided into many layers. Melanocytes are identified in the stratum germinativum (basale). (H&E stain.) **(C) Sweat glands** are localized in the dermis. The sweat gland has two parts: the secretory part and the duct (double-layered epithelium). Myoepithelial cells are associated with the secretory part. Adipose tissues fill up the dermis. (H&E stain.)

Cells of the epidermis: The epidermis contains four principal cell types: keratinocytes, melanocytes, Langerhans cells, and Merkel cells. Keratinocytes constitute the vast majority of epidermal cells, while the other three are specialized cell types dispersed among them. Keratinocytes arise from the stratum basale and produce keratin and lipids that form the protective epidermal water barrier. Melanocytes are found among the cells of stratum basale and synthesize melanin, the pigment responsible for skin colour and protection against ultraviolet (UV) radiation. Langerhans cells are dendritic cells and distributed predominantly in the stratum spinosum. They serve as the first line of immune defence in the epidermis and are crucial for antigen presentation **(Fig. 1.23)**. They are of mesenchymal origin and belong to the mononuclear phagocytic system. Merkel cells are specialized tactile epithelial cells located in the stratum basale. They serve as mechanoreceptors for light touch and are abundant in the palms, soles, and oral mucosa.

The epidermis is avascular and receives oxygen and nutrients by diffusion from the richly vascularized dermis. Sensory nerve fibers also extend into the epidermis as free nerve endings, which function primarily as nociceptors and thermoreceptors, with some contributing to light-touch sensation **(Fig. 1.23A, B)**. The cell bodies of these primary sensory neurons are located in the dorsal root ganglia or the sensory ganglia of cranial nerves.

Dermis (Fig. 1.23A, B; Fig. 1.24A, B)

The dermis is the connective tissue layer that supports and nourishes the epidermis. It consists of two layers: papillary layer and reticular layer. The papillary layer is the superficial layer composed of loose connective tissue. It projects into the epidermis as dermal papillae, which interdigitate with epidermal ridges to strengthen the attachment between the epidermis and dermis. Reticular layer is the deeper and much thicker layer composed of dense irregular connective tissue. This layer is rich in collagen and elastic fibers, providing tensile strength and elasticity to the skin. The dermis is rich in blood vessels, nerves, sensory receptors, hair follicles, and sweat glands.

A. **Blood vessels and nerves (Fig. 1.23 A, B)** The dermis contains numerous arteries, veins, and capillaries that supply nutrients and oxygen to the dermis and, by diffusion, to the avascular epidermis. In certain regions, arteriovenous shunts are present and play an important role in thermoregulation by regulating cutaneous blood flow.

B. The dermis is richly innervated by both sensory and postganglionic sympathetic nerve fibers **(Fig. 1.23A, B)**. Sensory fibers extend into the epidermis as free nerve endings (nociceptive), which detect pain, temperature, and itch. Other sensory fibers terminate in specialized receptors, including Meissner's corpuscles, located within the dermal papillae **(Fig. 1.25)**, and Pacinian corpuscles, located in the deep dermis and hypodermis **(Fig. 1.26A, B)**. Meissner's corpuscles detect light touch, whereas Pacinian corpuscles detect deep pressure and vibration. Postganglionic sympathetic nerve fibers innervate the arrector pili muscles, sweat glands, and vascular smooth muscle, thereby regulating piloerection, sweating, and cutaneous blood flow.

C. **Sweat glands (Fig. 1.23A, B; Fig. 1.24C)** These are simple coiled tubular glands consisting of secretory segment and a duct. Myoepithelial cells are associated with the secretory part of the gland. Contraction of these cells helps expel sweat into the duct. The secretory coils are located in the deep dermis or upper hypodermis, whereas the ducts pass through the dermis and epidermis to open onto the skin surface. The duct is lined by a double-layered stratified cuboidal epithelium.

D. **Hair follicles (Fig. 1.23B)** They are epithelial invaginations that extend from the epidermis into the dermis. Sebaceous glands are closely associated with hair follicles and secrete sebum into the follicular canal. The arrector pili muscle is a bundle of smooth muscle attached to the hair follicle and the superficial dermis. It is innervated by postganglionic sympathetic nerve fibers. Contraction of this muscle produces piloerection ("goosebumps") and also compresses the associated sebaceous gland, facilitating the release of sebum, which reduces transepidermal water loss.

Histological Differences between Thick and Thin Skin

1. **Thick skin** (Covers the palms of the hand and soles of the feet)
   - Hair follicles are absent.
   - Arrector pili muscles are absent.
   - Sebaceous glands are absent.
   - Sweat glands are numerous.
   - Epidermis is thick, with a very thick stratum corneum
   - Stratum lucidum is present

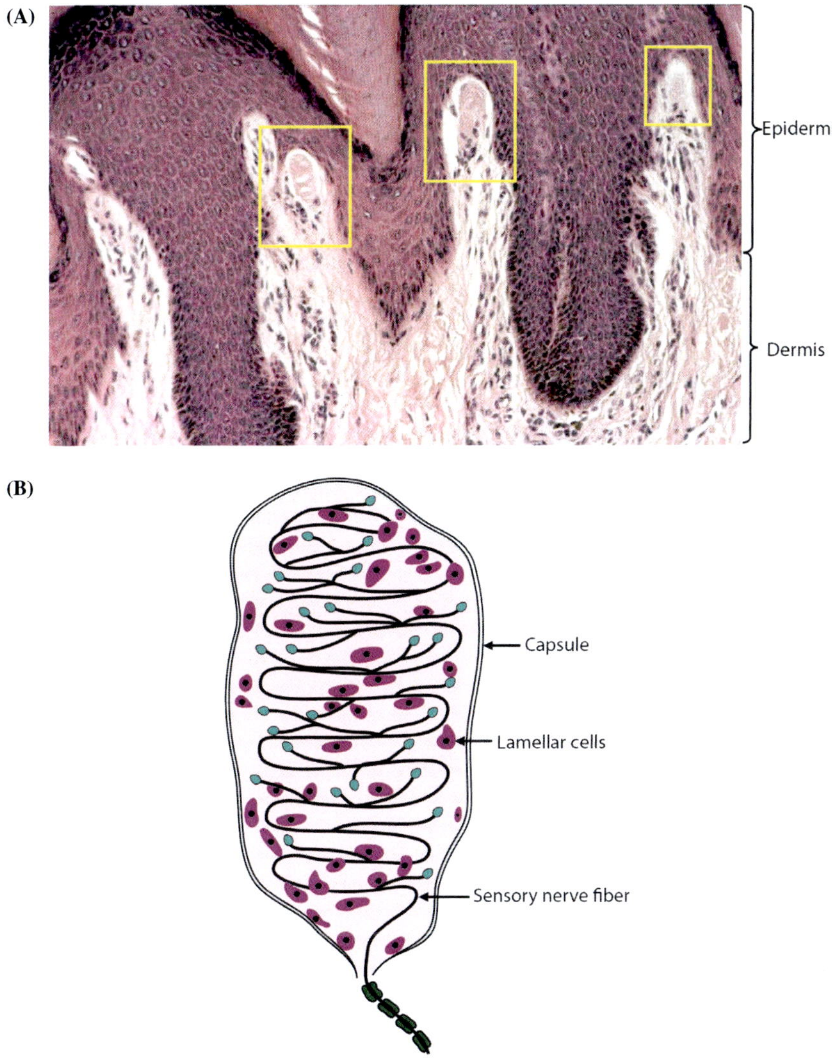

Figure 1.25. Meissner's corpuscle. (A) A section through the thick skin showing Meissner's corpuscles (yellow boxed area) localized in the dermal papilla. The receptors are sensitive to touch. The receptors are widely distributed at the skin of the fingertip. (H&E stain.) **(B)** A diagrammatic view of the mechanoreceptor Meissner's corpuscle. Note that the sensory nerve endings wind around the connective tissue cells (lamellar cells).

2. **Thin skin** (Covers most of the body surface)
   - Hair follicles are present.
   - Arrector pili muscles (smooth muscle supplied by sympathetic nerve fibres) are present; their contraction helps expel sebum from sebaceous glands and produces "goosebumps."

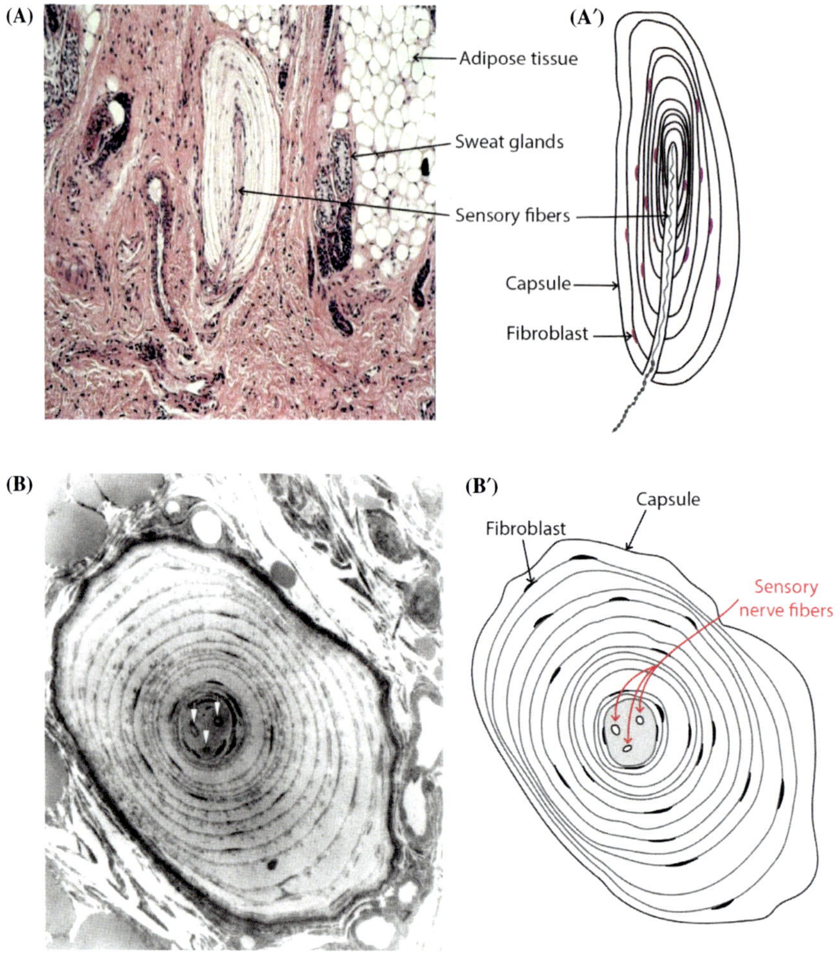

Figure 1.26. An encapsulated Pacinian corpuscle in the dermis stained by the H&E stain **(A, A')** and viewed by electron microscopy **(B, B')**. Note that the sensory nerve fiber is localized in the center of the receptor (arrows).

- Sebaceous glands are present; they secrete sebum, which lubricates the skin and helps reduce water loss.
- Sweat glands are present but are less numerous than in thick skin.
- Epidermis is thinner, with a relatively thin stratum corneum.
- Stratum lucidum is absent

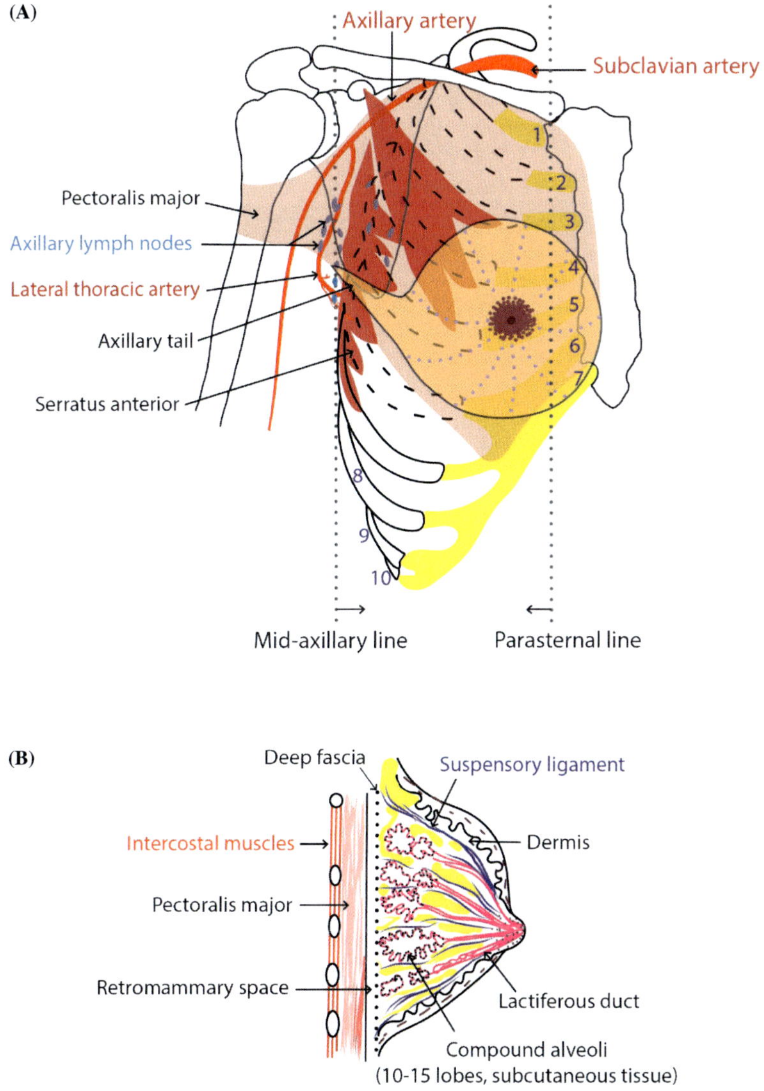

Figure 1.27. Mammary gland. (A) The mammary gland (breast) is a modified sweat gland. Histologically, it is considered a compound tubulo-aveolar gland. It extends from the 2nd to the 6th rib, from the parasternal line to the mid-axillary line. It lies on the pectoralis major and serratus anterior. **(B)** There are 10–15 lobes; each has a lactiferous duct leading to the nipple. The duct is dilated nearer to the nipple as the lactiferous sinus. The gland is mainly subcutaneous, containing adipose tissue and connective tissue. Fibrous bands extend from the deep fascia to the dermis — suspensory ligaments (Astley Cooper) that support the organ. Contraction of these ligaments due to the cancerous growth can cause "pitting of skin" over the gland.

- **Arterial supply:** Lateral thoracic artery, internal thoracic artery
- **Lymphatic drainage:** Axillary lymph nodes (mainly)

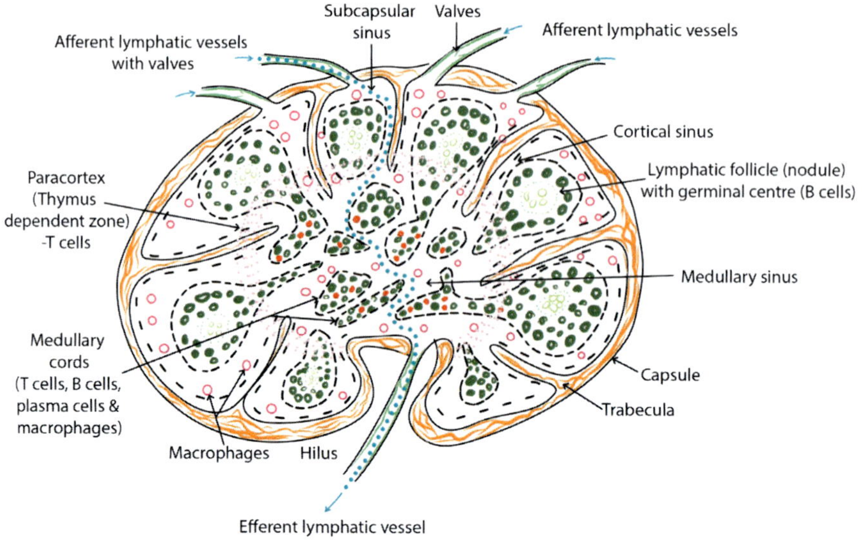

1. Site of immune response- the component cells respond vigorously to foreign antigens or pathogens that are brought in by tissue fluid (lymph fluid)in infection or inflammation. They also respond to cancer cells considered as non-self. The nodes serve like "police posts" and are in constant survelliance of invading pathogens.

2. Filtration of lymph or tissue fluid

   Afferent lymphatic vessel ⟶ Subcapsular sinus⟶ Cortical sinus ⟶ Medullary sinus

   ⟶ Efferent lymphatic vessel (valves)

3. Component cells

   - Lymphocytes: T & B lymphocytes
   - Macrophages: phagocytes - phagocytosis and antigen presentation
     (monocyte-derived) MHC I, MHC II, CR3

   T lymphocytes: T helper, cytotoxic, suppressor

   B lymphocytes $\xrightarrow{\text{on activation}}$ Plasma cells ⟶ antibodies

Figure 1.28. Lymph node. In a histological section, the lymph node is bean-shaped or concavo-convex. Its surface is covered by a layer of capsule with trabeculae (finger-like projections) extending into the parenchyma of the node. The outer part of the node is the cortex, and the inner part nearer to the hilus is the medulla. The cortex shows the presence of lymphatic nodules (follicles); each has a germinal center. The follicle contains mainly B lymphocytes and dividing cells. The medulla has many irregular medullary cords containing a mixture of cells. The paracortex (thymus-dependant zone) at the border area between the cortex and medulla contains predominantly T lymphocytes. The capsule on the convex surface of the node is pierced by afferent lymphatic vessels, whose valves guide the inflow of lymphatic fluid into the subcapsular sinus, cortical sinus, medullary sinus, and thence into the outflowing efferent lymphatic vessel. As the lymph fluid percolates or filters through the node, the lymphocytes, along with macrophages in the sinuses, are activated by potential pathogens, thus triggering an immune response.

(A)

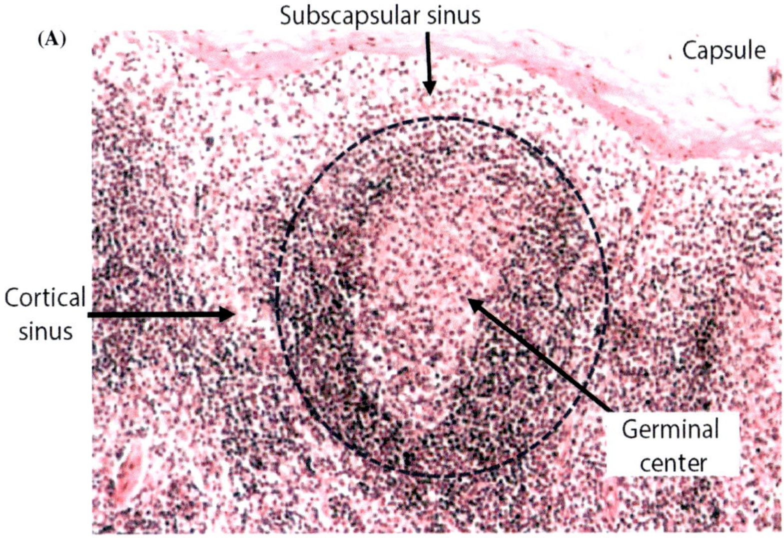

(B)

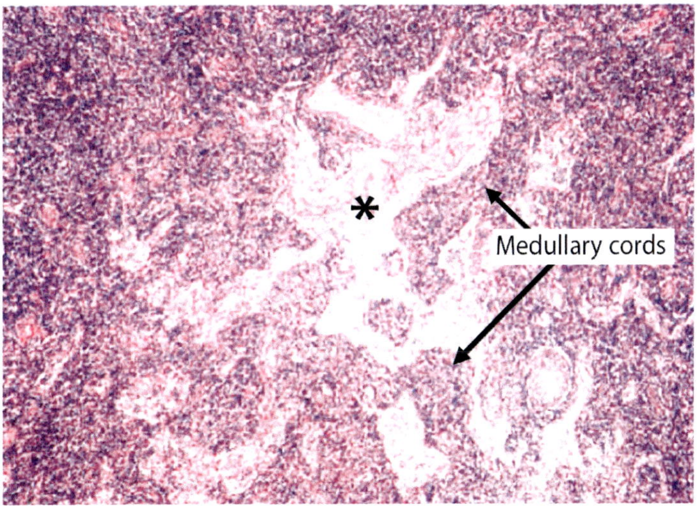

Figure 1.29. Lymph node. (A) Cortex. Showing its covering capsule, subcapsular sinus, cortical sinus, and a lymphatic follicle (nodule) (outlined) with its lighter area, the germinal center. **(B) Medulla.** Showing the medullary cords (arrows), and between them, the medullary sinuses (asterisk). (H&E stain.)

Chapter 2

RESPIRATORY SYSTEM

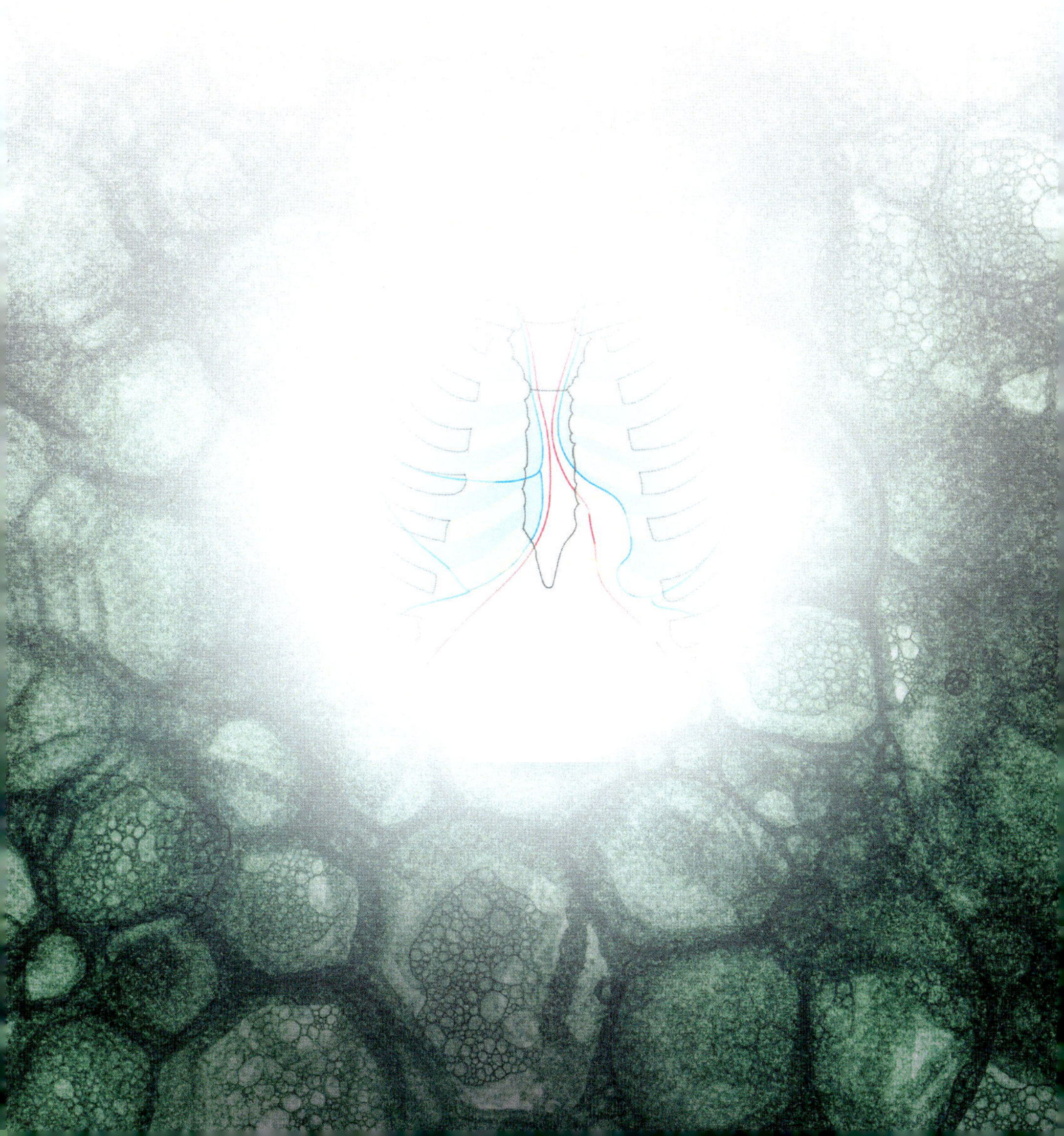

RESPIRATORY SYSTEM

The respiratory system facilitates gas exchange by taking in oxygen from the atmospheric air for metabolic activities and releasing carbon dioxide, which is transported via the blood circulation. The system consists of two main components: the respiratory passage, which conducts air, and the lungs, where gas exchange occurs. Further anatomically the respiratory system is divided into the upper and lower respiratory tracts. The upper respiratory tract begins at the two nostrils leading to the nasal cavity, nasopharynx and paranasal sinuses. The lower respiratory tract comprises larynx, trachea, primary bronchi, secondary bronchi, tertiary bronchi, bronchioles, alveolar ducts which lead to the pulmonary alveoli where gas exchange takes place. In addition to conducting the air, the nasal cavity filters, warms, and humidifies inspired air. The lungs are protected by the thoracic cage, which helps in respiration through movements of the ribs and the diaphragm.

The thoracic cage is made up of the following bony components **(Fig. 2.1A)**:

1. **Twelve Pairs of Ribs**: There are true ribs (1–7) and false ribs (8–12), of which 11 and 12 are called the floating ribs. The true ribs articulate with the thoracic vertebrae (body and intervertebral disc) at the costovertebral joint, posteriorly and with the sternum at the sternocostal joint via costal cartilages, anteriorly. The false ribs 8–10 articulate with the costal cartilage of the rib above at the interchondral joint. The floating ribs (11th and 12th ribs) do not have anterior attachments and end freely in the abdominal wall. All joints mentioned above are synovial joints except for the first sternocostal joint, which is a cartilaginous joint (with no movement).
2. **Twelve Thoracic Vertebrae**: A typical rib articulates with the body of the corresponding vertebra and the one above it, as well as with the intervertebral disc (intra-articular ligament).
3. **Sternum**: It includes the manubrium, body of the sternum and xiphoid process. Between the manubrium and the sternum is the manubriosternal joint, which presents an angulation of the sternal angle corresponding to the level of between T4 & T5 thoracic vertebrae which is at the plane of Louis, where many important structures, such as the bifurcation of the trachea and ligamentum arteriosum, are identified.

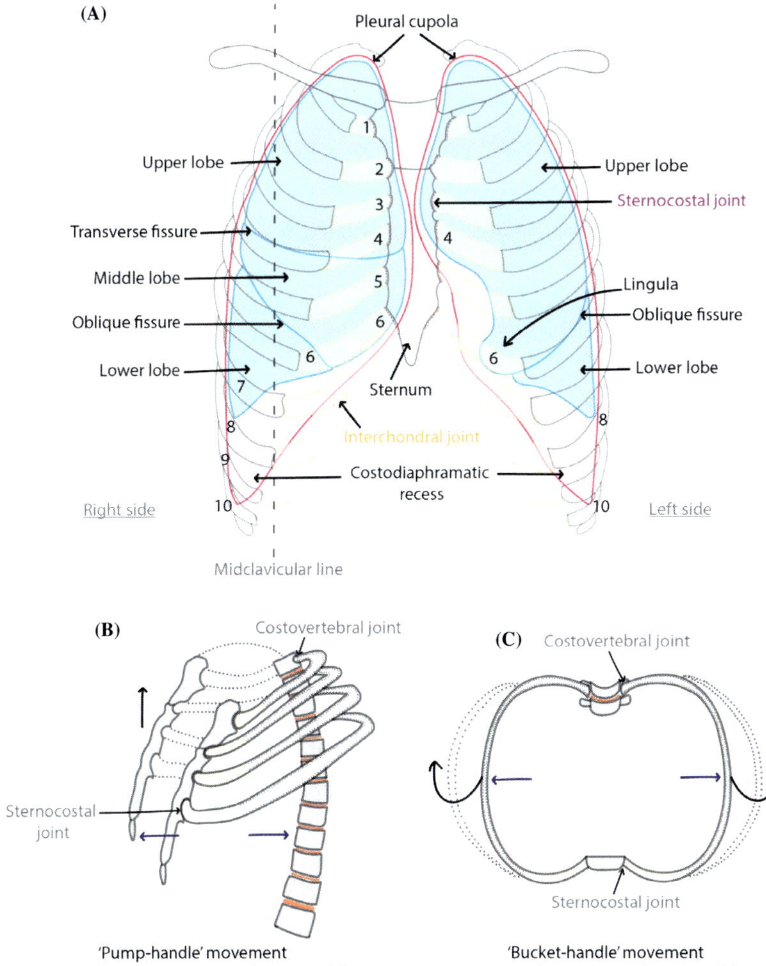

Figure 2.1. Thoracic cage, pleura and lung surface marking, and movements of the ribs. **(A)** The thoracic cage is made up of 12 ribs (numbered), a sternum, and 12 thoracic vertebrae. **(B)** The upper ribs are slanting downward and medially. They articulate with the vertebrae posteriorly at the costovertebral joint and anteriorly with the sternum at the sternocostal joint. The lower ribs articulate anteriorly with the costal cartilage above at the interchondral joint **(A)**. The parietal pleura (red line) lines the inner surface of the thoracic cavity, while the visceral pleura lines the surface of the lung (blue). Between the lung and parietal pleura below (diaphragmatic pleura) is the costodiaphragmatic recess — the lower part of the pleural cavity. Cupola **(A)** is the cervical part of the parietal pleura, which rises above the clavicle and 1st rib. **(A)**. In the right lung, the oblique and transverse fissures divide the right lung into three lobes. The oblique fissure is along the 5th rib, which intersects with the 6th costal cartilage. The transverse fissure extends from the 4th costal cartilage to the 5th rib laterally. In the left lung, the mediastinal surface is deviated to the left due to the heart. **(B)** "Pump-handle" movement in the upper ribs. **(C)** "Bucket-handle" movement in the lower ribs.

FEATURES OF A TYPICAL RIB

It consists of the head, neck, articular tubercle (articulates with the transverse process of the corresponding vertebra), non-articular tubercle (ligament attachment), angle, and shaft. Anteriorly, the bony rib articulates with the sternum via costal cartilage. Costal cartilage is made up of hyaline cartilage histologically. The shaft has a groove inferiorly (subcostal groove), in which lies the neurovascular bundle (intercostal vein, intercostal artery, and intercostal nerve which are arranged supero-inferiorly).

Intercostal Spaces (Fig. 2.2A, B, C)

Between the ribs are the intercostal spaces, which are occupied by intercostal muscles that aid in changing the volume of the thoracic cavity during inhalation (inspiration) and exhalation (expiration). The intercostal muscles and the overlying skin are supplied by the intercostal nerves, intercostal arteries, and veins.

Intercostal Muscles

1. **External intercostal muscle (Fig. 2.2C)**: The muscle fibers are attached to the inferior border of the rib above and the superior border of the rib below. The muscle fibers are oriented downward, forward and medially. They raise the ribs below, resulting in the expansion of the thoracic cage (volume) during inhalation (inspiration).
2. **Internal intercostal muscle (Fig. 2.2C)**: The muscle fibers are attached to the superior border of the rib below and attached to the inferior border of the rib above (costal groove). The muscle fibers are oriented downward, backward, and laterally. During contraction, they compress the thoracic cage and decrease the thoracic volume during exhalation.
3. **Intercostalis intimi (innermost layer muscle)**: The innermost muscular layer of the thoracic wall is incomplete and discontinuous. It comprises the innermost intercostal muscles, along with associated muscles such as the transversus thoracis (sternocostalis) anteriorly and the subcostal muscles posteriorly. (Note: Terminology varies among different textbooks — the muscle actions are not clearly defined.)

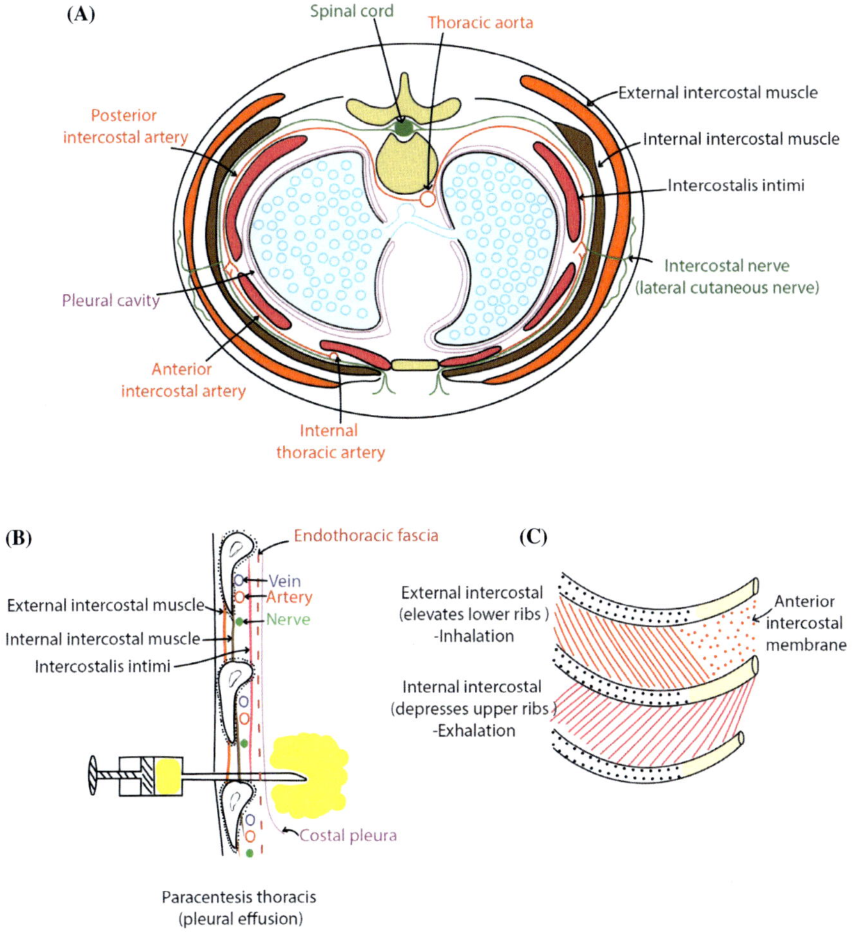

Figure 2.2. Intercostal spaces — muscles and neurovascular bundle. (A) Transverse section across the thorax showing the three layers of intercostal muscles between the ribs: external intercostal muscle, internal intercostal muscle, and intercostalis intimi (innermost layer) arranged from outside inward. The intercostal artery and intercostal nerve lie between the second and the third layers. Note the intercostal artery arises from the thoracic aorta. The intercostal nerve originates from the thoracic segment of the spinal cord. **(B)** A side view of the intercostal spaces showing the arrangement of the neurovascular bundle. Note the intercostal vein, intercostal artery, and intercostal nerve are arranged in this order from above downward; hence, when inserting a needle into the pleural cavity, e.g., paracentesis thoracis, it should be directed over the upper border of the rib to avoid damaging the nerve. **(C)** The muscle fibers of the external oblique are directed downward and medially. Contraction of the muscle fibers elevates the lower ribs, which increases the volume of the thoracic cavity during inhalation. The internal intercostal muscle fibers are directed upward; they compress the upper ribs and decrease the volume of the thoracic cavity during exhalation.

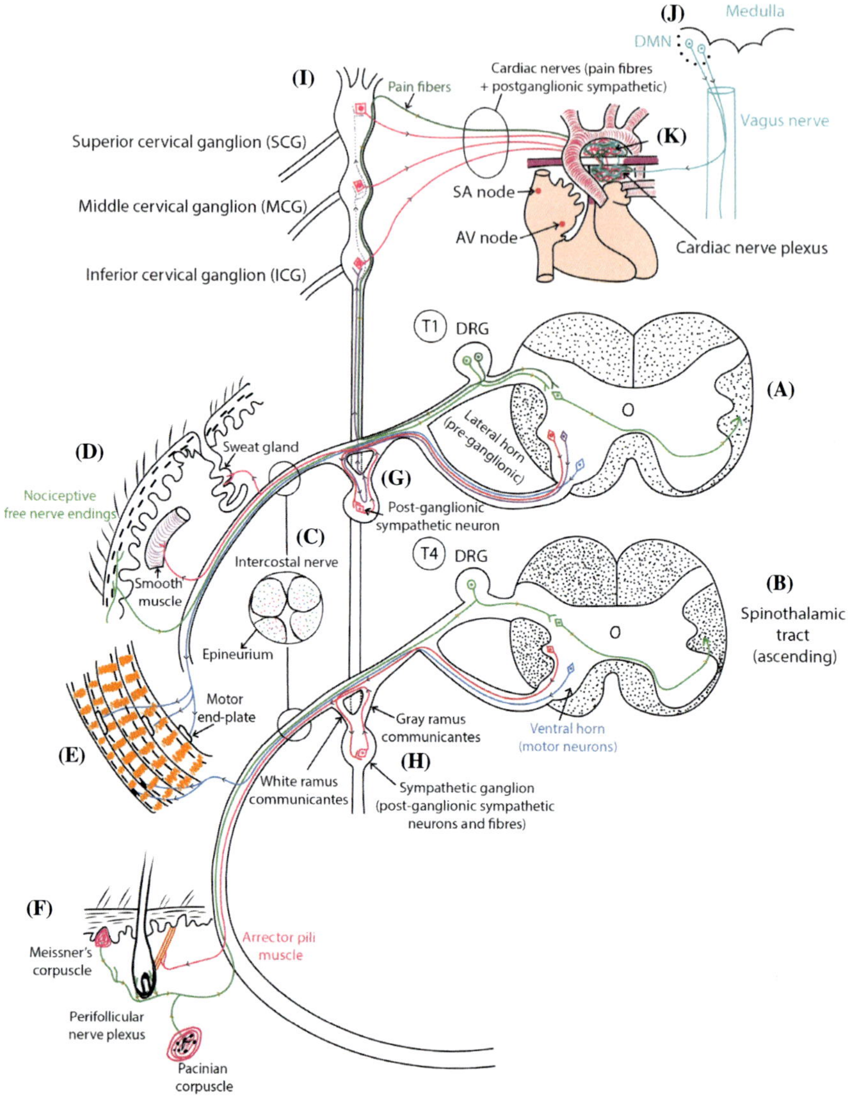

Figure 2.3. Intercostal nerves and autonomic nerves of the thorax. Organization and distribution of intercostal nerves **(A)** T1 and **(B)** T4. The intercostal nerve is enveloped in a layer of epineurium **(C)**. It is composed of sensory and motor nerve fibers. The sensory fibers represent the peripheral processes of the sensory neurons localized in the dorsal root ganglion (DRG) **(A, B)**. The sensory fibers (also called the afferents) terminate in the peripheral receptors: free nerve endings **(D)**, Meissner's corpuscle **(F)**, Pacinian corpuscle **(F)**, and perifollicular nerve plexus **(F)**. The central processes of the DRG neurons enter the spinal. After relay, the ascending axons constitute the spinothalamic tract **(B)**. (The neuroanatomical details can be explored further in the neuroanatomy.) The intercostal nerve also contains motor fibers, which represent the axons of motor or

Intercostal Nerves (Fig. 2.3)

There are 11 intercostal nerves, arising from the thoracic segment of the spinal cord. The intercostal nerve is a mixed (motor and sensory fibers) spinal nerve innervating the intercostal muscles, the overlying skin, and the adjacent parietal pleura. The nerve cell body of the sensory nerve fiber (afferent) is localized in the corresponding dorsal root (sensory) ganglion, while the cell body of the motor nerve fibers (axons or efferent fibers) is localized in the ventral horn of the spinal cord. In addition to the above, the intercostal nerve also contains the postganglionic sympathetic nerve fibers, which supply the blood vessels (smooth muscle in the vascular walls), sweat glands, and arrector pili.

Intercostal Arteries and Arterial Anastomoses at the Thoracic Walls (Fig. 2.4)

The intercostal spaces are supplied by the intercostal arteries, which originate from the internal thoracic artery and thoracic aorta.

There are two main sets of intercostal arteries — anterior and posterior intercostal arteries.

- Anterior intercostal arteries arise primarily from the internal thoracic artery, which originates from the subclavian artery. At the 6th intercostal space, the internal thoracic artery divides into the musculophrenic artery and the

Figure 2.3. (*Continued on facing page*) ventral horn neurons (blue neurons, **A**, **B**). The axon ends at the motor endplate supplying the skeletal muscle fibers **(E)**. The autonomic nerves have two parts: (i) sympathetic and (ii) parasympathetic. **(A, B)**. The preganglionic sympathetic neurons are localized in the lateral horn of the spinal cord (red neurons). The preganglionic sympathetic fibers synapse with the postganglionic sympathetic neurons in the sympathetic ganglion **(G)** and **(H)**. The postganglionic sympathetic fibers then enter the intercostal nerve to supply the sweat glands **(D)**, blood vessels **(D)**, and arrector pili muscle **(F)**. Axons of some preganglionic sympathetic neurons in the lateral horn (dark blue neurons) ascend along the sympathetic trunk to make synaptic contacts with postganglionic sympathetic neurons in the superior-, middle-, and inferior cervical ganglia **(I)**. The postganglionic sympathetic fibers from SCG, MCG, and ICG form the cardiac nerves. They are joined by the parasympathetic nerve fibers from the dorsal motor nucleus (DMN, green neurons) of the vagus nerve **(J)**, forming the cardiac nerve plexus **(K)** around the ligamentum arteriosum. The cardiac nerve plexus supplies the sinoatrial (SA) node and atrioventricular (AV) node that regulates the cardiac rhythm. Note that some pain fibers emanating from the heart travel along with the sympathetic nerves.

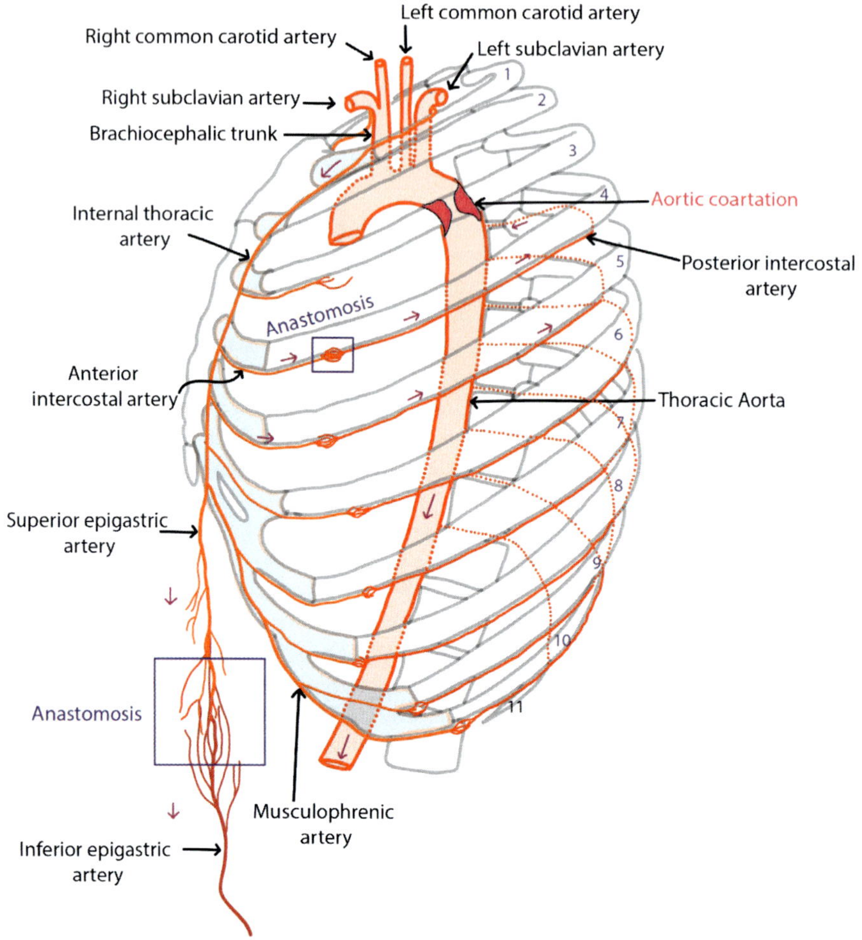

Arterial anastomoses [Collateral circulation]

1. Anterior intercostal artery↔ Posterior intercostal artery↔ Thoracic aorta
2. Superior epigastic ↔ Inferior epigastric↔ External iliac

Figure 2.4. Arterial anastomosis provides collateral circulation in the event of an aortic coartation. The intercostal spaces are supplied by the intercostal arteries: anterior intercostal arteries and posterior intercostal arteries. The posterior intercostal arteries arise directly from the thoracic aorta (except for the first posterior intercostal artery). The anterior intercostal arteries in the upper intercostal spaces (till the sixth intercostal space) arise from the internal thoracic artery from the subclavian artery. In the lower intercostal spaces, the anterior intercostal arteries arise from the musculophrenic artery, one of the two branches of the internal thoracic artery, the other branch being the superior epigastric artery. Arterial anastomosis is established between the anterior and posterior intercostal arteries at the intercostal spaces. This provides a collateral circulation for the lower part of the body in the event of an aortic coarctation. Also, the superior epigastric artery forms an arterial anastomosis with the inferior epigastric artery in the anterior abdominal wall.

superior epigastric artery (descends to the umbilical region). The anterior intercostal arteries in the upper intercostal spaces are derived directly from the internal thoracic artery, while those of the lower intercostal spaces arise from the musculophrenic artery.

- The majority of the posterior intercostal arteries are from the thoracic aorta.
- Arterial anastomosis is established between the anterior and posterior intercostal arteries, which provides a collateral circulation in the event of aortic coarctation (stenosis) distal to the arch of the aorta.
- Superior epigastric arteries establish an arterial anastomosis with the inferior epigastric arteries (branching from the external iliac artery) at the umbilical region. This provides a collateral circulation linking the subclavian artery with the external iliac artery supplying the lower limb.

THORACENTESIS (PLEURAL TAP) (Fig. 2.2B)

In emergency conditions such as pneumothorax or pleural effusion, a needle or catheter can be inserted into the pleural cavity to aspirate the air or fluid. To avoid damage to the neurovascular bundle, the needle is inserted into the lower part of the intercostal space.

DIAPHRAGM

The diaphragm is a musculotendinous partition that separates the thorax from the abdomen. Embryologically, it is derived from the (1) septum transversum, (2) body muscular walls, (3) dorsal meso-esophagus (mesentery), and (4) pleuroperitoneal membrane (minor). It receives motor and sensory innervation from the phrenic nerve (C3, 4, 5) and the lower intercostal nerves (sensory). During inspiration, the diaphragm contracts and descends, increasing the vertical diameter of the thoracic cavity. In phrenic nerve injury, the muscular part of the affected side of the diaphragm is paralyzed leading to hemidiaphragm.

MOVEMENTS OF RIBS DURING THE RESPIRATION (Fig. 2.1B, C)

1. **Pump-handle movement**: This occurs predominantly in the upper ribs during inspiration. The anterior ends of the ribs and the sternum move superiorly and anteriorly, increasing the anteroposterior diameter of the

thorax. The axis of rotation lies approximately along a transverse line passing through the costovertebral and costotransverse joints (near the neck of the rib).

2. **Bucket-handle movement**: This occurs mainly in the lower ribs. The ribs elevate laterally, increasing the transverse diameter of the thorax. The axis of rotation is more anteroposterior, extending roughly between the anterior and posterior ends of the rib.

Both types of movements of the ribs and contraction of the diaphragm increase the thoracic volume during the inspiration (inhalation).

RESPIRATORY PASSAGE (Fig. 2.5)

Nasal Cavity: The nasal cavity begins at the nostrils (vestibule) and is separated by the nasal septum. The surface of the nasal cavity is lined by the respiratory epithelium (ciliated pseudostratified columnar epithelium). Its main function is to warm, moisturize and humidify the inspired air. Nasal cavity opens into the nasopharynx, oropharynx, laryngopharynx which leads to larynx and trachea.

Trachea: It is made up of a series of C-shaped hyaline cartilage. Posteriorly, the free ends of the C-shaped cartilage are bridged by the trachealis muscle (smooth muscle). The C-shaped cartilage rings help maintain the patency of the windpipe. The trachea bifurcates into two primary bronchi at the level of T4, where a ridge, the carina, separates the openings of the two bronchi **(Fig. 2.5A)**. The mucous membrane is lined by the respiratory epithelium. Some seromucous glands are distributed in the submucosa of trachea **(Fig. 2.5B; Fig. 2.6A)**.

Bronchus: It contains broken-up hyaline cartilage and smooth muscle bundles as well as seromucous glands which are found in the submucosa **(Fig. 2.5C)**. It is lined by the respiratory epithelium. Viral or bacterial infection of the bronchi may cause obstruction to the airways. Chronic obstruction pulmonary disease (COPD) may result in the breakdown of the alveolar septa (bulla, emphysema) thereby resulting in difficulty in breathing.

Bronchiole (Fig. 2.5D; Fig. 2.6C): It divides into the terminal bronchiole and the respiratory bronchiole. The terminal bronchiole is lined by the simple cuboidal epithelium whereas the respiratory bronchiole is partly lined by alveolar

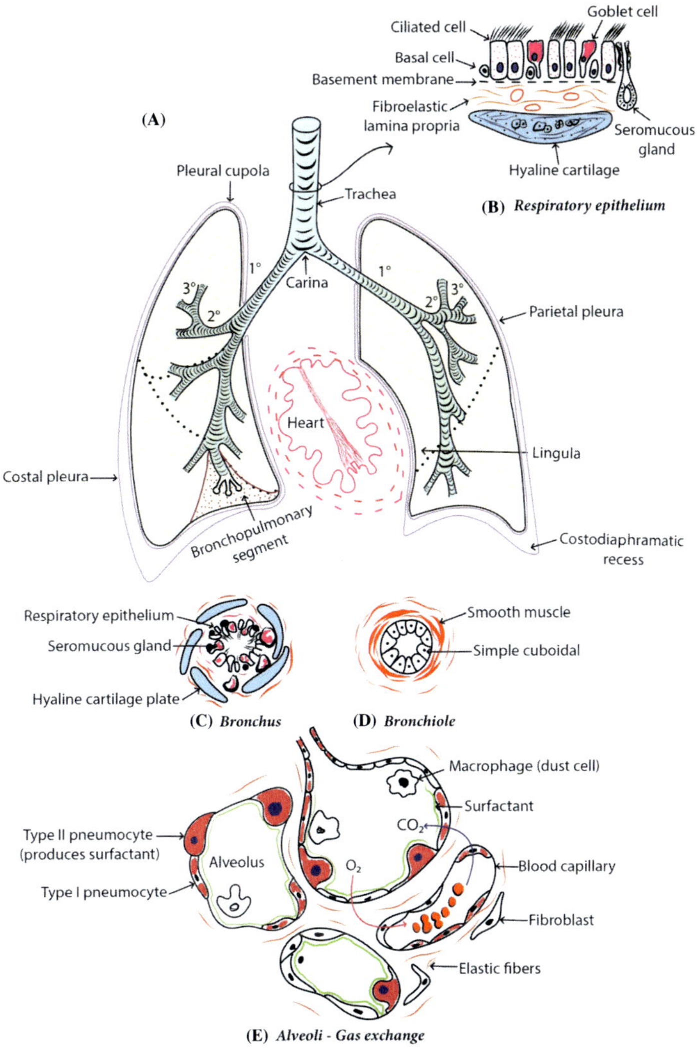

Figure 2.5. Respiratory passage and lungs. (A) The trachea bifurcates into the right and left primary bronchus (1°); each entering the hilus of the respective lung. The bronchus then divides further into the 2° and 3° bronchi. The area of the lung tissue supplied by a 3° bronchus is a "bronchopulmonary segment." **(B)** The trachea and bronchus are lined by a ciliated pseudostratified columnar epithelium (respiratory epithelium) composed of ciliated columnar cells, goblet cells, and basal cells resting on a basement membrane. Serous mucous glands and cartilage are present. The wall of the trachea has C-shaped cartilage rings (hyaline). **(C)** In the bronchus, overlapping cartilage plates are present. **(D)** Distal to the 3° bronchus is the terminal bronchiole lined by the simple cuboidal epithelium lacking cilia. Smooth muscle fibers encircle the lumen. **(E)** Further distal to the bronchiole is the alveolar duct that leads to pulmonary alveoli lined by simple squamous epithelial cells: Type 1 pneumocyte and Type II pneumocyte that secrete surfactant. In the interalveolar septum, elastic fibers, macrophages, fibroblasts, and blood capillaries for exchanges of gas are present.

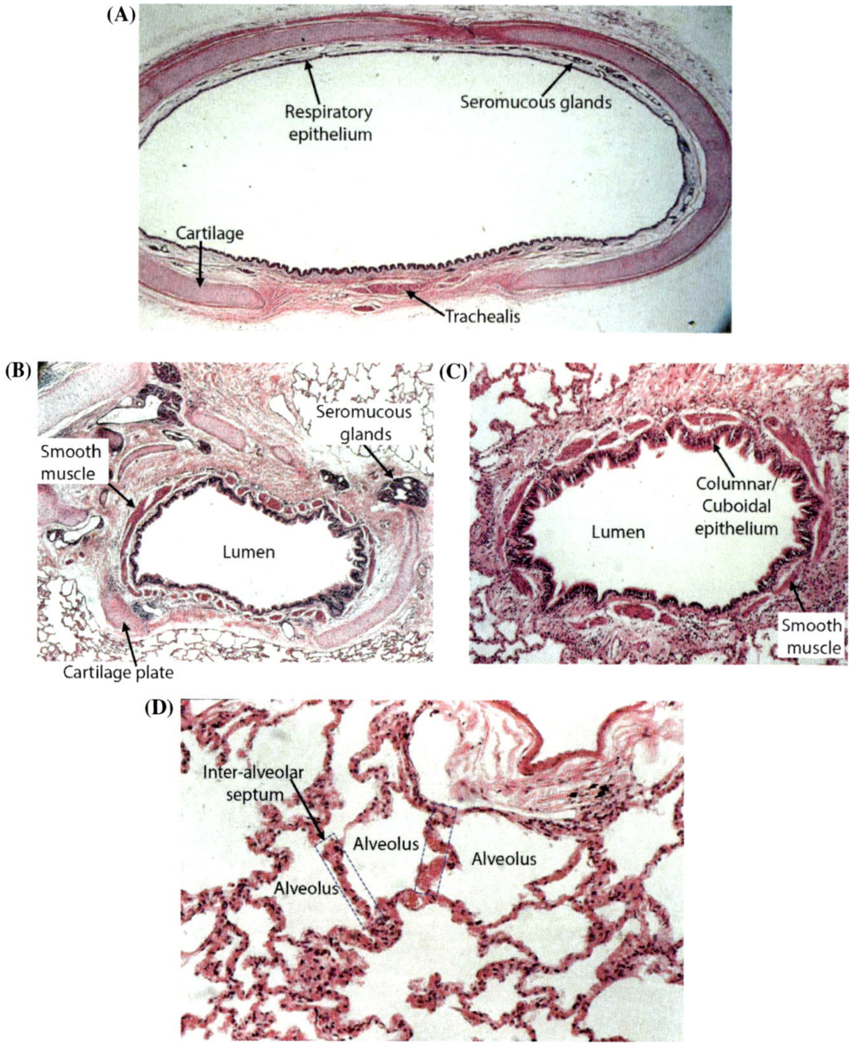

Figure 2.6. **(A) Trachea** in a transverse section showing its lumen and the C-shaped cartilage (hyaline), whose free ends are bridged by trachealis muscle (smooth). The mucosa of the lumen is lined by the respiratory epithelium. Deep to the epithelium are seromucous glands. (Hematoxylin and eosin (H&E) stain.) **(B) Bronchus** in a transverse section. The mucosa is lined by a respiratory epithelium. Some seromucous glands are beneath the epithelium. The wall shows overlapping cartilage plates. A thin, discontinuous layer of smooth muscle is present. (H&E stain.) **(C) Bronchiole** in a transverse section. The lumen is lined by the simple columnar/cuboidal epithelium. Note the absence of goblet cells in the epithelium; also, seromucous glands and cartilage plates are absent. A distinct layer of smooth muscle encircles the respiratory tube. (H&E stain.) **(D) Pulmonary alveoli**. The alveolus is lined by Type 1 pneumocytes (epithelial cells) and Type 2 pneumocytes (secrete surfactant). They are at too low a magnification to be identified. Between the alveoli is the inter-alveolar septum (boxed) containing blood capillaries, elastic tissue, and macrophages. The septum may break down in emphysema, causing breathlessness. (H&E stain.)

epithelium (simple squamous epithelium); hence, gas exchange can take place at the respiratory bronchiole. Cartilage plates, cilia, and seromucous glands are absent in the bronchiole. A conspicuous feature is the smooth muscle layer. Asthma is caused by bronchiolar smooth muscle spasm. Bronchodilators are therefore used for its treatment.

Pulmonary Alveolus (Alveoli) (Fig. 2.5E; Fig. 2.6D): It is lined by the simple squamous epithelium, composed of two cell types:

1. **Type 1 pneumocyte**: A thin-layered cell that facilitates gas exchange.
2. **Type 2 pneumocyte**: It produces pulmonary surfactant that decreases the surface tension for the expansion of the epithelial lining.

In respiratory distress syndrome in newborns, there is insufficient production of surfactant (premature birth), causing difficulty in breathing.

Interalveolar Septum (Fig. 2.5E; Fig. 2.6D): It contains blood capillaries (gas exchange), elastic fibers (aiding recoil of lung tissue after expansion), and macrophages (known as dust cells for phagocytosis of dust particles). Breakdown of the septum decreases the surface area for gas exchange in some diseases.

LUNGS (Fig. 2.1; Fig. 2.7)

The lungs are located within the thoracic cavity. The surface features of the right and left lungs are different due to the impressions or indentations caused by different organs or structures to which they are closely related. In general, each lung has an apex, base, costal surface, mediastinal surface, diaphragmatic surface (base), anterior border, and posterior border. The hilus (hilum) which is on the mediastinal surface, is the site of the entrance of the bronchus and pulmonary artery and exit of the pulmonary veins. The hilum together with the associated structures are called the root of the lung.

The right lung **(Fig. 2.7A)** has three lobes (upper, middle, and lower) separated by the oblique and the transverse fissures, whereas the left lung **(Fig. 2.7B)** has only two lobes (upper and lower) separated by oblique fissure. There is a small projection called the lingula in the upper lobe.

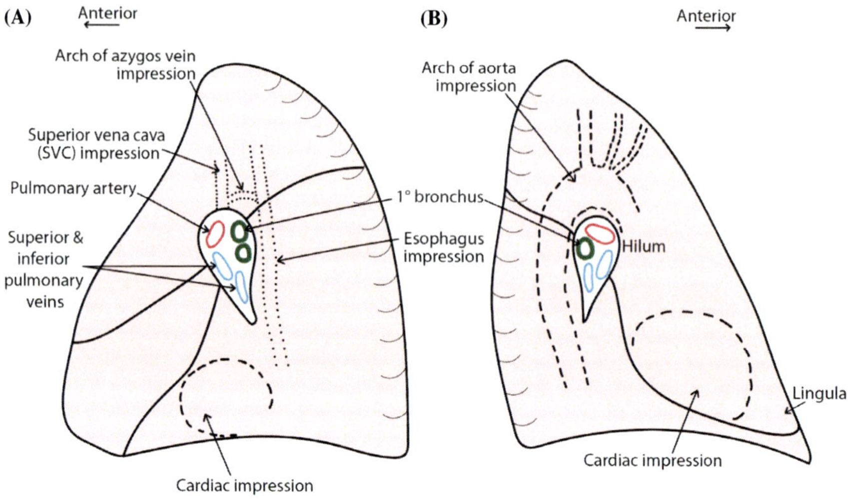

Figure 2.7. Mediastinal surface of lungs. (A) Right lung. **(B)** Left lung. The mediastinal surface of the right lung is related to the arch of the azygos vein, superior vena cava (SVC), esophagus, and heart (cardiac impression). The mediastinal surface of the left lung is related to the arch of the aorta and its branches and thoracic aorta. At the hilus of the lung are superior and inferior pulmonary veins (most anterior and inferior), pulmonary artery (superior), and the bronchus (primary), which is placed most posteriorly.

Pleura (Fig. 2.1; Fig. 2.2A; Fig. 2.5A)

The lung is covered by the visceral and parietal pleura. Lining the immediate surface of the lung is the visceral layer of the pleura, which may be traced to the hilus, where it becomes continuous with the parietal layer at the root of the lung (pulmonary ligament). The parietal pleura is closely adherent to the inner surface of the thoracic cavity (deep to the endothoracic fascia), and lines the mediastinal surface over the fibrous pericardium (mediastinal pleura) and the superior surface of the diaphragm (diaphragmatic pleura). The pleural cavity, which is between the parietal and the visceral pleura, contains a small amount of fluid that provides lubrication to the lung surfaces. The cupola (cervical pleura) is the apical part of the parietal pleura that projects above the first rib (or clavicle) **(Fig. 2.1A)**.

The parietal pleura, in relation to the ribs, is innervated by the intercostal nerves. The mediastinal pleura, along with the fibrous pericardium (to be explained later), is innervated by the phrenic nerve.

In traumatic chest injuries (stab wound) or other diseases, air may enter the pleural cavity, causing pneumothorax resulting in collapse of the lung.

Surface marking of the parietal pleura (Fig. 2.1A)

1. Right lung: A line is drawn from a point 2.5 cm above the medial third of the clavicle (cervical pleura) then passing through the sternoclavicular joint, manubriosternal joint up to the 6th costal cartilage. This line further extends to the 8th costal cartilage at the mid-clavicular line, to the 10th costal cartilage at mid-axillary line and finally to the 12th costal cartilage at the paravertebral line.
2. Left lung: Similar to the right side, except at the manubriosternal joint, the line is drawn to the 4th costal cartilage after which the line is deviated to the 8th costal cartilage at the mid-axillary line, which is due to the presence of the heart (cardiac notch).

Surface marking of the lungs (Fig. 2.1A)

The surface markings of the lungs generally follow those of the parietal pleura but lie approximately two rib levels higher at the inferior border. For example, at the midclavicular, midaxillary, and paravertebral lines, the inferior border of the lung lies at the 6th, 8th, and 10th ribs, respectively, whereas the pleura extends to the 8th, 10th, and 12th ribs.

The oblique fissure follows the course of the 5th rib, directed medially toward the 6th costal cartilage. The transverse fissure of the right lung is marked by a line drawn from the 4th costal cartilage at the sternum extending laterally to meet the oblique fissure at the level of the 5th rib in the midaxillary line.

The space between the inferior border of the lung and the inferior limit of the parietal pleura is known as the costodiaphragmatic recess, which allows for lung expansion during deep inspiration.

Innervation of the lungs

The lungs are innervated by the pulmonary nerve plexus, which is located at the root (hilum) of each lung. This plexus contains both sympathetic and parasympathetic nerve fibers.

Parasympathetic fibers are derived from the vagus nerve (cranial nerve X) and are responsible for bronchoconstriction, vasodilation, and stimulation of glandular secretion. The vagus nerve also carries visceral afferent fibers, including those involved in the cough reflex.

Sympathetic fibers arise from the thoracic sympathetic trunk and produce bronchodilation, vasoconstriction, and inhibition of glandular secretion.

Chapter 3

CARDIOVASCULAR SYSTEM

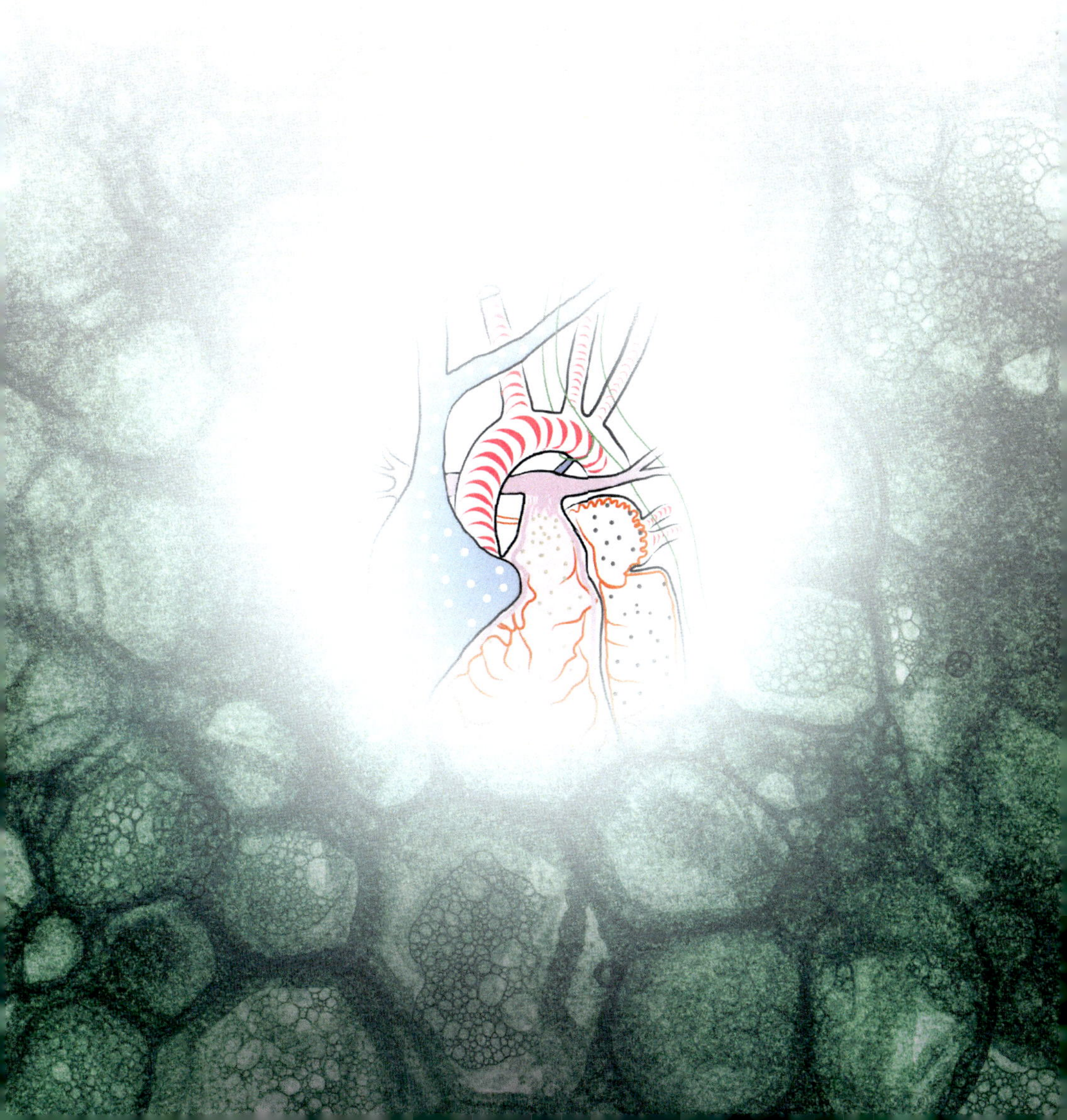

CARDIOVASCULAR SYSTEM

The cardiovascular system (CVS) is composed of structural and functional components: the heart and the circulatory system (**Fig. 3.1; Fig. 3.2; Fig. 3.3**).

1. **Heart:** It acts as a muscular pump delivering the oxygenated blood to different parts of the body (systemic circulation) for cellular metabolism. It also pumps the deoxygenated blood to lungs (pulmonary circulation) for oxygenation.
2. **Circulatory System:** The circulatory system is made up of many blood vessels, namely, arteries and veins. The arteries (excluding the pulmonary arteries) carry oxygenated blood to different parts of the body from the heart (systemic circulation). The veins (excluding the pulmonary veins) carry deoxygenated blood from different parts of the body to the heart and thence to the lungs through the pulmonary arteries for oxygenation (pulmonary circulation). Exchange of oxygen and carbon dioxide and nutrients/metabolites takes place in capillaries in the lung tissues or body tissues (where relevant).

HEART AND BLOOD CIRCULATION

The heart is a muscular organ with four chambers: right atrium, left atrium, left ventricle, and right ventricle (**Fig. 3.2**). The right atrium receives deoxygenated blood from different parts of the body *via* the superior and inferior vena cava, and from the heart itself *via* the coronary sinus. From the right atrium, the blood enters into the right ventricle via the right atrioventricular opening which is guarded by the tricuspid valve. Contraction of the right ventricle forces the blood into the pulmonary trunk through the pulmonary valves. It then enters into the lungs via pulmonary arteries for oxygenation (pulmonary circulation). After oxygenation, the blood is returned to the left atrium via the pulmonary veins (superior and inferior). Contraction of the left atrium forces the oxygenated blood into the left ventricle via the left atrioventricular opening guarded by

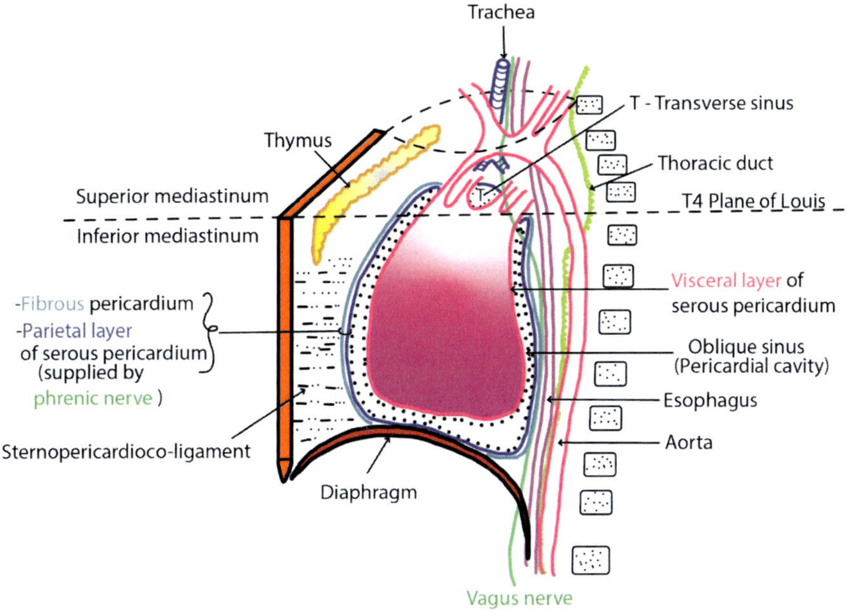

Superior mediastinum - Aorta (arch), cardiac nerve plexus
- Great vessels
- Trachea
- Esophagus
- Thymus(remnant)
- Vagus and phrenic nerves

Inferior mediastinum - Sternopericardioco-ligament
- Heart
- Vagus and phrenic nerves
- Thoracic duct
- Sympathetic trunk & ganglia
- Splanchnic nerves
- Azygos & hemiazygos veins

Figure 3.1. Mediastinum. The mediastinum between the two lungs is divided into the superior and inferior mediastinum, above and below the level of T4 (plane of Louis). The superior mediastinum contains mainly the great vessels, trachea, and esophagus. The inferior mediastinum is occupied by the heart, pericardial cavity, esophagus, thoracic aorta, etc.

bicuspid or mitral valve. The left ventricle, which has a thicker muscular wall than the right ventricle, contracts to pump the blood into the ascending aorta guarded by the aortic valves and the arch of the aorta and its branches to various parts of the body. This constitutes the systemic circulation.

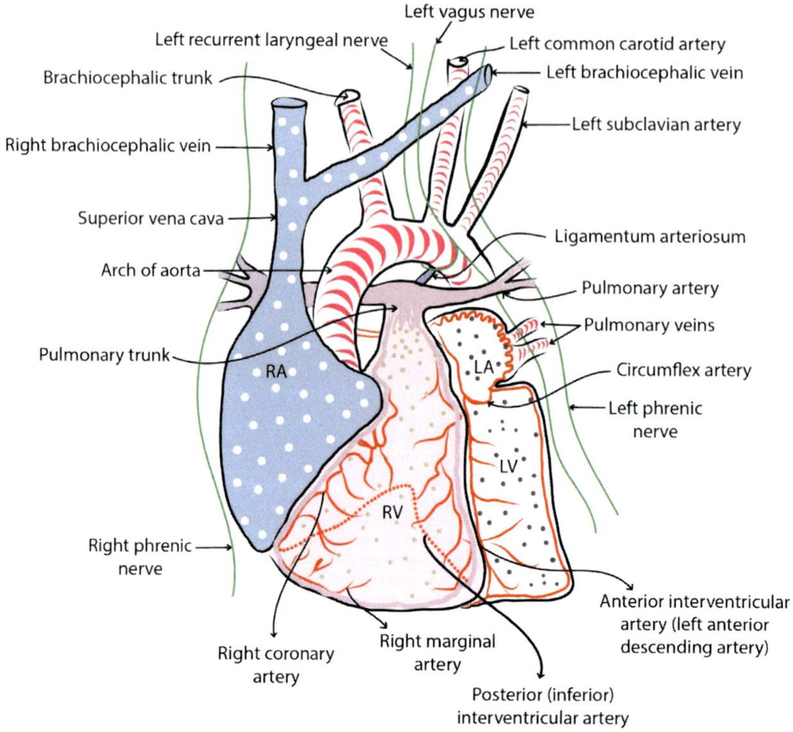

Figure 3.2. Heart (external features). The heart has four chambers: right atrium (RA), right ventricle (RV), left atrium (LA), and left ventricle (LV). The right coronary artery lies in the atrioventricular groove between the RA and RV. It gives rise to the right marginal artery and continues to terminate posteriorly (inferiorly) as the posterior (inferior) interventricular artery. The left coronary artery lies between the pulmonary trunk (RV) and LV. It gives rise to the anterior interventricular artery (left anterior descending artery) and circumflex artery. Both the phrenic and vagus nerves are closely related to the heart. Note that the left vagus gives off the left recurrent laryngeal nerve that hooks around the ligamentum arteriosum; it ascends to supply the larynx (muscles and mucous membrane).

HEART AND THE PERICARDIUM

The heart is located in the inferior mediastinum, while the great vessels (Branches of arch of aorta, pulmonary arteries and veins and superior vena cava) associated with it are located in the superior mediastinum above the plane of Louis (T4/T5) **(Fig. 3.1)**. The heart is enclosed by the fibrous and serous pericardium. The visceral layer of the serous pericardium closely covers the heart and is continuous with the parietal layer, which lines the inner surface of the fibrous pericardium. The pericardial sac which is the closed cavity between the two layers of serous pericardium, contains a small amount of pericardial fluid for lubrication purposes. In pathological conditions, excess fluid accumulation in this sac may compress the heart and compromise normal contraction. This condition is known as "cardiac tamponade".

The oblique sinus is a cul-de-sac of the main pericardial sac, located posterior to the left atrium and anterior to the esophagus. Therefore, enlargement of the left atrium may compress the esophagus. The transverse sinus lies posterior to the ascending aorta and pulmonary trunk of the heart, and anterior to the superior vena cava and communicates with the main pericardial sac.

The fibrous pericardium, the outer most layer, is anchored to the central tendon of the diaphragm inferiorly and blends with the tunica adventitia of the great vessels superiorly.

HEART AND ITS EXTERNAL FEATURES (Fig. 3.2)

The right and left atria are separated externally from the ventricles by the atrioventricular (coronary) sulcus. The irregular part (slightly serrated) of the atrium is the auricular appendage. The anterior and posterior (inferior) interventricular sulci mark the two ventricles. The right border of the heart is formed mainly by the right atrium, with contributions from the superior and inferior vena cava. The left border of the heart is formed by the left ventricle and left auricle (part of left atrium), while the inferior border of the heart is formed mainly by the right ventricle with some contribution from the left ventricle. The heart has four surfaces: sternocostal (anterior), diaphragmatic (inferior), and right and left pulmonary surfaces. The base of the heart is formed by both the atria, mainly by the left atrium. The apex of the heart is formed by the left ventricle and is located in the left 5th intercostal space at the midclavicular line where the apex beat is palpable.

ARTERIAL SUPPLY AND VENOUS DRAINAGE OF THE HEART (Fig. 3.2; Fig. 3.3)

The wall of the heart is made up of three layers: endocardium (innermost), myocardium, and epicardium (outermost). These layers are supplied by the coronary arteries, which are histologically muscular arteries **(Fig. 3.3E; Fig. 3.4C)**. The left and right coronary arteries arise from the corresponding

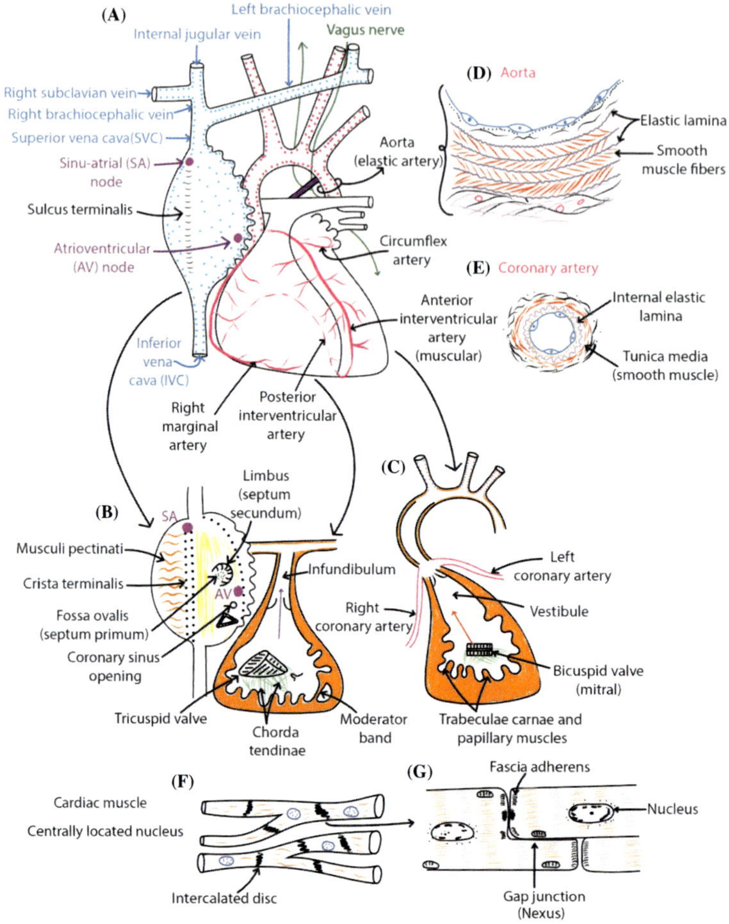

Figure 3.3. Heart (internal features). (A) The right atrium (outlined in blue), forming the right border of the heart, receives the returning venous blood from the superior and inferior vena cava. On its surface is a vertical groove, the sulcus terminalis. **(B)** In the right atrial chamber, the crista terminalis separates the rough from the smooth part. The rough area shows the musculi pectinati. Medially is the interatrial septum showing the limbus, fossa ovalis, and coronary sinus opening. The right atrioventricular opening guarded by the tricuspid value leads to the right ventricle. The right ventricular wall (shaded in light brown) shows trabeculae carnae, papillary muscles, and chorda tendinae attached to the tricuspid valve. The moderator (septomarginal) band extends from the interventricular septum to the base of the anterior papillary muscle. **(C)** The left ventricle has a thicker muscular wall (myocardium) when compared to the right ventricle. It has prominent trabeculae carnae. **(D)** The aorta is histologically an elastic artery with conspicuous elastic laminae. **(E)** The coronary artery is histologically a muscular artery with a prominent tunica media (smooth muscle). It arises from the ascending aorta above the aortic sinus **(C)**. **(F)** The myocardium is composed of branched cardiac muscle fibers (cells). The left ventricle receives oxygen from the left atrium through the left atrioventricular opening guarded by the mitral valve **(C)**. **(G)** The cardiac muscle fibers are connected by intercalated discs made up of fascia adherens and the gap junction (nexus).

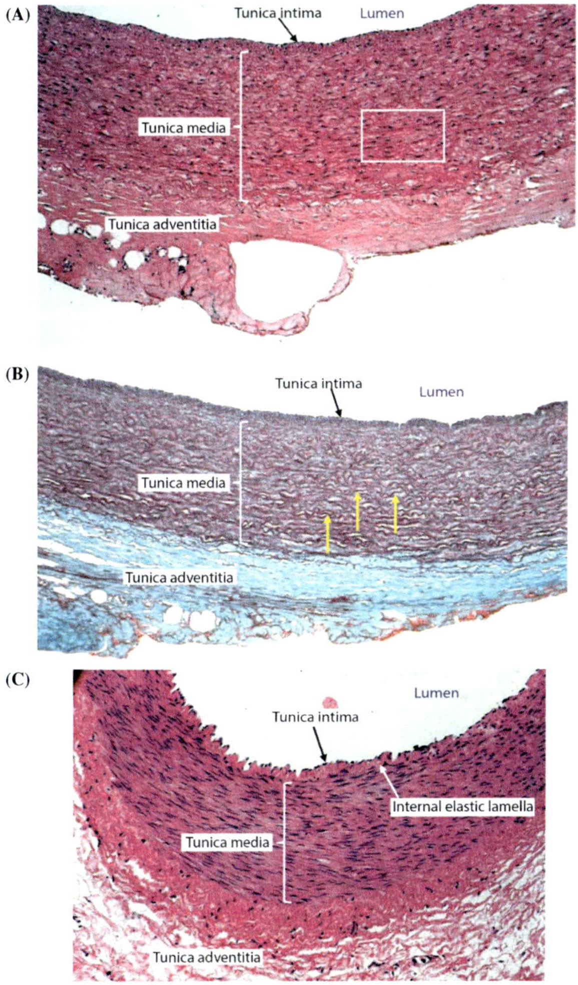

Figure 3.4. **(A) Elastic artery** in a transverse section. Note it has three layers: tunica intima, media, and adventitia. The tunica intima facing the lumen is lined by the endothelial cells (black arrow). The tunica media contains many smooth muscle cells whose nuclei appear as dense dots (white boxed area). The tunica adventitia is mainly composed of connective tissue. Examples of elastic arteries include the aorta, pulmonary trunk, carotid arteries, etc. (H&E stain.) **(B) Elastic artery** in a transverse section. The tunica media shows multi-layers of wavy elastic lamellae (yellow arrows) made up of elastic materials. Sandwiched between the elastic lamellae are smooth muscle fibers. The elastic lamellae provide elasticity to the vessel, e.g., during diastolic recoil. (Verhoeff's Masson trichrome stain (for elastic materials).) **(C) Muscular artery** in a transverse section. Like in the elastic artery, it has three layers: tunica intima, media, and adventitia. The intima is lined by endothelial cells (endothelium) (black arrow). The tunica media is the thickest layer and has prominent smooth muscle cells (spindle-shaped nuclei as dense dots). Between the intima and media is the internal elastic lamella, which is not readily identifiable in this staining. Examples of muscular arteries include the coronary arteries and most distributing arteries, such as the radial and ulnar arteries. (H&E stain.)

aortic sinus in the ascending aorta. The right coronary artery, embedded in the epicardium, courses along the atrioventricular groove between the right atrium and right ventricle. It then winds around the right margin of the heart to continue as the posterior interventricular artery (clinically referred to as posterior descending artery (PDA)) in the posterior interventricular groove. At the right margin of the heart, it gives off the marginal artery.

The left coronary artery runs along the atrioventricular groove between the left atrium and left ventricle. It gives off the anterior interventricular artery or left anterior descending (LAD) artery that lies in the interventricular groove. The left coronary artery also gives off the circumflex artery, which winds around the left side of the heart in the atrioventricular groove.

The coronary arteries are terminal arteries with limited anastomoses, which are often insufficient to compensate for sudden occlusion. Narrowing or blockage (e.g., due to atherosclerosis) can lead to myocardial ischemia and infarction (heart attack). Pain is typically retrosternal and may be referred to the medial aspect of the left arm, neck, or jaw.

Venous drainage of the heart is via cardiac veins that accompany the coronary arteries, including the great, middle, and small cardiac veins, which drain into the coronary sinus opening into the right atrium. The anterior cardiac veins drain directly into the right atrium.

GREAT VESSELS ASSOCIATED WITH THE HEART (Fig. 3.2; Fig. 3.3)

1. **Superior and Inferior Vena Cava:** The superior vena cava (SVC) drains the deoxygenated blood from the head, neck, upper limbs and thorax, while the inferior vena cava (IVC) drains the deoxygenated blood from the rest of the body below the diaphragm. Both SVC and IVC open into the right atrium.
2. **Pulmonary Trunk and Arteries:** The right ventricle pumps deoxygenated blood into the pulmonary trunk, which divides into the right and left pulmonary arteries which carry blood to the lungs for oxygenation.
3. **Aorta:** The left ventricle ejects oxygenated blood into the ascending aorta through the aortic valves. Both coronary arteries arise from the ascending

aorta. The arch of the aorta gives rise to the brachiocephalic trunk, left common carotid artery, and left subclavian artery. The aorta is histologically an elastic artery **(Fig. 3.3D; Fig. 3.4A, B)**.

INTERNAL FEATURES OF THE HEART CHAMBERS

1. Right Atrium

The atrial chamber has a smooth part and a rough part separated by a vertical ridge, crista terminalis **(Fig. 3.3B)**. The rough part shows the musculi pectinati (muscular ridges) which is derived from the primitive atrium. The smooth part is derived from the sinus venosus. The SVC, IVC and coronary sinus open into the right atrium. The right atrium is separated from the left atrium by the interatrial septum, which contains the limbus (derived from septum secundum) and the fossa ovalis (derived from septum primum). The sinoatrial (SA) node is located in its wall at the superior part of the crista terminalis (near the opening of SVC). The atrioventricular (AV) node is located near the opening of the coronary sinus. The right AV foramen, guarded by the tricuspid valve, opens into the right ventricle.

2. Right Ventricle (Fig. 3.3B)

The right ventricle receives blood through the right AV foramen, guarded by the tricuspid valve. Each valve is connected to the papillary muscle via the chorda tendinae (fibrous structure), which prevent the prolapse of the valve during ventricular systole. The interventricular septum separates the two ventricles; its upper part is membranous, while the lower part is muscular. The septomarginal trabecula (moderator band) connects the interventricular septum with the base of the anterior papillary muscle. It conveys the right bundle of conducting fibers.

3. Left Ventricle (Fig. 3.3C)

The internal surface of the chamber shows musculi pectinati and papillary muscles. Left ventricle receives oxygenated blood from the left atrium through the left AV foramen, guarded by the bicuspid or mitral valve. Each valve is connected to the papillary muscle *via* the chorda tendineae. The valve is a fibrous structure and contains no cardiac muscle.

The left ventricle has the thickest muscular wall of all the four heart chambers. This facilitates its forceful contraction during ventricular systole to pump oxygenated blood into the ascending aorta, arch of the aorta, and its branches through the aortic valves, thus constituting systemic circulation.

HISTOLOGY OF THE CARDIAC MUSCLE FIBERS (INCLUDING THE PURKINJE FIBERS) (Fig. 3.3F, G; Fig. 1.9A, B)

The heart wall consists of three layers: endocardium (innermost), myocardium, and epicardium (outermost). The endocardium is lined by the simple squamous epithelium, deep to which is the subendocardial region, with small amounts of connective tissues. The myocardium is composed of cardiac muscle cells, which are branched cells. Each cardiac muscle cell contains a single nucleus that is centrally located. A distinguishing feature of the cardiac muscle cells is the presence of intercalated discs, which represent the cell junctions between cells. The disc is composed of fascia adherens (desmosome) and gap junctions. The gap junction allows the direct passage of ions, e.g., Na^+, between cells for the depolarization or propagation of impulses. The cardiac muscle cells show striations representing the staggering and orderly arrangement of the contractile myofilaments: actin and myosin. Compared with the skeletal muscle cells, which are under voluntary control, the cardiomyocytes are under involuntary control. Motor endplates are absent in cardiac muscle.

Conducting System of the Heart (Fig. 3.5A, B)

The sinoatrial (SA) node, located in the superior part of the crista terminalis near the opening of the superior vena cava, acts as the pacemaker of the heart. It initiates the electrical impulses responsible for rhythmic contraction of the heart. Following the depolarization of the right atrium, the electrical impulse is transmitted to the AV node located near the opening of coronary sinus. From the AV node, the impulse is transmitted to the AV bundle or "bundle of His" and thence to the Purkinje fibers (in the subendocardial region) (also refer to **Fig. 1.9A, B**), resulting in depolarization of both the ventricles. The SA, AV, and Purkinje fibers are modified cardiac muscle cells.

Electrocardiogram (Fig. 3.5C)

Electrocardiogram (ECG) is the graphical representation of cardiac activities of the heart during contraction, which is denoted as PQRS. "P" wave represents

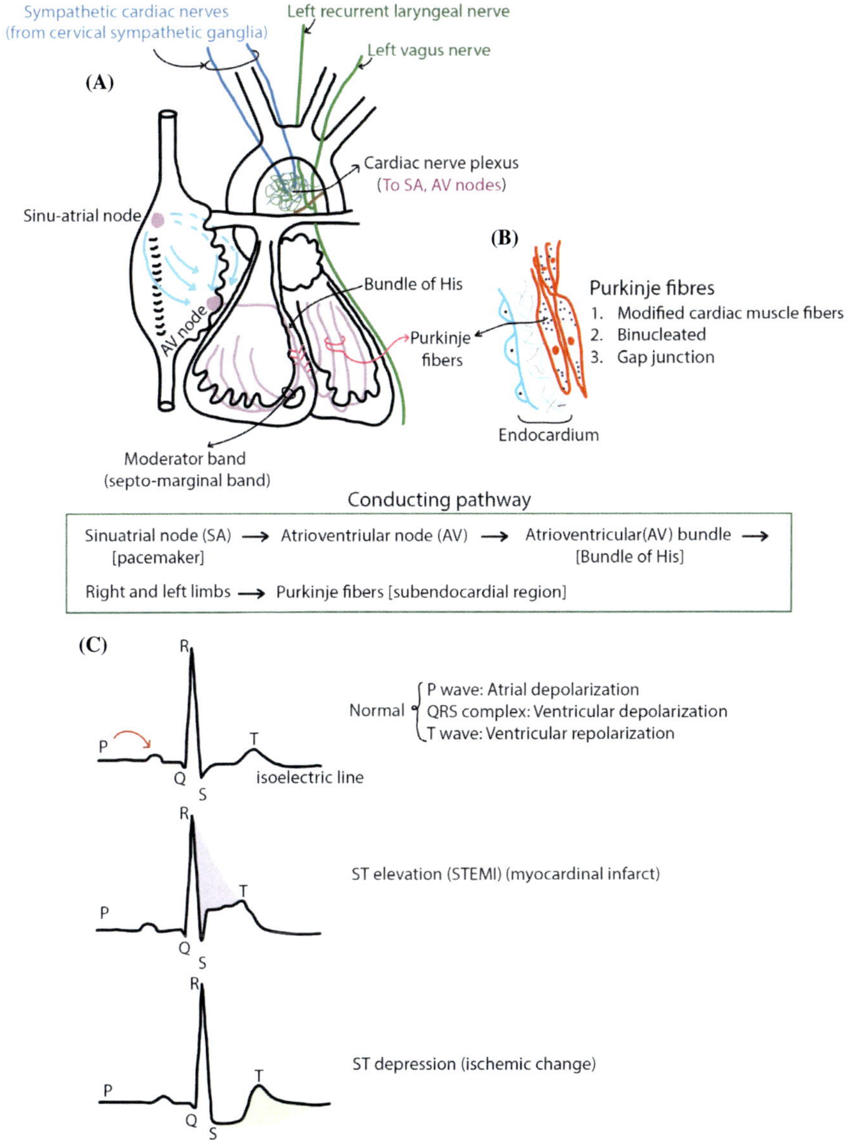

Figure 3.5. Conducting system of the heart. **(A)** The sinoatrial (SA) node or pacemaker is located at the upper pole of the crista terminalis. It initiates the depolarization of an electrical impulse, which is passed on to the atrioventricular (AV) node near the opening of the coronary sinus. From the AV node, the electrical impulse is transmitted to the lower part of the heart via the bundle of His and Purkinje fibers localized in the subendocardial region. **(B)** The sinus rhythm is regulated by the cardiac nerve plexus below the arch of the aorta. The cardiac plexus is composed of both the parasympathetic nerve (vagus) and sympathetic nerve fibers from the cervical sympathetic ganglia **(A)**. **(C)** Electrocardiogram (ECG) is a graphical representation of cardiac activities — either normal or abnormal.

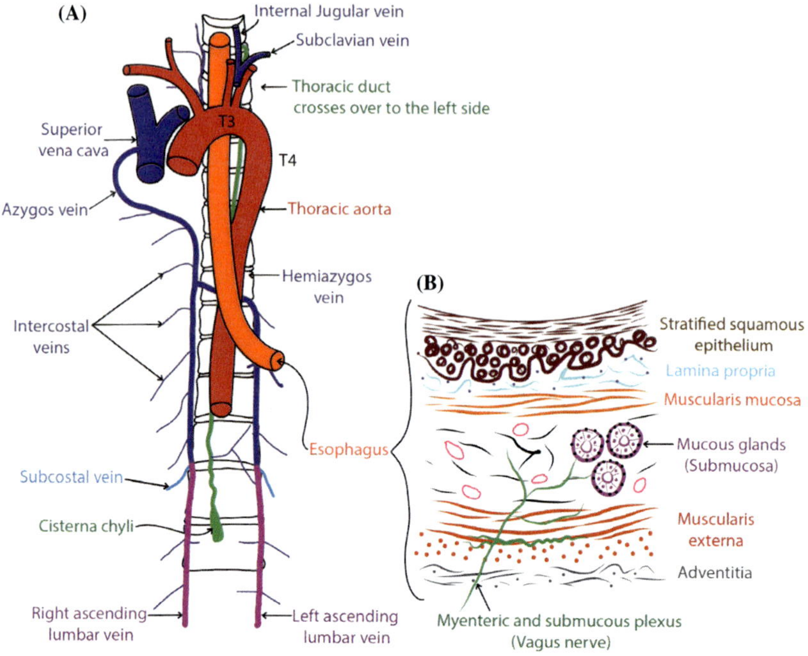

Esophagus (outlines)

1. It begins at C6 (cricoid cartilage) and terminates where it enters the cardia of stomach (in the upper part; it lies posterior to the trachea).
2. It is a muscular tube, 25cm in length.
3. It has three constrictions: at the site where pharnyx continues as the esophagus; where it is crossed by the arch of aorta; and at the cardia (where esophagus enters into stomach) .
4. It is lined by stratified squamous epithelium; mucous glands are present in submucosa in the lower esophagus.
5. Upper 1/3 is composed of skeletal muscles, middle 1/3 is composed of mixture of both skeletal & smooth muscles, and lower 1/3 contains inner circular and outer longitudinal smooth muscle.
6. Innervation is by the vagus nerve(X) - DMN and Nucleus Ambiguus (NA).
7. It is related to the left atrium, separated by the oblique sinus. In left atrium hypertrophy, it may cause dysphagia.
8. Gastroesophageal reflex disease(GERD) - Barretts' esophagus (Simple columnar epithelium - metaplasia).

Figure 3.6. Posterior mediastinum. (A) The posterior mediastinum contains the following: thoracic aorta, esophagus, azygos vein, and hemiazygos vein. The azygos vein is formed by the union of the ascending lumbar vein and subcostal vein. The esophagus descends through the posterior mediastinum. Detailed description of the esophagus, including its histology **(B)**, is given along with the figure.

the depolarization of the atria, "QRS" complex represents the depolarization of the ventricles, and "T" wave represents the repolarization of the ventricles. Abnormal patterns of PQRS may indicate myocardial ischemia or infarction.

Innervation of the Heart (Fig. 3.1; Fig. 3.2; Fig. 3.3; Fig. 3.5)

Both the phrenic and the vagus (CN X) nerves are closely associated with the heart.

- The phrenic nerve (C3-C5) provides sensory innervation to the fibrous pericardium and the parietal layer of the serous pericardium.
- The parasympathetic component of the vagus nerve supplies the SA and AV nodes, regulating the heart rate. Vagal stimulation decreases the heart rate.
- The left vagus nerve crosses the arch of the aorta anterolaterally and gives off the left recurrent laryngeal nerve that hooks around the ligamentum arteriosum.
- Sympathetic nerve fibers, arising from cervical and upper thoracic sympathetic ganglia, innervate the SA and AV nodes and myocardium, increasing the heart rate.

Both the parasympathetic and sympathetic nerves form the cardiac nerve plexus (around the ligamentum arteriosum) together with some visceral afferent fibers (pain). The referred cardiac pain is typically felt in left shoulder, neck, jaw and medial side of left arm and forearm.

Chapter 4

RENAL SYSTEM

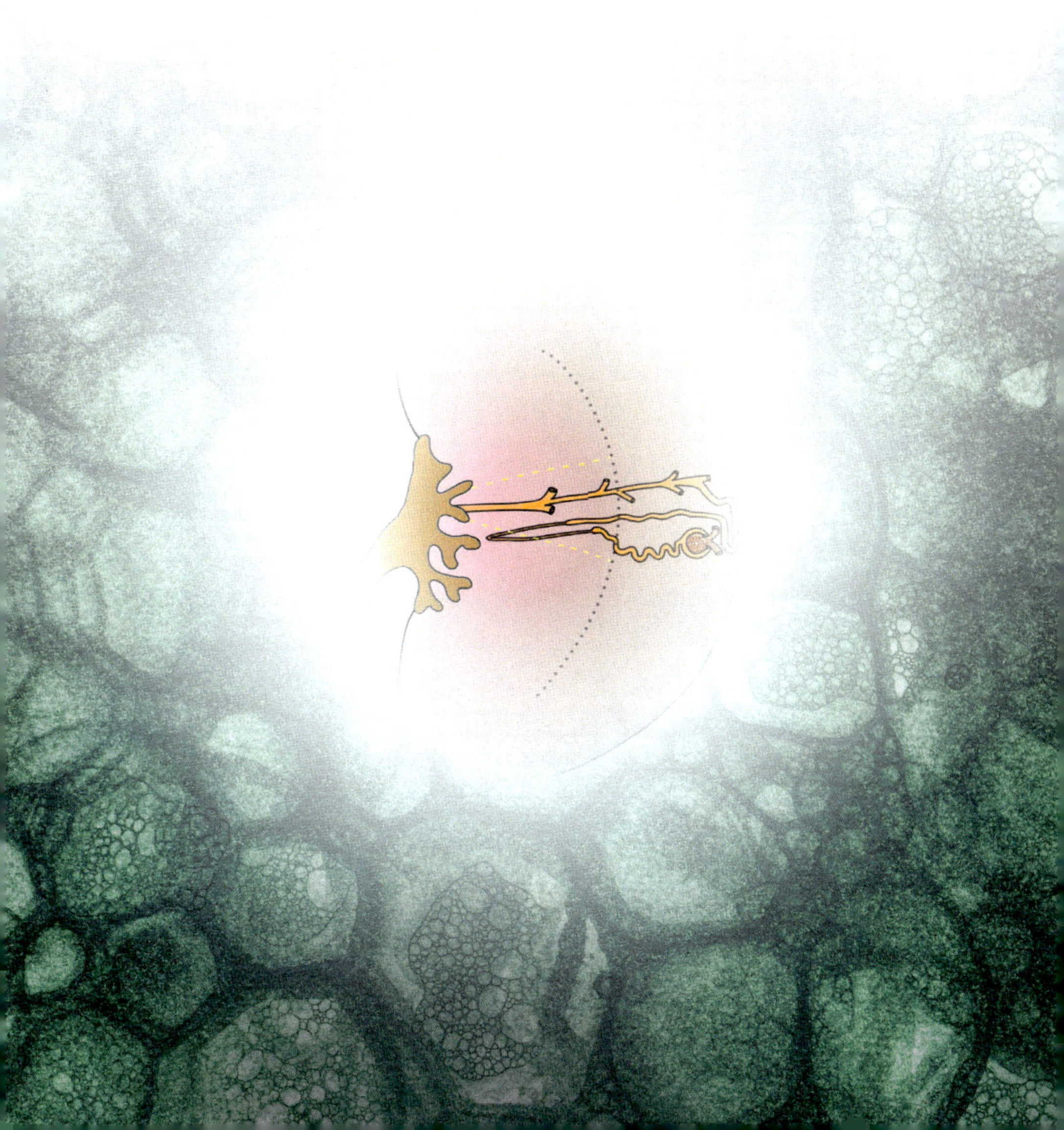

RENAL SYSTEM

The main function of the renal (urinary) system is to maintain the homeostasis of the body by eliminating the metabolic wastes such as bicarbonate ions, excess water, creatinine, uric acid, and ammonia, from the blood. The renal system consists of a pair of kidneys and two ureters, the urinary bladder and the urethra (**Fig. 4.1**).

KIDNEY

The kidneys (about 5 × 12 cm in size) are retroperitoneal organs located on the posterior abdominal wall (**Fig. 4.2**). The superior pole of the left kidney is at a higher level than right kidney, due to the presence of liver on the right side. Each kidney is supplied by the renal artery, which arises from the abdominal aorta at the level of L1–L2 and enters the kidney at the hilus (**Fig. 4.3**). The renal vein and ureter are also located at the hilus. The kidney is protected by three layers: a fibrous capsule which directly surrounds the kidney (**Fig. 4.4; Fig. 4.5**), perinephric fat that serves as a cushion for protection (**Fig. 4.6**) and renal fascia which is the outermost layer anchoring the kidney in position.

Functions

1. Excretion of urine — removal of metabolic waste products.
2. Regulation of pH of body fluids — maintains acid-base balance in body fluids.
3. Regulation of level of ions (electrolytes) in the body fluids.
4. Control of blood volume by regulating the volume of urine output.

Relations

A. **Posterior (Fig. 4.2):** Both the right and left kidneys are related posteriorly to the diaphragm, which separates them from the costo-diaphragmatic recess of the pleura. Inferior to this, they are related to the psoas major (medially), quadratus lumborum (intermediate) and transversus abdominis (laterally)

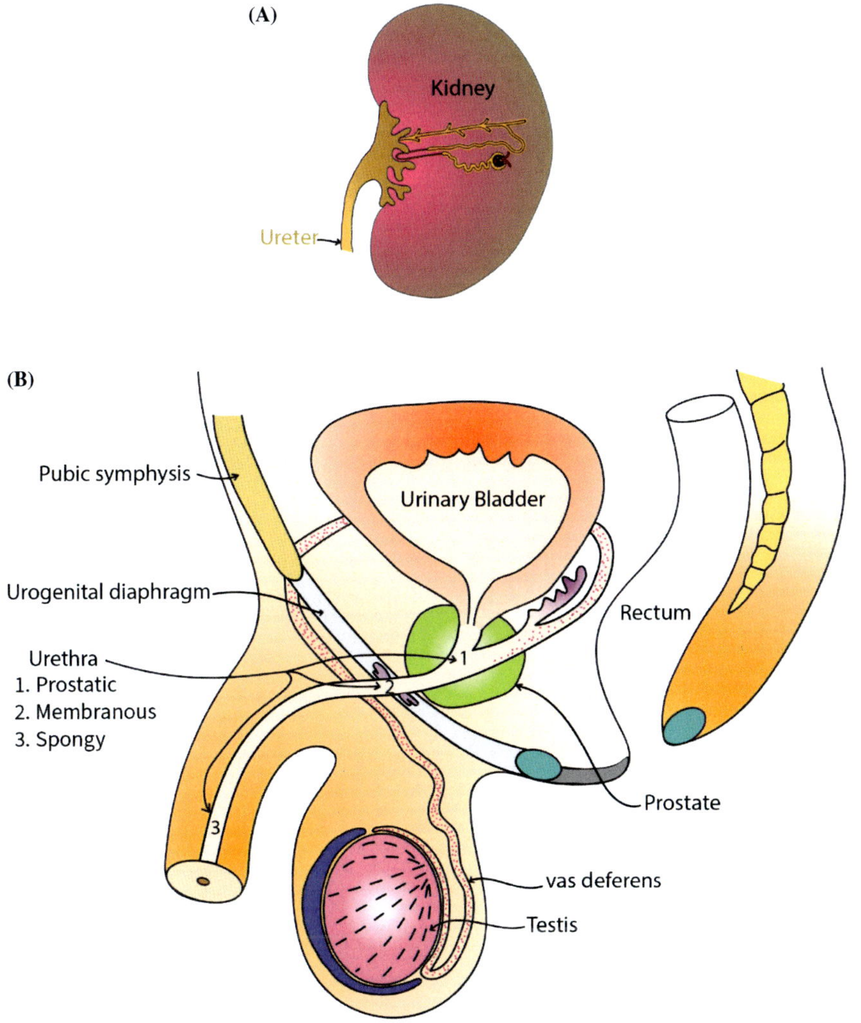

Figure 4.1. Urinary system (Male). It is made up of paired kidneys **(A)** and ureters, urinary bladder, and urethra. **(B)** Note the urethra has three parts:

1. Prostatic urethra (surrounded by the prostate),
2. Membranous urethra (through the urogenital (UG) membrane/diaphragm),
3. Spongy or penile (spongy) urethra.

muscles. The superior pole of the right kidney is related to the 12th rib whereas the left kidney is related to both the 11th and 12th ribs. They are also related to three nerves which include the subcostal nerve (T12), the ilioinguinal nerve (L1), and the iliohypogastric nerve (L1). The subcostal nerve innervates

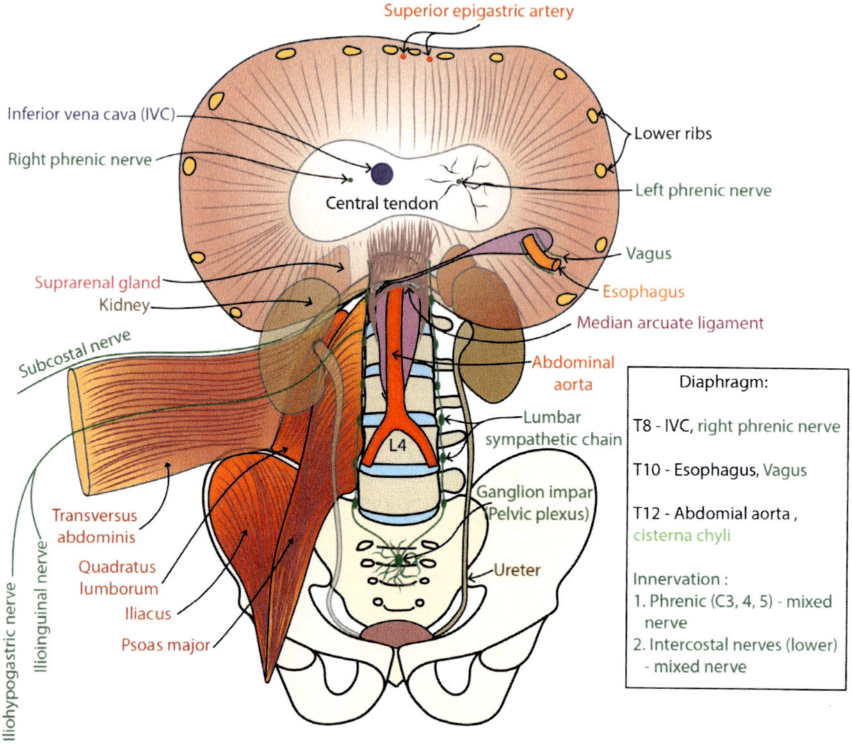

1. Kidney posterior relations: 12th rib, diaphragm, costodiaphragmatic recess
: Subcostal nerve(T12), Iliohypogastric and Ilioinguinal (L1)
: Transversus abdominis, Quadratus lumborum, Psoas major

2. Ureter: Muscular tube, 25 cm in length, three constrictions (site of stone impact) at
(a) the pelvi-ureteric junction, (b) sacroiliac joint, and (c) entry to the bladder.
Course - along the tip of transverse processes of lumbar vertebrae.
Stone impact - Pain is referred to L1 dermatome - " Loin to groin".
Urothelium - Transitional epithelium (muscle layers: inner longitudinal and outer circular muscles)
Arterial supply - renal artery, gonadal artery and superior vesical artery.

Figure 4.2. Kidney-posterior relations. The kidney lies on the posterior abdominal wall related to these muscles: quadratus lumborum, transversus abdominis, and psoas major, 12th rib, diaphragm, and three nerves (subcostal nerve, ilioinguinal nerve, iliohypogastric nerve). The ureter lies on the psoas major muscle along the tip of the transverse processes of the lumbar vertebrae.

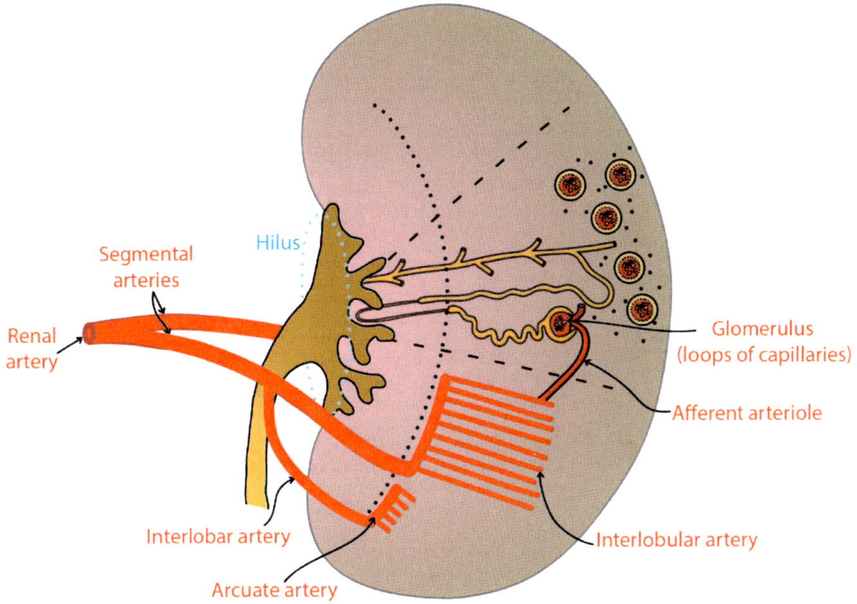

Figure 4.3. Kidney — arterial supply. The kidney is supplied by the renal artery, which enters the kidney at the hilus. It first divides into segmental arteries, each continuing as the interlobar artery, arcuate artery, interlobular artery, and afferent arteriole. The afferent arteriole gives rise to the glomerulus (capillary loops). After ultrafiltration, the blood flows into the efferent arteriole, vasa recta, and veins (not shown). Crush syndrome: injury to a lower limb (reflex action) result in arteriolar spasm in kidney-renal failure.

the abdominal wall muscles and skin of the lower abdominal wall. The iliohypogastric nerve innervates the internal oblique and transversus abdominis muscles and provides cutaneous innervation to the suprapubic region. The ilioinguinal nerve innervates the skin of the upper medial thigh and parts of the external genitalia.

B. **Anterior:** It is related to the greater sac (peritoneum) and abdominal viscera. The right kidney is related to the liver, duodenum (mainly 2nd part), and right colic flexure. The left kidney is related to the stomach, spleen, pancreas, jejunum, and left colic flexure. On lateral side, they are related to the paracolic gutters adjacent to the ascending (right side) and descending (left side) colons.

C. **Superior pole:** Each kidney is capped by the suprarenal gland (adrenal gland).

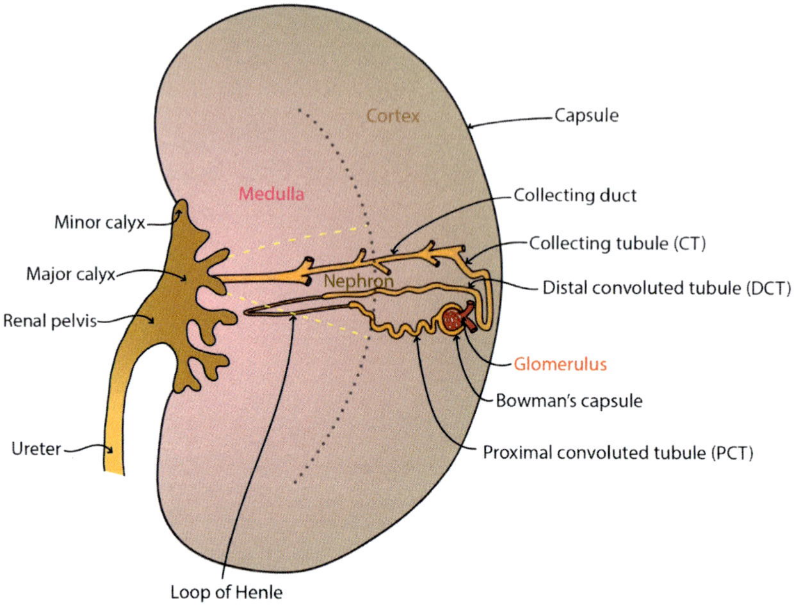

Figure 4.4. Kidney. In a section, the kidney is divided into the cortex and medulla, as marked by the dotted line. A nephron with its parts: Bowman's capsule, proximal convoluted tubule (PCT), loop of Henle (LH), distal convoluted tubule (DCT), and collecting tubule lies partly in the cortex and partly in the medulla. The collecting ducts and loop of Henle are closely packed in the medulla like a pyramid (outlined by the yellow lines), the renal (medullary) pyramid. The collecting ducts open into the minor calyx, which leads to the major calyx, renal pelvis, and ureter.

D. **Inferior pole:** The inferior pole of the right kidney lies lower than that of the left kidney due to the presence of the liver. The inferior pole of the right kidney may be palpable in thin individuals.
E. **Medial:** The hilum of right kidney medially is directed towards the inferior vena cava whereas the hilum of the left kidney faces the abdominal aorta.

Blood supply to the kidney (Fig. 4.3)

The renal arteries arise from the abdominal aorta at the level of L1–L2, just inferior to the superior mesenteric artery. The right renal artery is longer than the left because it passes posterior to the inferior vena cava. At the hilum, each renal artery divides into five segmental arteries (they are end arteries). The segmental arteries give rise to interlobar arteries, which pass through the renal columns between the pyramids.

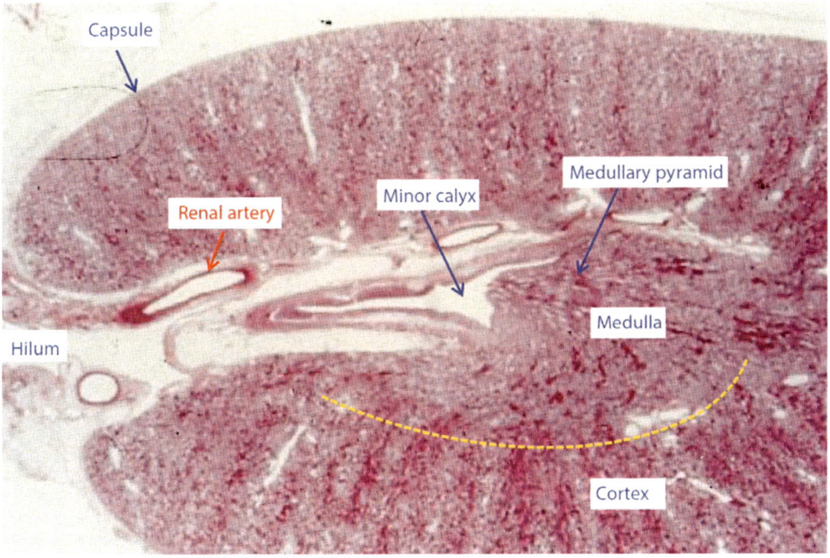

Figure 4.5. **Kidney.** A section through the hilum of the kidney showing its cortex and medulla, medullary pyramid, minor calyx, and renal vessels. The dotted line demarcates the cortex and medulla. (Hematoxylin and eosin (H&E) stain.)

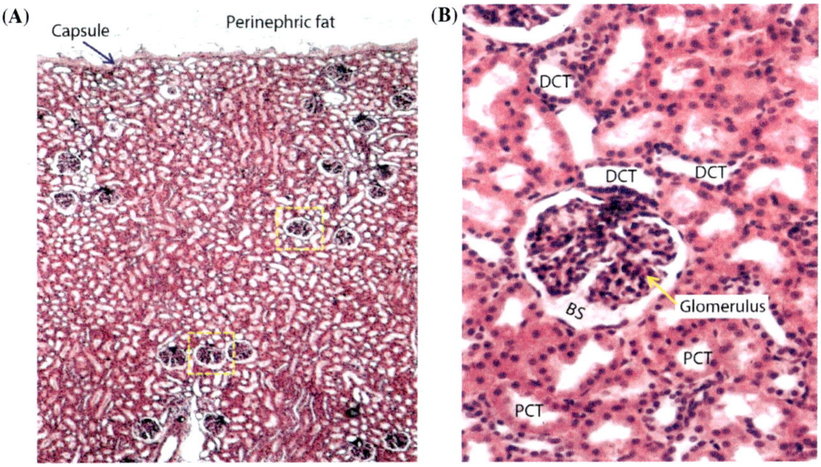

Figure 4.6. **Kidney — cortex.** **(A)** The surface is covered by a layer of capsule (arrow). External to the capsule is the perinephric fat (adipose tissue). The cortex is occupied by closely packed profiles of renal tubules in different planes of section. Renal corpuscles (yellow boxed area) are widely distributed. **(B)** An enlarged view of a renal (Malpighian) corpuscle. It is formed by a tuft of capillaries — glomerulus (arrow). Capping the glomerulus is Bowman's capsule with Bowman's space (BS). Both the proximal convoluted tubules (PCT) and distal convoluted tubules (DCT) are lined by the simple cuboidal epithelium. Note that the lumen of the DCT is more regular in outline compared to the PCT. (H&E stain.)

At the corticomedullary junction, the interlobar arteries continue as the arcuate arteries that give rise to a series of interlobular arteries. From the interlobular arteries arise afferent arterioles, each forming a glomerulus (a tuft of capillaries) which is involved in filtration of metabolic wastes. The glomerulus is encapsulated by the Bowman's capsule. After ultrafiltration, the blood circulation exits the glomerulus via the efferent arteriole.

At the corticomedullary junction, capillaries arising from the efferent arterioles of juxtamedullary nephrons form straight vessels that descend into the medulla as vasa recta. These vessels run in parallel bundles, loop within the medulla, and ascend back toward the cortex, where they drain into the arcuate veins, and ultimately into the renal vein and inferior vena cava. The vasa recta are essential for the countercurrent exchange system and help maintain the medullary osmotic gradient required for urine concentration. (*Details of this will be described in renal physiology.*)

Histological Features

In a histological section stained with hematoxylin and eosin (H&E), the kidney is surrounded by an outer fibrous capsule **(Fig. 4.5; Fig. 4.6A)**. Beneath this capsule lies the parenchyma, which constitutes the outer cortex and inner medulla. The cortex is readily identifiable by the presence of spherical structures called the renal (Malpighian) corpuscles **(Fig. 4.6A)**. In contrast, the medulla, located closer to the hilum, lacks these corpuscles. The medulla is composed of parallel arrays of collecting ducts arranged into cone-shaped structures known as medullary pyramids **(Fig. 4.5)**. The apex of each pyramid extends into a minor calyx, while its base is covered by the overlying cortical tissue. Together, a medullary pyramid and its associated cortex form a structural unit called a renal lobe.

Nephron (Fig. 4.7)

Nephron which is the functional unit of the kidney, consists of two parts:

1. **Renal tubule**, which begins at the renal capsule and ends at the collecting tubule.
2. **Glomerulus**, which is a tuft or network of capillaries in the form of capillary loops.

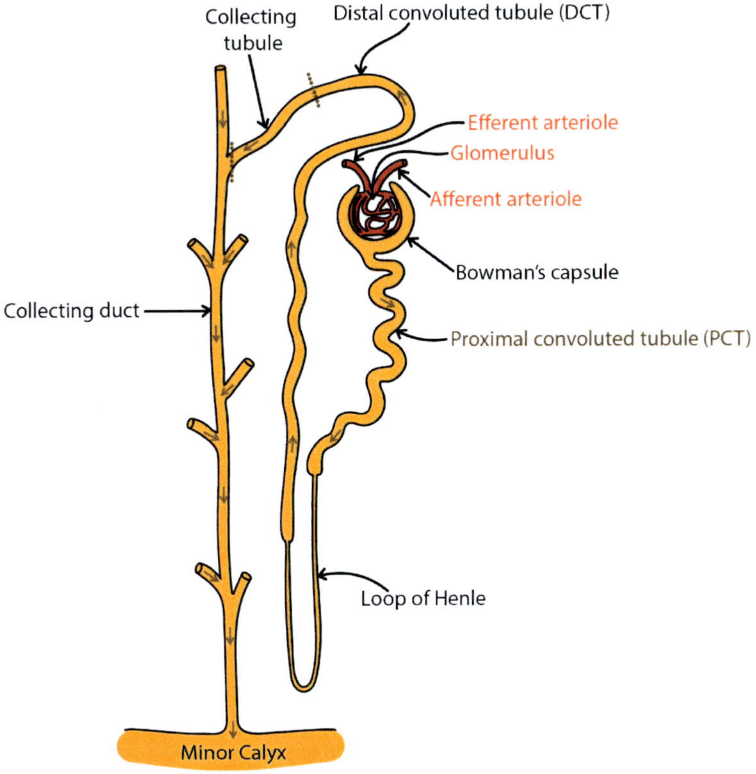

Figure 4.7. A nephron. The nephron begins at Bowman's capsule, which caps the glomerulus (tufts of blood capillaries linking the afferent and efferent arterioles). The ultrafiltrate in Bowman's space (in Bowman's capsule) drains into the proximal convoluted tubule, loop of Henle, distal convoluted tubule, and collecting tubule. Many collecting tubules open into a collecting duct containing hyperosmotic urine that ultimately drains into the minor calyx (arrow).

Glomerular Filtration and Passage of Filtrate

The renal tubule begins as an expanded bulb called the Bowman's capsule, which encloses the glomerulus **(Fig. 4.7)**. The glomerulus, together with Bowman's capsule, is the renal (Malpighian) corpuscle **(Fig. 4.6; Fig. 4.7)**.

The Bowman's capsule has two layers of lining cells: (a) the visceral layer with its lining cells, podocytes, covers the outer surfaces of glomerular capillaries, and (b) the parietal layer, which is continuous with the visceral layer of the Bowman's capsule and with the proximal convoluted tubule (PCT). Between the two layers of the Bowman's capsule is Bowman's space, which receives filtrate from the glomerular capillaries upon ultrafiltration. From Bowman's space, the filtrate enters the PCT, lined by the simple cuboidal epithelium with a prominent brush border **(Fig. 4.8)** and then into the U-shaped loop of Henle. This loop consists of a thick descending, thin loop, and thick ascending and is lined by the simple squamous epithelium that facilitates the transport of ions such as Na^+ and K^+ across the lining cells. The filtrate then passes to the distal convoluted tubule (DCT) **(Fig. 4.8)** and collecting tubule, the last segment of the nephron. Both the DCT and collecting tubule are lined by simple cuboidal epithelium **(Fig. 4.9)**.

Many nephrons drain their filtrate (now hyperosmotic urine) into a common collecting duct and then into the minor calyx, which caps the apex of the medullary pyramid **(Fig. 4.4; Fig. 4.7)**. From the minor calyx, the urine flows into the major calyx, renal pelvis, and the ureter. All these structures are lined by the transitional epithelium (urothelium).

Ultrafiltration (Fig. 4.10; Fig 4.11)

At the glomerular capillaries, the filtrate passes through the thin-layered endothelial cells, the basal lamina of the endothelium, the basal lamina of the visceral layer of the Bowman's capsule, and the filtration slits with a diaphragm between the pedicels of podocytes to reach Bowman's space.

Both the basal lamina of the endothelium and the basal lamina of podocytes form the glomerular basement membrane (GBM).

Selective Reabsorption by the Renal Tubule

Glucose and amino acids are primarily reabsorbed at the PCT. Approximately 65% of water together with sodium, potassium, and chloride ions, is reabsorbed by the PCT lining cells. Additional water is reabsorbed by the lining cells of the collecting duct which is regulated by the anti-diuretic hormone (ADH) from the pars nervosa (neurohypophysis), resulting in the production of hyperosmotic urine. The loop of Henle plays a key role in establishing a graded hyperosmotic environment in the medullary interstitium through a counter-current multiplier mechanism, which is essential for urine concentration and dilution (*Further details are covered in renal physiology.*)

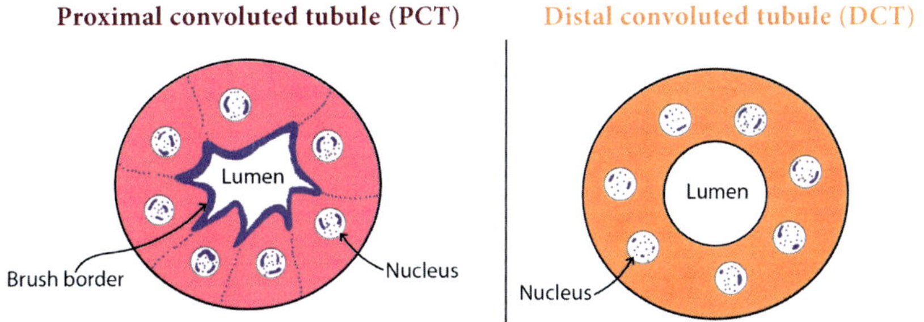

Proximal convoluted tubule (PCT)

- It absorbs 7/8 of H_2O passing through
- It absorbs sodium and other metabolites
- It absorbs all amino acids & glucose
- It has well-developed brush border
- It has a star-shaped lumen
- Its lining cells have extensive lateral walls
- These cells show eosinophilic cytoplasm
- Basal infoldings of plasma membrane that facilitate transport

Distal convoluted tubule (DCT)

- It is shorter in length than PCT
- It has a regular lumen
- Brush border is indistinct
- Its lining cells are lighter in staining
- It absorbs water through the action of anti-diuretic hormone (ADH). This helps form hypertonic urine.

Figure 4.8. Diagrammatic figures depicting the histological differences between the proximal convoluted tubule (PCT) and distal convoluted tubule (DCT), as visualized by H&E staining.

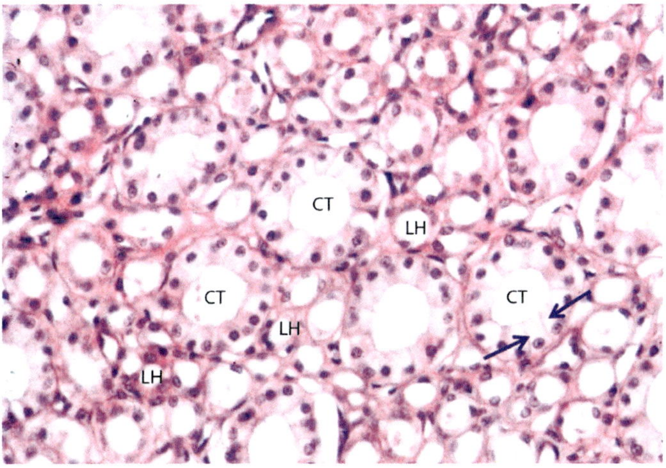

Figure 4.9. Kidney — medulla. The medulla is occupied by closely packed profiles of collecting tubules (CTs), mostly in the transverse section. The collecting tubule is lined by the simple cuboidal epithelium. Note that the lining cells have distinct cell boundaries (arrows). The cytoplasm is lightly stained. Between the CTs are profiles of the thin loop of Henle (LH), lined by the simple squamous epithelium. (H&E stain.)

- Collecting tubule — absorption of water (target of ADH)
- Loop of Henle — production of hyperosmotic urine

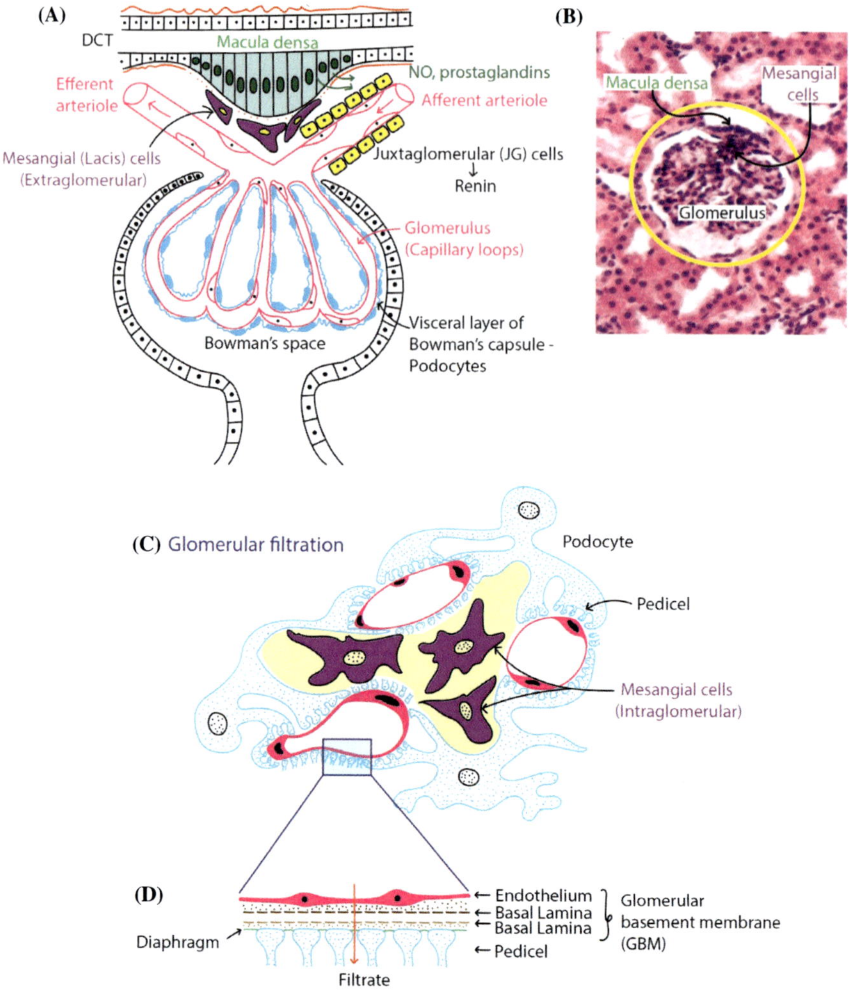

Figure 4.10. Kidney — juxtaglomerular apparatus (JG). (A) A diagrammatic figure showing the various components of JG apparatus: JG cells (modified smooth muscle cells) of afferent arteriole that secrete renin. Also showing the macula densa (modified lining cells of the distal convoluted tubule (DCT)), a chemoreceptor for the detection of changes of Na^+ in the DCT. The extra-glomerular mesangial cells are phagocytic and the production of erythropoietin. **(B)** A portion of the renal corpuscle (circled) showing its associated macula densa and mesangial cells. (H&E stain.) **(C)** Podocytes and their foot processes (pedicels). The foot processes rest on the outer surface of the capillary endothelial cells. **(D)** Enlarged view of the boxed area in "C" showing various components of the glomerular basement membrane (GBM). Arrow indicates the passage of the filtrate. N.B. New GBM is added onto it on the epithelial side; old GBM is removed on the endothelial side by mesangial cells (intraglomerular); and escaped products may trigger an antigen — an antibody autoimmune response that can cause glomerular damage.

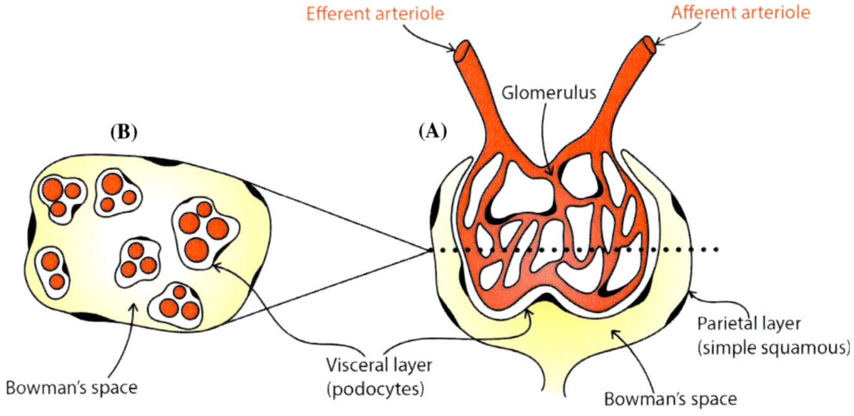

Figure 4.11. Renal (Malpighian) corpuscle. (A) It is composed of loops of capillaries (glomerulus), which receive incoming blood from the afferent arteriole. After ultrafiltration through the capillaries, the blood leaves by the efferent arteriole. The glomerulus is capped by Bowman's capsule, composed of the visceral layer (podocytes) and the parietal layer. Between them is Bowman's space, which receives the filtrate. **(B)** Showing the corpuscle in a transverse section (dotted line in A).

Juxtaglomerular Complex (Fig. 4.10 A, B)

This complex is involved in regulation of blood flow and maintaining blood pressure. It has three main components:

1. **Juxtaglomerular (JG) cells:** They are modified smooth muscle cells located in the wall of the afferent arteriole. They secrete renin, which converts angiotensinogen (from the liver) into angiotensin I and subsequently into angiotensin II via the angiotensin-converting enzyme (ACE) in the lungs. Angiotensin II acts to increase blood pressure.
2. **Lacis cells (extraglomerular mesangial cells):** The exact function of these cells is not fully understood, although they may be involved in the secretion of erythropoietin.
3. **Macula densa:** This is a specialized epithelium in the DCT adjacent to the vascular pole of the renal corpuscle. These lining cells act as chemoreceptors, constantly monitoring the changes in Na^+ concentrations in the filtrate in the DCT.

URETER (Fig. 4.2; Fig. 4.12)

1. It is a muscular tube about 25 cm in length.
2. It lies on the psoas major muscle, along the tips of transverse processes of the lumbar vertebrae (as seen on X-ray) **(Fig. 4.2)**. In the pelvis, it runs along the lateral wall of the pelvic cavity towards the ischial spine, then turns obliquely forward to enter the posterosuperior aspect of the urinary bladder.
3. The ureter has three constrictions: at the pelvi-ureteric junction, at the pelvic brim (where it crosses the external iliac artery) and at the ureterovesical junction (where it enters the urinary bladder). These are the common sites for ureteric stone impaction.
4. **Arterial supply:** The ureter has a segmental arterial supply: the upper part is supplied by branches of the renal artery; the middle part by branches from the gonadal artery, abdominal aorta, and common iliac arteries; and

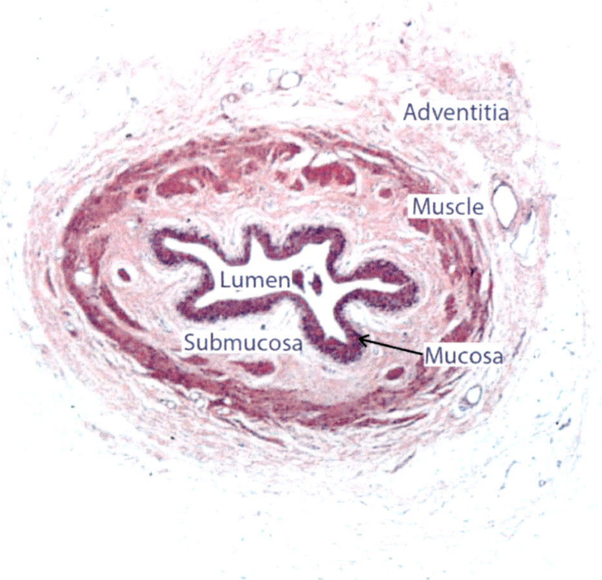

Figure 4.12. Ureter. The star-shaped lumen is lined by a transitional epithelium (urothelium). Beneath the mucosa is the submucosa. External to this is the muscle coat consisting of inner longitudinal/outer circular muscles. The outermost layer is the adventitia. (H&E stain.)
N.B. Stone impact in the ureter can cause excruciating pain (ureteric colic) that is referred to as L1 dermatome (from "loin to groin"). Pain fibers that originate from the ureter travel with the sympathetic nerves.

the lower part by branches of the superior vesical artery (with additional contributions from the inferior vesical artery in males or the uterine artery in females).

5. **Innervation:** The ureter is innervated by the autonomic nerves that supply the smooth muscles in its walls. Spasmodic muscle contraction causes severe pain (ureteric colic), typically referred from "loin to groin". The visceral pain fibers originating from the ureter travel with sympathetic nerves (T11–L2).
6. **Histology (Fig. 4.12):** The ureter has a thick wall with characteristic star-shaped lumen (due to mucosal folds). The wall has three main layers: mucosa, muscularis layer, and adventitia. The mucosa is lined by the transitional epithelium (urothelium). The muscularis layer is composed of an inner longitudinal and an outer circular muscle. At the lower one third of the ureter, an outer longitudinal layer may be present.

URINARY BLADDER

The urinary bladder consists of an apex, body (main part), dome (superior surface), fundus (base), and neck **(Fig. 4.13A)**. The apex continuous with the median umbilical ligament (remnant of urachus).

A. Relations

1. Male (Fig. 4.13A)

a. Anterior: It is related to the pubic symphysis and retropubic space.
b. Superior: The "dome" is covered by peritoneum and related to the peritoneal cavity.
c. Posterior: The upper part of the base is separated from the rectum by the rectovesical pouch (peritoneal reflection). Inferior to this, the base is related to a pair of seminal vesicles and vas deferens **(Fig. 4.13A)**.
d. Inferior: The bladder neck rests on the prostate gland and is surrounded by the sphincter vesicae which is composed of smooth muscle **(Fig. 4.13A)** (*Details are described in the chapter on the Male Reproductive System*).

2. Female

a. The relations of the urinary bladder in the female differ from that of the male due to the absent of prostate gland and the presence of uterus and vagina.

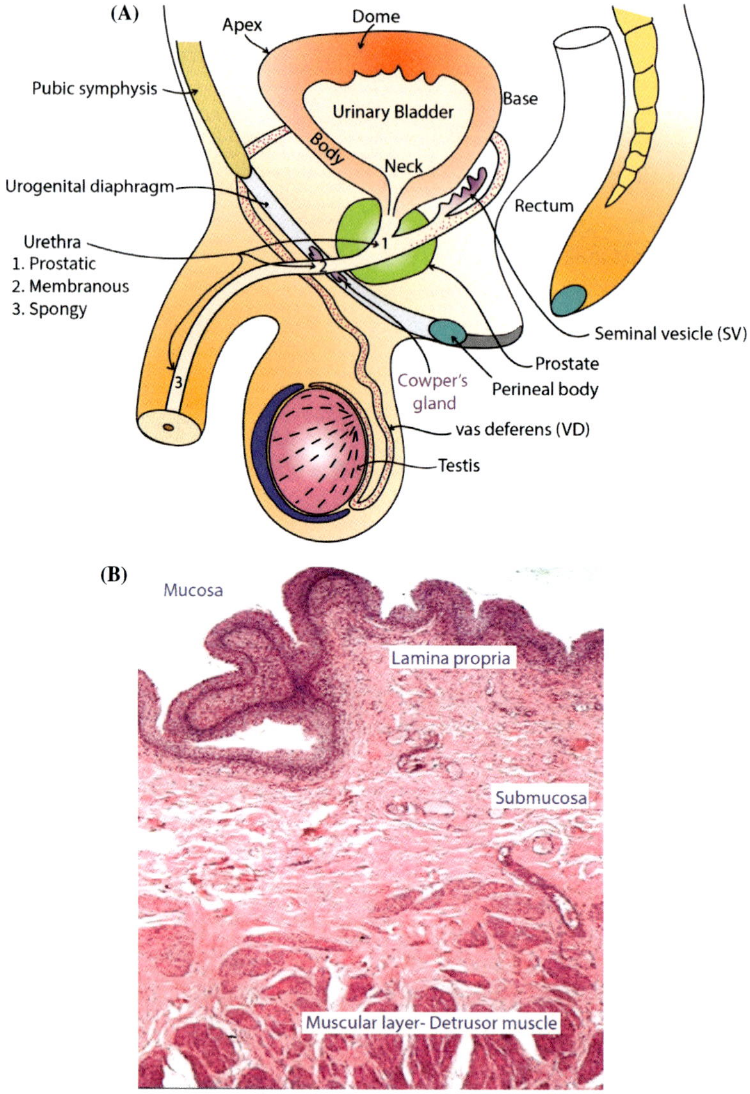

Figure 4.13. Urinary bladder and urethra (Male). (A) A sagittal section through the urinary bladder, prostate gland, and urethra. The bladder has a body, dome, apex, base, and neck. SV: seminal vesicle, VD: vas deferens. **(B)** The wall has mucosa (transitional epithelium), lamina propria, submucosa, and muscular layers (detrusor). The muscle layer is composed of smooth muscle cells (detrusor muscle) supplied by the pelvic splanchnic nerves (S2–4) (parasympathetic). Detrusor contraction facilitates micturition. (H&E stain.)

b. Posterior: It is separated from the uterus by the vesicouterine pouch.
c. Inferior: It continues as the short urethra that opens into the vestibule anterior to the vaginal opening. The bladder neck rests on pelvic floor (urogenital diaphragm).

B. Peritoneal Relations

The dome of the urinary bladder is covered by a layer of peritoneum, which is reflected over the rectum as the rectovesical pouch in the male; in the female, the peritoneum is reflected over the uterus, posteriorly forming the vesicouterine pouch.

C. Arterial Supply

The urinary bladder is supplied by branches of the internal iliac arteries, mainly superior vesical arteries, inferior vesical arteries (male) and vaginal arteries (female).

D. Histology (Fig. 4.13B)

The wall of urinary bladder has four layers: mucosa, submucosa, muscularis layer, and serosa (adventitia, an area where it is devoid of peritoneal covering). The mucosa is thrown into many folds except over the trigone (triangular-shaped) area at the base **(Fig. 4.14A)**. The trigone is bounded by the two ureteric openings and one internal urethral orifice at the bladder neck. Between the two ureteric openings is the interureteric ridge (bar). The function of the trigone is uncertain, but its contraction has been described to prevent the reflux of urine into the ureters and bladder. The mucosa is lined by the transitional epithelium (urothelium). The submucosa contains loose connective tissue rich in blood vessels and nerves. The muscle fibers (detrusor) are not arranged in true distinct layers.

E. Innervation

The urinary bladder is innervated by parasympathetic, sympathetic, and somatic fibers, which together regulate bladder function. The bladder receives its parasympathetic innervation from the pelvic splanchnic nerves (S2–S4) **(Fig. 4.14A)**. The preganglionic parasympathetic nerve fibers originate from the sacral spinal cord and synapse in ganglia which are located in the bladder wall **(Fig. 4.14A, B)**. The postganglionic parasympathetic nerve fibers stimulate the contraction of the detrusor muscle in the bladder wall and relax the internal urethral sphincter thereby facilitating urination. Visceral afferents responsible for physiological reflex (sensation of fullness or distension) follow the parasympathetic pathways to the sacral spinal cord.

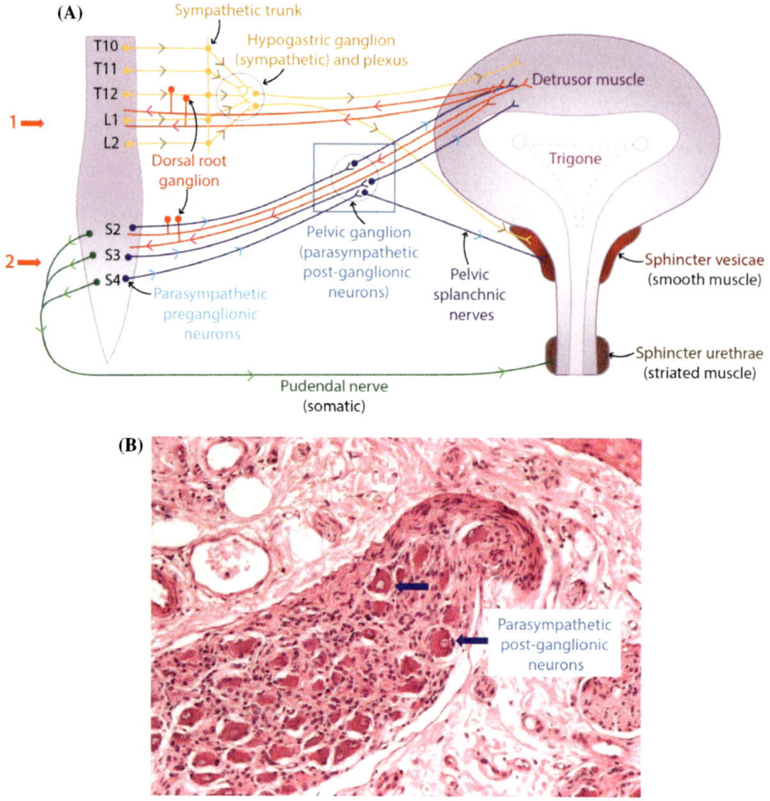

Figure 4.14. Urinary bladder — innervation. (A) The urinary bladder is innervated by both parasympathetic and sympathetic nerves. For convenience of description, the sympathetic innervation is omitted. The parasympathetic supply is by the pelvic splanchnic nerves from the spinal cord segments at the S2, 3, 4 levels (sacral outflow). The preganglionic parasympathetic neurons are localized in the lateral horn of the cord. The preganglionic parasympathetic axons synapse with the postganglionic neurons in the pelvic ganglion (boxed). The postganglionic parasympathetic neurons, with their axons, then supply the muscles of the bladder walls (detrusor muscle) as well as the sphincter vesicae (internal sphincter). The pelvic splanchnic nerves also carry sensory fibers, whose cell bodies are localized in the dorsal root ganglion at S2, 3, 4. They mediate sensory inputs from the bladder, such as fullness or distension. S2, 3, 4 also give rise to the pudendal nerve, which supplies the sphincter urethrae (striated muscle) that is under voluntary control.

Spinal cord injury at 1 — Spinal cord injury at a higher level — reflex bladder — automatic bladder
Spinal cord injury at 2 — Sacral cord is crushed — autonomous bladder — no reflex — bladder fills to empty.

(B) A parasympathetic ganglion in the bladder wall. The ganglion contains a cluster of postganglionic parasympathetic neurons. They are postsynaptic to the preganglionic neurons in the lateral horn of the sacral spinal cord (S2–S4). Passing through the ganglion are S2, 3, 4 sensory fibers (for registration of bladder distension or fullness sensation), whose cell bodies are in the dorsal root ganglia. (H&E stain.).

Sympathetic fibers arise from T11–L2 spinal segments and reach the bladder via the hypogastric plexus. Stimulation of these sympathetic nerve fibers relaxes the detrusor muscle and contracts the internal urethral sphincter thereby promoting bladder filling. In addition, somatic fibers from the pudendal nerve (S2–S4) innervate the external urethral sphincter, which contracts during bladder filling and provides voluntary control over urination.

F. Clinical Considerations (Fig. 4.14A)

1. **Reflex (spastic) bladder:** This occurs due to injury to the spinal cord above the sacral segments (S2–S4), for example at T10. The sacral reflex arc remains intact, and the bladder empties automatically via spinal reflexes (involuntary micturition).
2. **Autonomous (flaccid) bladder:** This occurs due to damage to the sacral spinal cord segments (S2–S4) or pelvic nerves, involving both the motor and sensory pathways. There is a complete disruption of the neural circuitry. The bladder becomes overdistended and flaccid. Urine retention occurs, often with overflow incontinence. The bladder must be emptied manually or by catheterization.

URETHRA

1. Male Urethra

The urethra is divided into three parts: prostatic urethra, membranous urethra, and penile or spongy urethra **(Fig. 4.1B)**.

a. **Prostatic urethra:** This is surrounded by the prostate gland. It is lined by transitional epithelium. It is the widest and most dilatable part of the urethra. On the posterior wall, there is a raised ridge (urethral crest) and a prominent elevation, colliculus seminalis (verumontanum). On both sides of the seminal colliculus are the openings of common ejaculatory ducts, and above it is the prostatic utricle (a vestigial structure). Enlargement of the prostate (e.g., benign prostatic hyperplasia) can compress the urethra and obstruct urine flow.
b. **Membranous urethra:** It passes through the urogenital (UG) diaphragm, which encloses the deep perineal pouch. It is the shortest and least distensible part of the urethra. It is lined by transitional epithelium. The membranous

urethra is surrounded by the external urethral sphincter, composed of skeletal muscle innervated by the pudendal nerve (S2–S4).

c. **Penile or spongy urethra:** This is the longest part of the urethra. In the proximal part, it is lined by transitional epithelium, which changes progressively to become stratified squamous epithelium distally and nearing the external urethral orifice. Pain or irritable sensation of the entire length of the urethra is mediated by the pudendal nerve (S2–S4).

2. Female Urethra

It is short and opens into the vestibule anterior to the vaginal opening. It is lined by transitional epithelium (proximal)/stratified squamous epithelium (distal). It is prone to infection (urinary tract infection), due to its short length. Pain and burning sensation arising from this is mediated by the pudendal nerve (S2–S4).

Chapter 5

DIGESTIVE SYSTEM

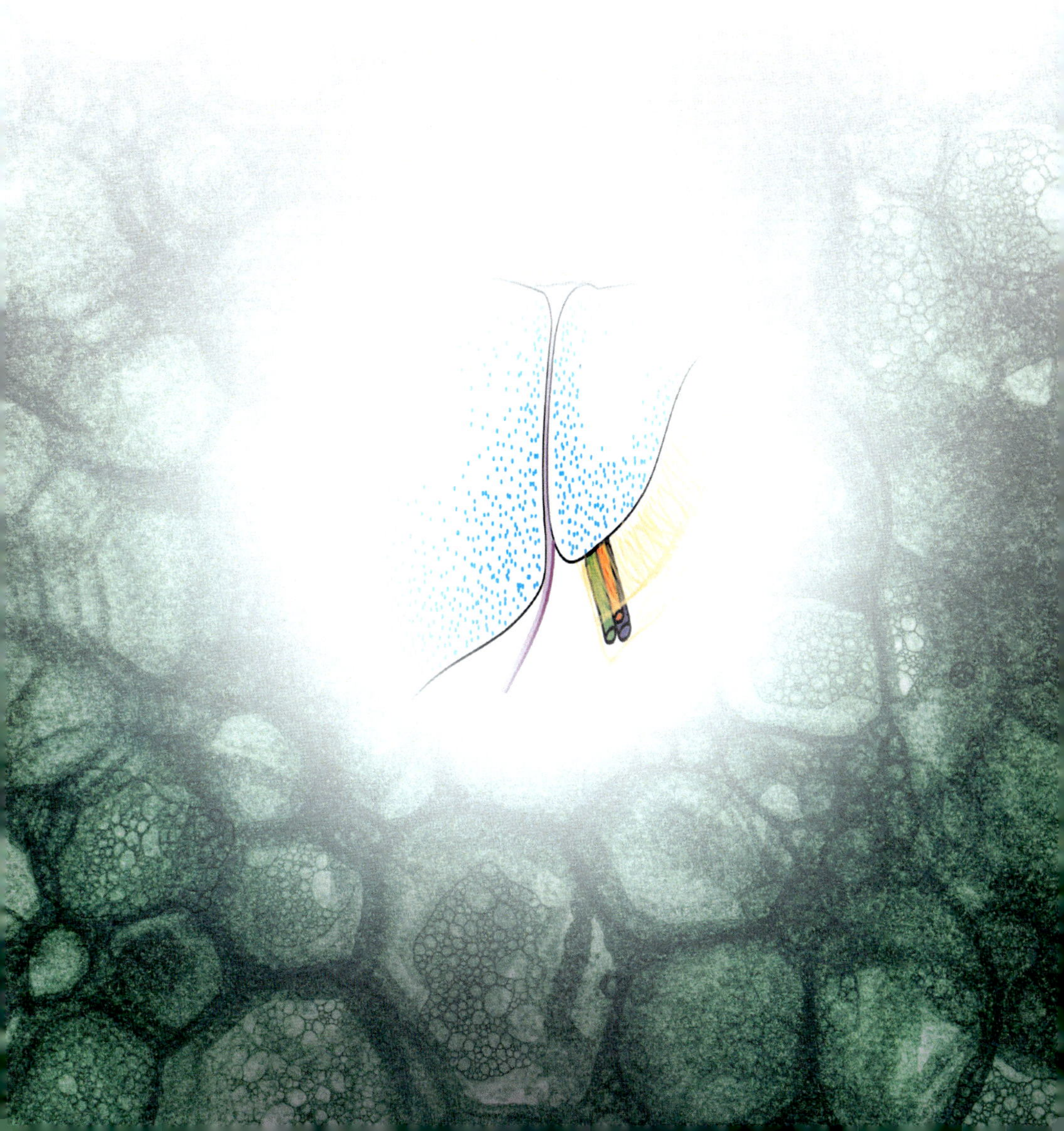

DIGESTIVE SYSTEM: UPPER GASTROINTESTINAL TRACT

ABDOMINAL WALL

It consists of the anterior (anterolateral) and posterior abdominal wall. The abdominal wall encloses the abdominal and peritoneal cavities and the abdominal viscera, including the digestive organs, providing them with protection and support. In this chapter, the anterior abdominal wall is described whereas the posterior abdominal wall is described in the chapter of renal system (Chapter 4), **Fig. 4.2.**).

Anterior (Anterolateral) Abdominal Wall

The anterior abdominal wall is a multi-layered musculotendinous structure. The abdominal wall muscles contract, increasing the intra-abdominal pressure which aids in forceful expiration (coughing), defecation, micturition, and parturition. These muscles also contribute to movements of the trunk, including flexion and lateral flexion.

Structurally, the abdominal wall is made up of skin, superficial fascia, muscles with their aponeurosis, transversalis fascia, pre-peritoneal fat, and parietal peritoneum. Superiorly, the anterior abdominal wall is bounded by the subcostal margin (along the lower costal cartilages) and xiphoid process; inferiorly, it is bounded by the iliac crest, inguinal ligament (attached to the anterior superior iliac spine and pubic tubercle), pubic crest, and pubic symphysis.

Nine regions of the abdominal wall (Fig. 5.1)

For descriptive purposes, the anterior abdominal wall is divided into nine regions by two vertical and two horizontal planes. The vertical planes are the midclavicular lines, extending from the midpoint of the clavicle to the midpoint of the inguinal ligament. The horizontal planes include the subcostal plane, which passes through the inferior border of the 10th costal cartilage at the level of the L3

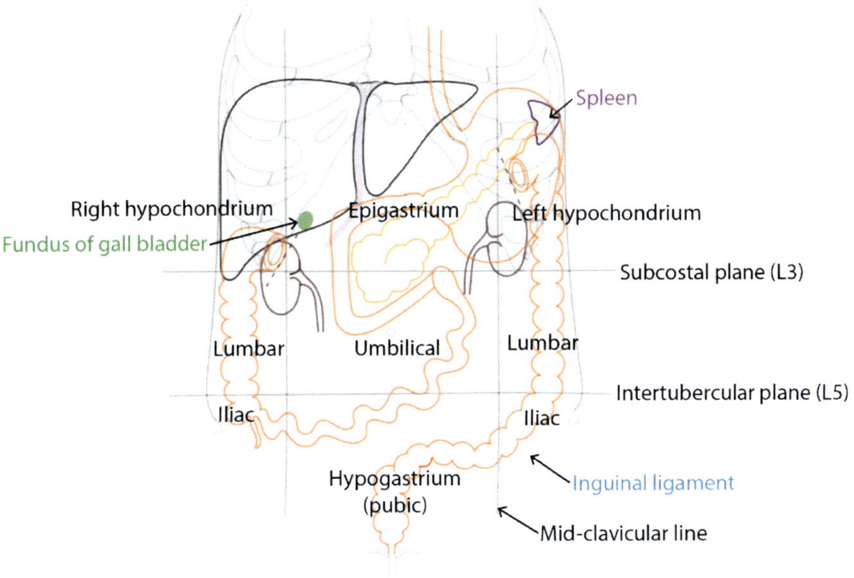

Figure 5.1. Anterior abdominal wall. For the purpose of clinical or physical examination (inspection, auscultation, percussion, and palpation), the anterior abdominal wall is divided into nine regions demarcated by two horizontal planes and two vertical lines. The horizontal planes are the subcostal plane (L3) and intertubercular plane (L5). The two vertical lines are the mid-clavicular lines; each intersects with the mid-inguinal line. The nine abdominal areas outlined are: right and left hypochondrium, right and left lumbar, right and left iliac, epigastrium, umbilical, and hypogastrium (pubic region). All abdominal organs or viscera may be related to one of the nine regions.

vertebra, and the intertubercular (transtubercular) plane, which passes through the iliac tubercles at the level of the L5 vertebra. These regions include the right hypochondrium, epigastrium, and left hypochondrium; the right lumbar region, umbilical region, and left lumbar region; and the right iliac region, hypogastrium (pubic region), and left iliac region. This regional division is clinically important for describing the location and surface marking of various internal organs during physical examination (inspection, auscultation, percussion, and palpation) as well as in surgical procedures.

Skin & Surface Markings

The anterior abdominal wall receives sensory innervation from the thoracoabdominal nerves (T7–T11) and the subcostal nerve (T12), with additional contribution from the L1 nerve via the iliohypogastric and ilioinguinal nerves **(Fig. 5.2)**.

Clinically, specific dermatomes correspond to characteristic areas of referred pain. Dermatome **T7** corresponds to the epigastric region (e.g., referred pain from gastric ulcer), **T10** corresponds to the umbilical region (referred pain from the appendix during early-stage appendicitis), and **L1** extends from the "loin to groin" region (as in ureteric colic caused by a stone in the ureter).

The abdominal wall is supplied by the superior and inferior epigastric arteries **(Fig. 5.2)**. The superior epigastric artery is a terminal branch of the internal

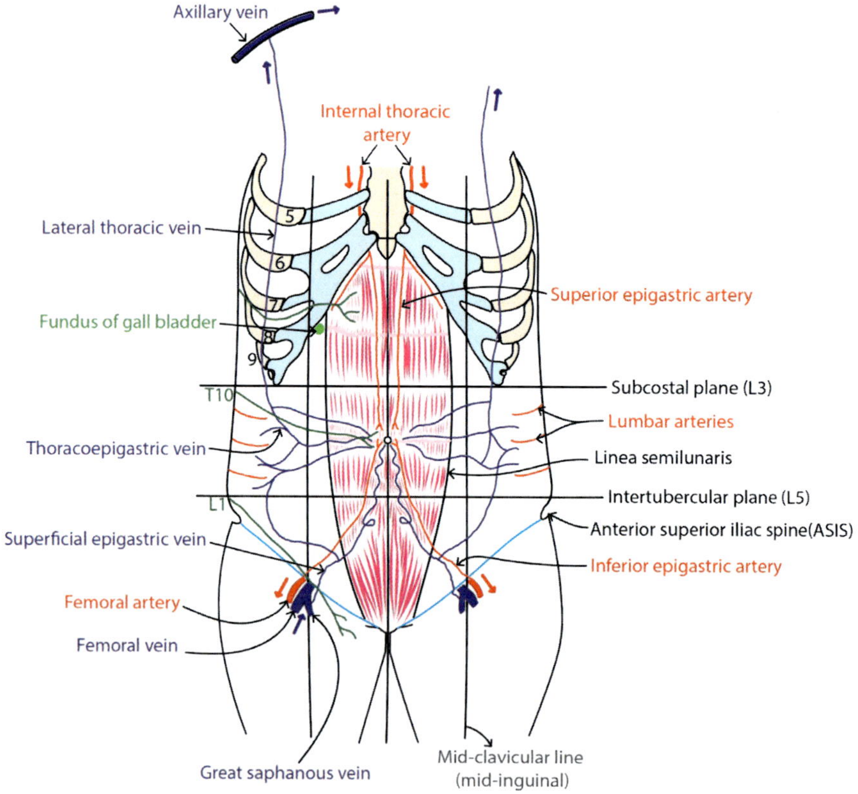

Figure 5.2. Anterior abdominal wall. Innervation: It is by the thoracoabdominal nerves: T1 supplies the muscles and skin over the epigastrium, T10 over the umbilicus region, and L1 over the region from the "loin to groin." **Arterial supply:** It is mainly by the superior and inferior epigastric arteries; in addition to these are the lumbar arteries. **Venous drainage:** It is drained into the lateral thoracic vein and superficial epigastric vein. Note that the surface marking of the fundus of the gall bladder is at the tip of the ninth costal cartilage on the right.

thoracic artery whereas the inferior epigastric artery arises from the external iliac artery. This anastomosis provides an important collateral pathway between the subclavian and external iliac arterial systems, which may help maintain blood flow to the lower limb in conditions such as coarctation of the aorta. Additional blood supply to the abdominal wall is provided by the lumbar arteries, which arise from the abdominal aorta.

Venous drainage **(Fig. 5.2)** of the anterior abdominal wall occurs through both superficial and deep veins. The superficial veins include the lateral thoracic vein and the superficial epigastric vein, the latter draining into the great saphenous vein.

Lymphatic drainage **(Fig. 5.3)** of the anterior abdominal wall depends on the level of the umbilicus. Above the umbilicus, lymph drains primarily into the axillary lymph nodes, whereas below the umbilicus, lymph drains into the superficial inguinal lymph nodes.

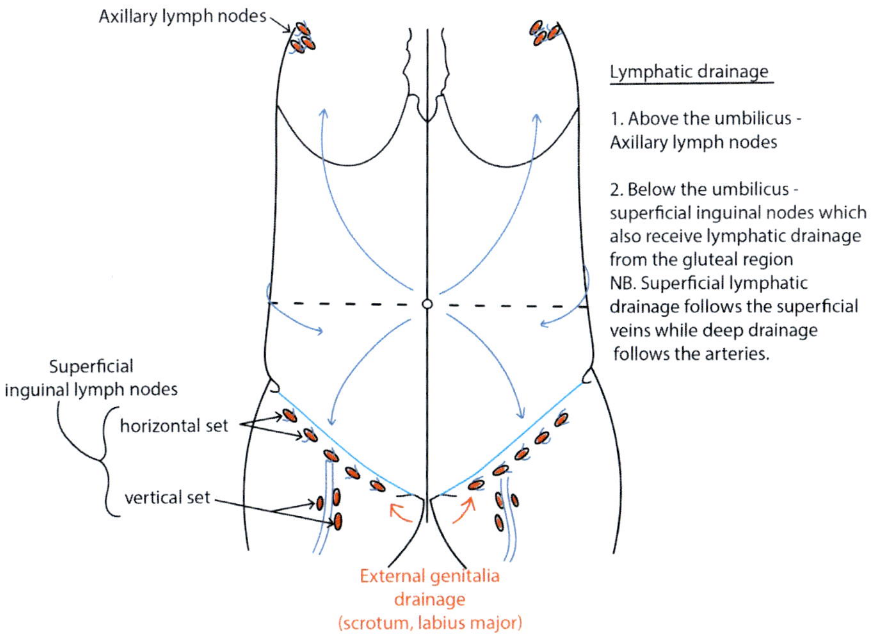

Figure 5.3. Anterior abdominal wall — lymphatic drainage. Above the level of the umbilicus, the lymphatic drainage is to the axillary lymph nodes. Below this, it is drained into the superficial inguinal lymphatic nodes. The superficial inguinal lymph nodes also receive lymphatic drainage from the gluteal region as well as the external genitalia.

Surface features:

- Linea alba is a fibrous structure that extends from the xiphoid process to the public symphysis.
- Linea semilunaris **(Fig. 5.2)** is a groove along the lateral border of the rectus abdominis muscle. Its intersection with the tip of the 9th costal cartilage denotes the surface marking of the fundus of the gall bladder.
- Langer's lines represent the natural orientation of parallel bundles of collagen fibers in the reticular layer of the dermis. Surgical incisions made parallel to these lines tend to heal better and produce less scarring.
- McBurney's point: It is located at the junction of the lateral one-third and middle one-third of a line joining the umbilicus and the right anterior superior iliac spine (ASIS). This point corresponds to the site of maximal tenderness in acute appendicitis.

Superficial fascia

This lies deep to the skin and is composed of two distinct layers: a superficial fatty layer (Camper's fascia) and a deep membranous layer (Scarpa's fascia). The fatty layer contains mainly fatty tissues, while the membranous layer is fibrous, which extends downward into the thigh and fuses with the fascia lata just below the inguinal ligament. Medially, it is continuous with the Colles' fascia in the perineum. Because Scarpa's fascia is continuous with Colles' fascia, fluids such as urine or blood from injuries can spread from the abdominal wall to the perineum, but not into the thigh due to its attachment to the fascia lata.

Muscles of the anterior abdominal wall

These include the external oblique, internal oblique, transversus abdominis, and rectus abdominis. They are supplied by the thoracoabdominal nerves (T7– T11) and the ilioinguinal nerve (L1). These muscles are involved in flexion, lateral flexion, and rotation of the trunk.

1. External oblique (Fig. 5.4)

The muscle originates from the outer surface of the lower ribs (5–12). The muscle fibers are directed downward and medially (similar to the direction of placing hands into pockets). About halfway toward the midline, the muscle fibers

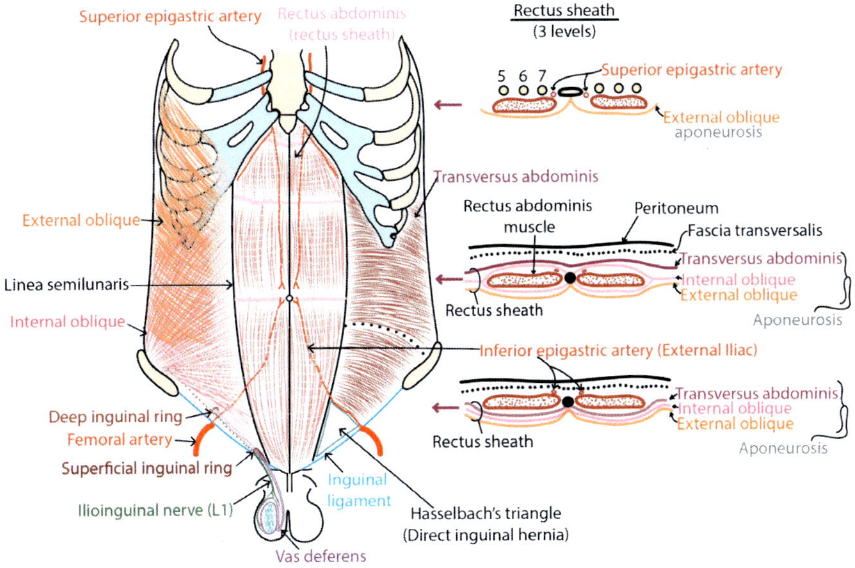

1. Langer's line: Due to the parallel bundles of collagen bundles in the reticular layer of dermis, incisions made along this orientation heal better with less scarring.
2. Inguinal hernia (direct and indirect) - differentiate them.
3. Non-descent testis - may result in sterility
(scrotal sac temperature < body temperature)

Figure 5.4. Anterior abdominal wall muscles. External oblique: the muscle fibers are directed downward and medially; internal oblique: muscle fibers are directed upward and medially. Transversus abdominus: muscle fibers are directed horizontally. The rectus abdominis muscle in the midline is attached above to the 5th, 6th, and 7th ribs; below, it is attached to the pubic crest. Three tendinous intersections are present in the muscle. The muscle is enclosed by the rectus sheath formed by the aponeurosis of the oblique muscles and transversus abdominis. (*Refer to the text for a detailed description of rectus sheath formation.*) Embedded in the paired rectus muscles are the superior and inferior epigastric arteries, which form an arterial anastomosis.

transition into a broad aponeurosis (a flat tendinous sheet). This aponeurosis attaches to the xiphoid process, linea alba, pubic symphysis, pubic tubercle, anterior superior iliac spine (ASIS), and the iliac crest.

Between the ASIS and the pubic tubercle, the inferior free margin of the aponeurosis folds inward to form the inguinal ligament. Near the pubic crest, the aponeurosis splits to create the superficial inguinal ring, which allows passage of the spermatic cord (or the round ligament of the uterus in females).

At the linea semilunaris, the aponeurosis passes anterior to the rectus abdominis to form the anterior layer of the rectus sheath.

2. Internal oblique (Fig. 5.4)

The muscle arises from the lateral two-thirds of the inguinal ligament, the iliac crest and the thoracolumbar fascia. Its fibers are directed upward and medially crisscrossing those of the external oblique muscle fibers. Superiorly, it is attached to the lower three ribs (10–12). At the linea semilunaris, the muscle is replaced by a layer of aponeurosis, which splits into the anterior and posterior lamellae, enclosing the rectus abdominis. Medially, the lamellae are attached to the linea alba. Together with the aponeurosis of the external oblique and transversus abdominis, they form the rectus sheath.

3. Transversus abdominis (Fig. 5.4)

The muscle arises from the lateral third of the inguinal ligament, the thoracolumbar fascia, the iliac crest and the lower ribs (7–12). The muscle fibers are oriented horizontally like a belt or corset. At the linea semilunaris, the muscle is replaced by a layer of aponeurosis, which contributes to form the posterior lamella of the rectus sheath (above the arcuate line).

4. Rectus abdominis (Fig. 5.4)

This muscle originates from the pubic crest and the pubic symphysis and inserts superiorly into the costal cartilages of ribs (5–7). The muscle is enclosed by the rectus sheath which is formed by the aponeurosis of external oblique, internal oblique, and transversus abdominis. The rectus sheath contains three tendinous intersections located at the tip of xiphoid process, at the umbilicus level, and midway between them. Lying posterior to the muscle are the superior and inferior epigastric arteries, which form an anastomosis at the umbilical region.

Fascia transversalis and peritoneum (Fig. 5.4)

Deep to the abdominal muscle layers lies the fascia transversalis. Beneath this layer is the parietal peritoneum, which forms the inner lining of the abdominal cavity.

INGUINAL CANAL (Fig. 5.5)

The inguinal canal is an oblique passage located just above the inguinal ligament which forms the boundary between abdomen and thigh. It transmits the vas deferens in the male and the round ligament in the female. The canal has two

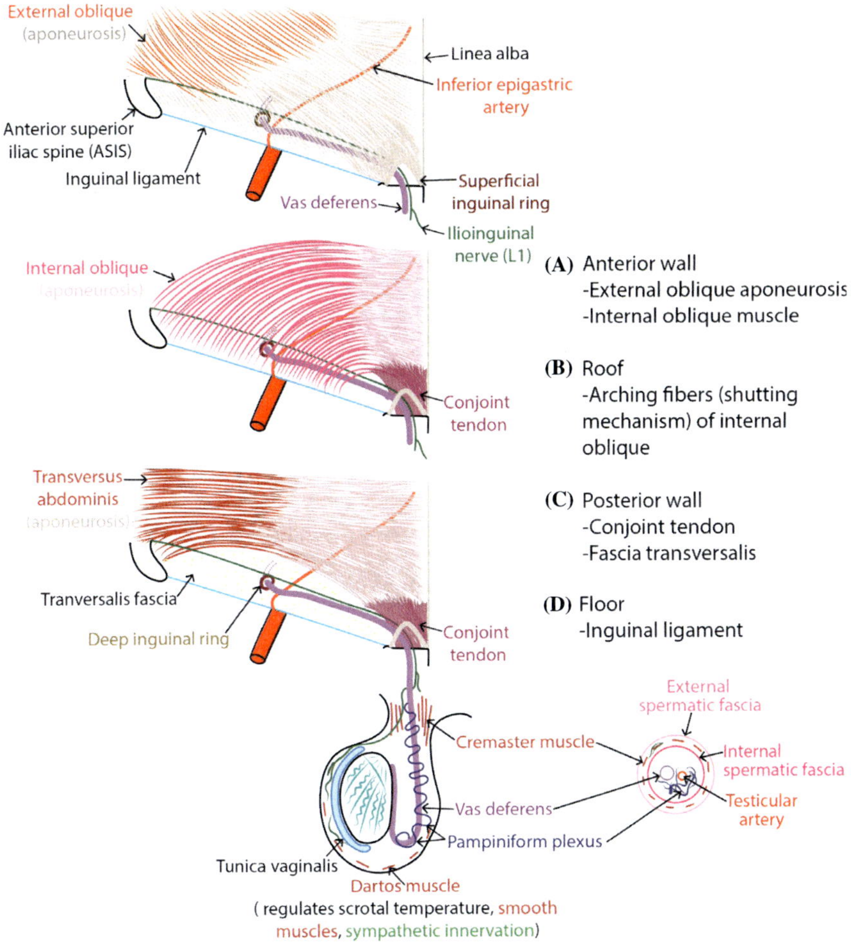

Figure 5.5. Inguinal canal — its boundaries and contents. The inguinal canal allows the passage of the vas deferens in the male and the round ligament of the uterus in the female. **(A) Anterior wall:** aponeurosis of the external oblique; medially it is "slit open," forming the superficial inguinal opening. Note that the opening allows the exit of the ilioinguinal nerve (L1). **(B) Roof:** lower arching fibers of the internal oblique. **(C) Posterior wall:** conjoint tendon and fascia transversalis. Floor: inguinal ligament. **(D) Spermatic cord.** In this, the vas deferens and its accompanying testicular artery and veins (pampiniform plexus) are surrounded by the internal spermatic fascia, cremasteric muscle/fascia, and external spermatic fascia.

openings: a deep inguinal ring and a superficial inguinal ring. The deep inguinal ring is an opening at the fascia transversalis, approximately 2.5 cm above the midpoint of the inguinal ligament. The vas deferens enters the deep inguinal ring, winding lateral to the inferior epigastric artery and exits at the superficial inguinal ring located above the public crest.

A. Boundaries of the Inguinal Canal (Fig. 5.5):

1. **Anterior wall:** Aponeurosis of the external oblique muscle
2. **Roof:** Lower arching fibers of internal oblique and transversus abdominis muscles — they serve like a "shutter mechanism".
3. **Posterior wall:** Transversalis fascia, reinforced medially by the conjoint tendon, which is formed by the fused tendons of the internal oblique and transversus abdominis muscles.
4. **Floor:** Inguinal ligament

B. Contents:

It transmits vas deferens (as part of the spermatic cord) in the male and round ligament in the female. The ilioinguinal nerve (L1) arises from the lumbar plexus, runs between the external and internal oblique and emerges at the superficial inguinal ring with the spermatic cord. It provides sensory innervation to the scrotal skin. Note that the ilioinguinal nerve does not enter the deep inguinal ring.

C. Clinical Considerations

A segment of the small intestine may protrude through the posterior wall of the inguinal canal, resulting in an inguinal hernia **(Fig. 5.4)**. There are two main types of inguinal hernia:

- **Direct inguinal hernia:** It occurs when abdominal contents push directly through a weakened area of the posterior wall of the inguinal canal, usually within Hesselbach's triangle, medial to the inferior epigastric vessels, often associated with weakness of the conjoint tendon.
- **Indirect inguinal hernia:** It occurs when abdominal contents enter the deep inguinal ring, lateral to the inferior epigastric vessels, pass through the inguinal canal, and may emerge through the superficial inguinal ring.

In some newborn males, the testis may fail to descend completely, resulting in an undescended testis (cryptorchidism) that may be located within the inguinal canal.

Cremasteric reflex

Stroking of the skin on the medial side of the upper thigh may elicit the cremasteric reflex. In response, the cremaster muscle contracts and elevates the testis. The reflex is mediated by the genitofemoral nerve (L1–L2).

DIGESTIVE SYSTEM

The digestive system is responsible for the digestion of food and absorption of nutrients essential for metabolic activities. It consists of two main components: the gastrointestinal tract (GIT) (digestive tube or alimentary canal) and the accessory digestive organs (liver, gallbladder, and pancreas).

The gastrointestinal tract is a long muscular and glandular tube extending from the mouth to the anus and lined by epithelium that varies along its length. The muscular wall propels food along the tract by peristalsis, which is coordinated rhythmic contractions of smooth muscle. These muscles fibers are arranged in an inner circular layer and an outer longitudinal layer.

The movement of food along the tract allows gradual digestion and absorption of nutrients such as amino acids, glucose, fatty acids, and water. Most nutrient absorption occurs in the small intestine, while the large intestine plays an important role in water absorption.

The accessory digestive organs such as the pancreas and liver secrete their secretions into the lumen of GIT. While pancreas secretes a variety of digestive enzymes into the intestinal lumen, the liver produces bile, which is stored and concentrated in the gallbladder and released into the intestine to aid in the digestion and absorption of fats.

Gastrointestinal Tract (Fig. 5.1; Fig. 5.6)

The gastrointestinal tract begins at the oral cavity, followed by the oropharynx, laryngopharynx, esophagus, stomach, small intestine (duodenum, jejunum, and ileum), large intestine (caecum, ascending colon, transverse colon, descending colon, sigmoid colon, rectum), and anal canal. Mostly, GIT is lined by the simple columnar epithelium except the oral cavity, oropharynx, laryngopharynx, esophagus and distal anus. This epithelium is composed of simple columnar cells (absorptive) and goblet or surface mucous cells (mucus secretion). Cilia are absent throughout the GIT.

In the oral cavity, the mucosa is lined by the stratified squamous non-keratinized epithelium, which protects against abrasion from solid food. In this epithelium, superficial cells are continuously shed and replaced by new cells produced by mitosis in the basal layer. The oropharynx, laryngopharynx, and esophagus are mainly for the passage of food from oral cavity to the stomach.

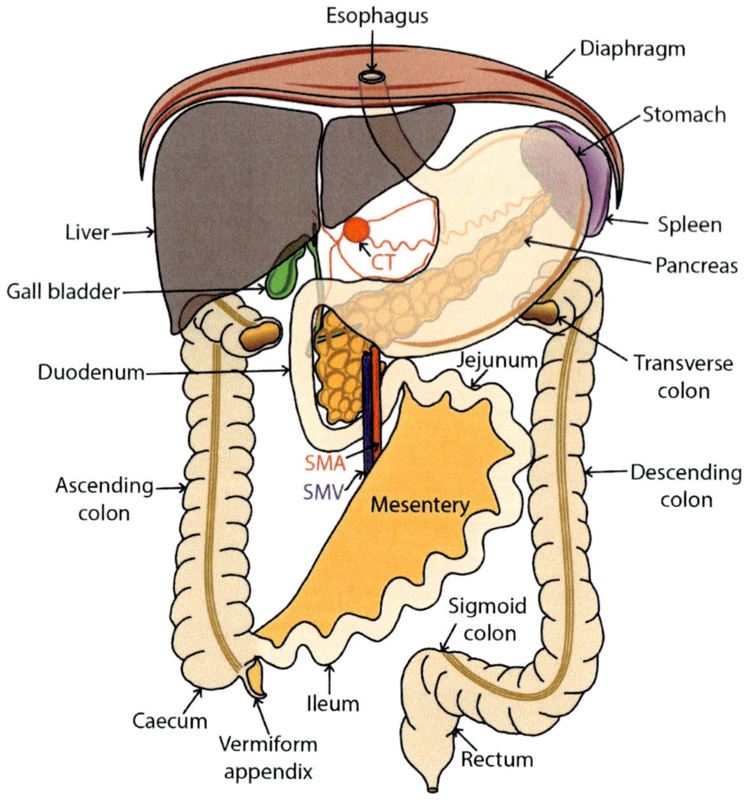

Figure 5.6. Gastrointestinal tract and glands. A diagrammatic picture showing the general arrangement of the digestive tract and associated glands (liver, gall bladder, pancreas). Red arrow indicates the coeliac trunk (CT) arises from the abdominal aorta. **SMA**: superior mesenteric artery.

Embryological division (Fig. 5.7)

The embryonic gut is divided into the foregut, midgut, and hindgut, each of which gives rise to different derivatives. The foregut begins at the pharnyx extending to the major duodenal papilla in the second part of the duodenum; the midgut extends from the the major duodenal papilla in the second part of the duodenum to the proximal two-thirds of the transverse colon. Hindgut extends from the distal one-third of the transverse colon to the upper part of the anal canal. The arterial supply and parasympathetic innervation are based on this division.

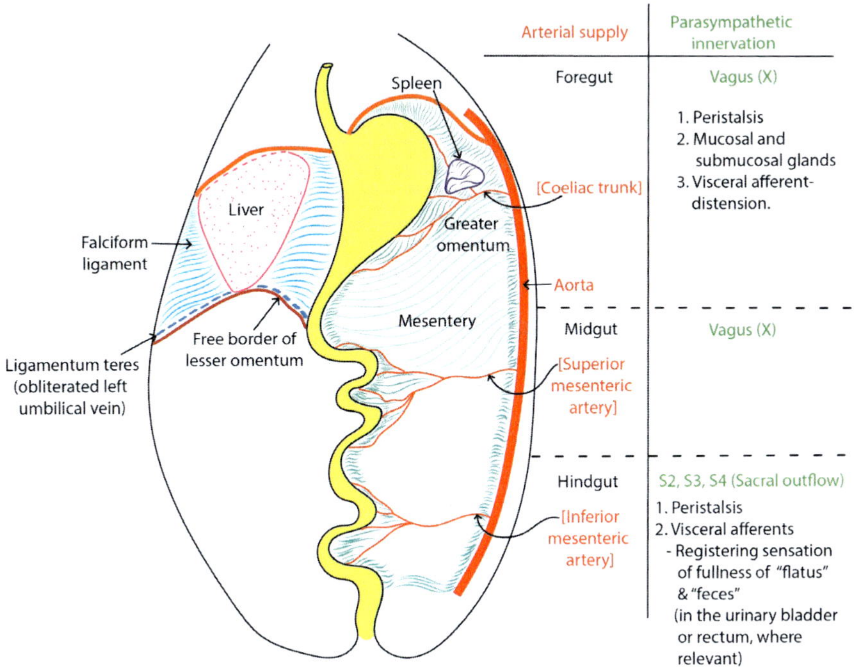

Embryological origins:
1 Foregut - up to opening of bile duct and derivatives (bile duct, pancreas).
2. Midgut - up to proximal 2/3 of transverse colon.
3. Hindgut - up to anal canal (upper part).

Figure 5.7. Development of the gut. The gut is divided into three parts: foregut, midgut, and hindgut. It is suspended to the dorsal wall by the dorsal mesentery, which coveys the arterial and nerve supplies. Note that the spleen is formed in the dorsal mesentery in relation to the stomach. The dorsal mesentery is divided into three parts: gastrosplenic ligament, greater omentum, and lienorenal ligament. A ventral mesentery extends between the foregut to the anterior wall. With the development of the liver, it is divided into two parts: falciform ligament and lesser omentum, which has a free border. Note that the coeliac trunk, superior mesenteric artery, and inferior mesenteric artery supply the foregut, midgut, and hindgut, respectively. The foregut and midgut are supplied by the vagus nerve, whereas the hindgut is supplied by the pelvic splanchnic nerves (S2, 3, 4). Both nerves are parasympathetic.

Arterial supply: While the foregut derivates are supplied by the coeliac trunk and its branches, the midgut and hindgut derivatives are supplied by the superior mesenteric artery and the inferior mesenteric artery, respectively.

Parasympathetic innervation: Both the foregut and midgut derivates receives parasympathetic innervation from the vagus nerve (cranial nerve X), which synapses in the myenteric (Auerbach) and submucosal plexuses of the gut wall. On the other hand the derivates of the hindgut, receives parasympathetic innervation from the pelvic splanchnic nerves (S2, 3, 4) which, like the vagus nerve, supply the muscles and glands of the gastrointestinal tract.

Upper Gastrointestinal Tract

1. Oral cavity

The oral cavity, which is responsible for ingestion and fragmentation of foods, is lined predominantly by the stratified squamous epithelium. Three salivary glands (parotid, submandibular, and sublingual) secrete saliva into the oral cavity **(Fig. 5.8)**. The saliva contains mainly water, some minerals, enzymes (e.g., salivary amylase), mucins, and IgA which aid in digestion, moisturization and immune defense. The tongue plays an important role in this process, bolus formation and deglutition (swallowing) **(Fig. 5.9)**. *(Details of this will be given in the chapter on the Head and Neck.)*

2. Oropharynx and laryngopharynx

Both the oropharynx and laryngopharynx mainly serve as passageways for food during swallowing. They are lined by stratified squamous epithelium (non-keratinized). The walls are composed of striated (skeletal) muscles supplied by the pharyngeal nerve plexus. Inflammation (red or swollen) of the pharynx commonly seen in infections such as influenza, is known as pharyngitis or "sore throat."

3. Esophagus (Fig. 5.10)

The esophagus, which, is a muscular tube approximately 25 cm long, begins at the lower border of the cricoid cartilage at the level of C6 and extends to the cardiac orifice of the stomach after passing through the oesophageal hiatus of the diaphragm (at the level T10). At the gastroesophageal junction, a physiological lower esophageal sphincter helps prevent reflux of gastric contents.

The esophagus initially lies in the midline posterior to the trachea and deviates to the left as it descends through the thorax. It consists of three constrictions: where it begins (pharyngoesophageal junction), where it is crossed by the arch of the aorta on its left side, and at the cardia (gastroesophageal junction).

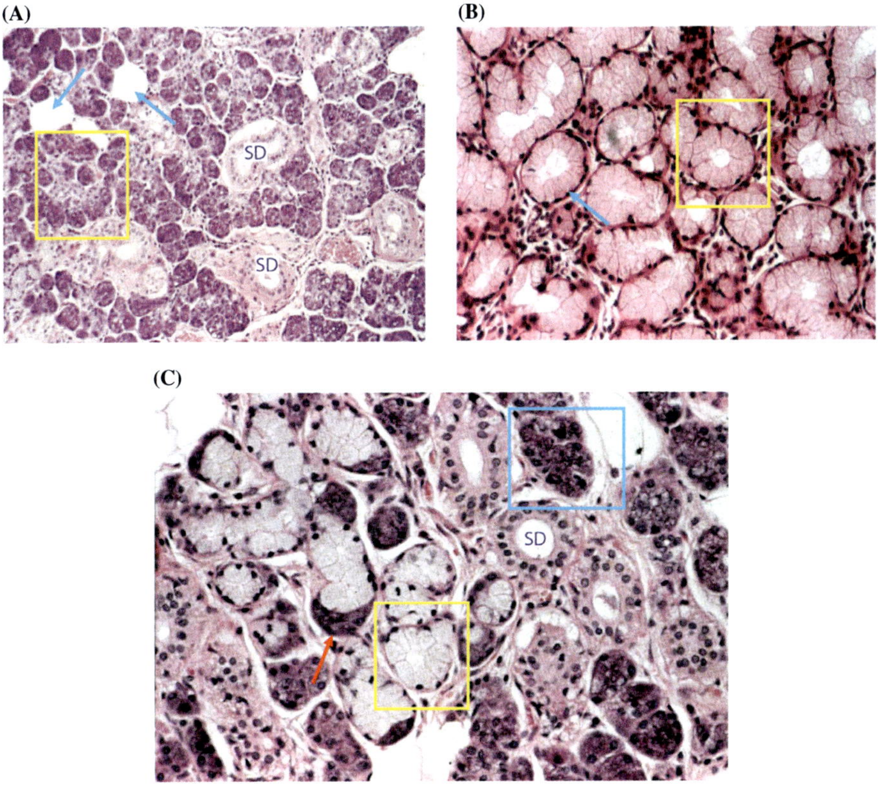

Figure 5.8. **(A) Parotid gland.** The parotid gland is composed of exclusively serous acini (darkly stained, boxed area) with some adipocytes (arrows) distributed in the parenchyma. Intralobular striated duct (SD) is lined by the simple cuboidal epithelium. **(B) The sublingual gland** is mainly composed of mucous acini (palely stained, boxed area). Note that the flattened nucleus of the mucous cells is compressed to the base of the cells. (Hematoxylin and eosin (H&E) stain.) **(C) Submandibular gland.** It is a mixed salivary gland composed of mucous (yellow box), serous acini (blue box), and mixed acini (a mucous acinus capped by a crescent-shaped serous semilune (red arrow)). The striated ducts (SD, intralobular) are lined by the simple cuboidal epithelium. (H&E stain.)

These constrictions are common sites where foreign bodies, such as fish bones, may become lodged and occasionally pierce the esophageal wall, potentially damaging adjacent structures such as the arch of the aorta and leading to severe internal bleeding. Posteriorly, the esophagus is related to the left atrium, separated by the oblique sinus. Enlargement of the left atrium may compress the esophagus and cause difficulty in swallowing (dysphagia).

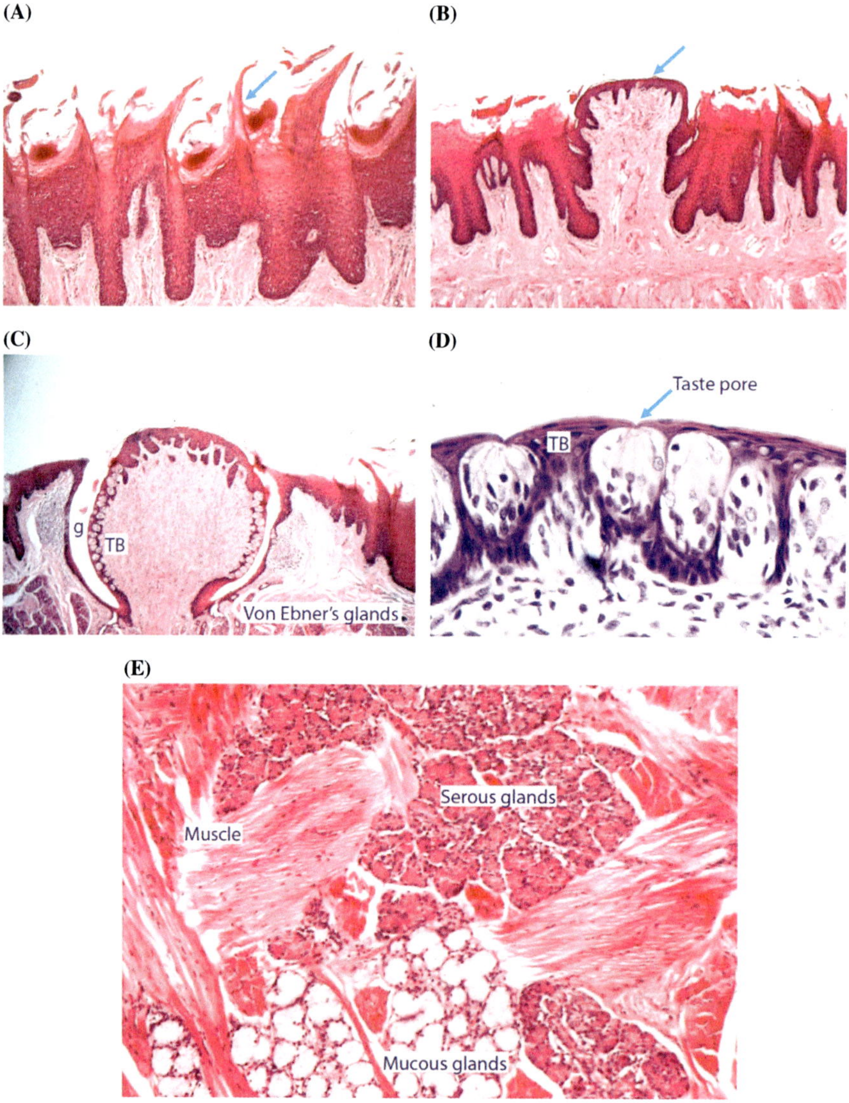

Figure 5.9. Lingual papillae. There are three main types of papillae (arrows): **(A) Filiform papillae, (B) Fungiform papillae, and (C) Circumvallate papillae.** Note the lack of taste buds on filiform papillae. The fungiform papilla has taste buds on its top. The circumvallate papillae are surrounded by a groove (g) whose taste buds (TB) are at the sides **(C, D)**. The taste bud has a small taste pore (arrow). Note that von Ebner's glands open into the groove. (H&E stain.) **(E) Tongue.** The tongue is composed of both intrinsic and extrinsic muscles arranged in bundles. All tongue muscles are striated, mainly supplied by the hypoglossal nerve (XII nerve). Between the muscles are mucous and serous glands. (H&E stain.)

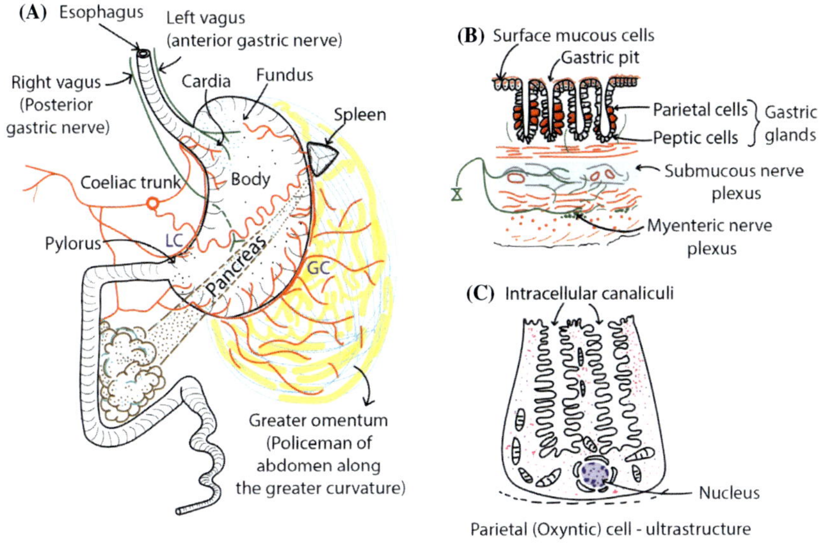

- Parts - Cardia, Fundus, Body & Pylorus
- Arterial supply - Coeliac trunk (Left gastric, Right gastric, Left & Right gastroepiploic and Short gastric)
- Posterior relation - Pancreas (posterior gastric ulceration may involve pancreas)
- Vagus nerves supply muscles, glands, pyloric sphincter (relaxation), hunger, distension & vomiting reflex.
- Cell types: 1. Surface mucous epithelial cells
  2. Parietal (oxyntic cells) -HCl, intrinsic factor (glycoprotein , Vitamin B12 uptake)
  3. Zymogenic cells - Pepsinogen
- Peptic ulcer - *Helicobacter pylorii*
- Gastroesophageal reflux disease (GERD) - metaplasia in esophagus
- Lymphatic drainage - follows the arteries - aortic lymph nodes

Figure 5.10. Esophagus and stomach. (A) The stomach receives the opening of the esophagus at the cardia. It is divided into different parts: fundus, cardia, body, and pylorus. It presents the lesser curvature (LC) and greater curvature (GC). Attached to the greater curvature is the greater omentum, which receives its arterial supply from the coeliac trunk. Parasympathetic innervation is by the vagus nerves (anterior and posterior gastric nerves). **(B)** The mucosa shows gastric pits, which receive the gastric glands from below. The gastric mucosa lining is simple columnar epithelial cells (surface mucous epithelial cells). The gastric gland lining cells are the parietal (oxyntic) cells and peptic (zymogenic) cells. **(C)** Electron microscopic features of a parietal cell. Note the presence of intracellular canaliculi and abundant mitochondria.

The esophageal wall consists of four main layers: mucosa, submucosa, muscularis externa, and adventitia/serosa **(Fig. 5.11)**. The mucosa is lined by the stratified squamous epithelium. Some mucous glands may be present in the submucosa at the lower end. The muscularis externa shows regional variation:

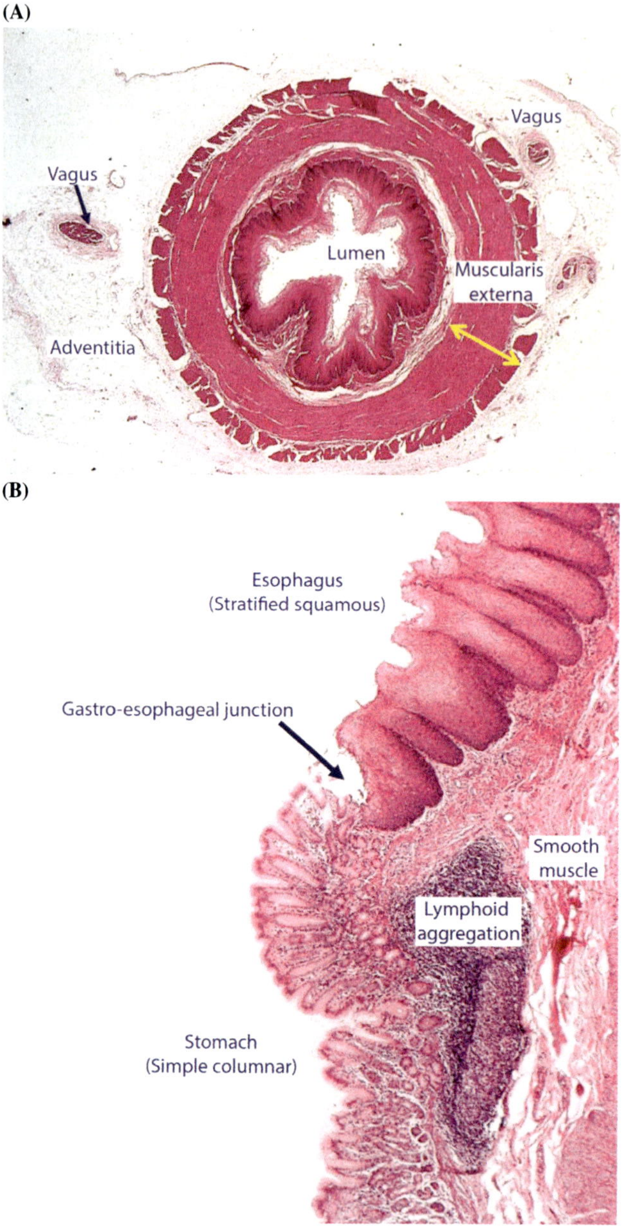

Figure 5.11. **(A) Esophagus in transverse section.** The lumen is lined by the stratified squamous epithelium. Beneath it is the submucosa and the muscularis externa (inner circular and outer longitudinal). On both sides are the left and right vagus nerves, which supply the muscles. (H&E stain.) **(B) Gastroesophageal junction.** Note the abrupt change in the epithelium from stratified squamous (esophagus) to the simple columnar epithelium (cardia). A lymphoid aggregation is seen at the junction in the submucosa. (H&E stain.)

the upper third contains skeletal muscle, the middle third contains both skeletal and smooth muscle, and the lower third contains smooth muscle only.

The esophagus is innervated by the vagus nerve (both nucleus ambiguus and dorsal motor nucleus are involved in this). Arterial supply is provided by the inferior thyroid artery, left gastric artery, and esophageal branches from the thoracic aorta.

Gastroesophageal reflex disease (GERD) results from reflux of acidic gastric contents into the esophagus. Chronic reflux may lead to metaplasia of the esophageal epithelium.

4. Stomach

The esophagus joins the stomach at the gastroesophageal junction where the epithelium changes abruptly from the stratified squamous epithelium (of esophagus) to the simple columnar epithelium (of stomach) **(Fig. 5.11)**. In the abdomen, the stomach lies mainly in the left hypochondrium beneath the left dome of the diaphragm. It consists of four main parts: cardia, fundus, body, and pylorus. The pyloric canal which is guarded by a pyloric sphincter, leads to the first part of the duodenum at the level of the transpyloric plane (L1 vertebral level). The stomach presents two curvatures: the greater and the lesser curvatures. Attached to the greater curvature is the greater omentum **(Fig. 5.10)** which is considered as the "policeman of the abdomen" as it limits the spread of infection. Along the lesser curvature is the lesser omentum, which extends to the porta hepatis of the liver. The free border of the lesser omentum contains the hepatic artery, bile duct, and portal vein, forming the anterior border of the epiploic foramen (foramen of Winslow).

(A) Relations (Fig. 5.10): The posterior surface of the stomach rests on the "stomach bed," which is formed by the diaphragm, spleen, left kidney, left suprarenal gland, pancreas, splenic artery, and transverse mesocolon, with the omental bursa (lesser sac) separating these structures from the stomach. A posterior gastric ulcer may erode into the splenic artery, leading to profuse internal bleeding, and may also involve the pancreas.

(B) Arterial supply (Fig. 5.10): The arterial supply of the stomach is mainly derived from the coeliac trunk (T12) and its branches. The greater curvature of the stomach is supplied by the left gastroepiploic (gastro-omental) artery, a branch of the splenic artery, anastomosing with the right gastroepiploic

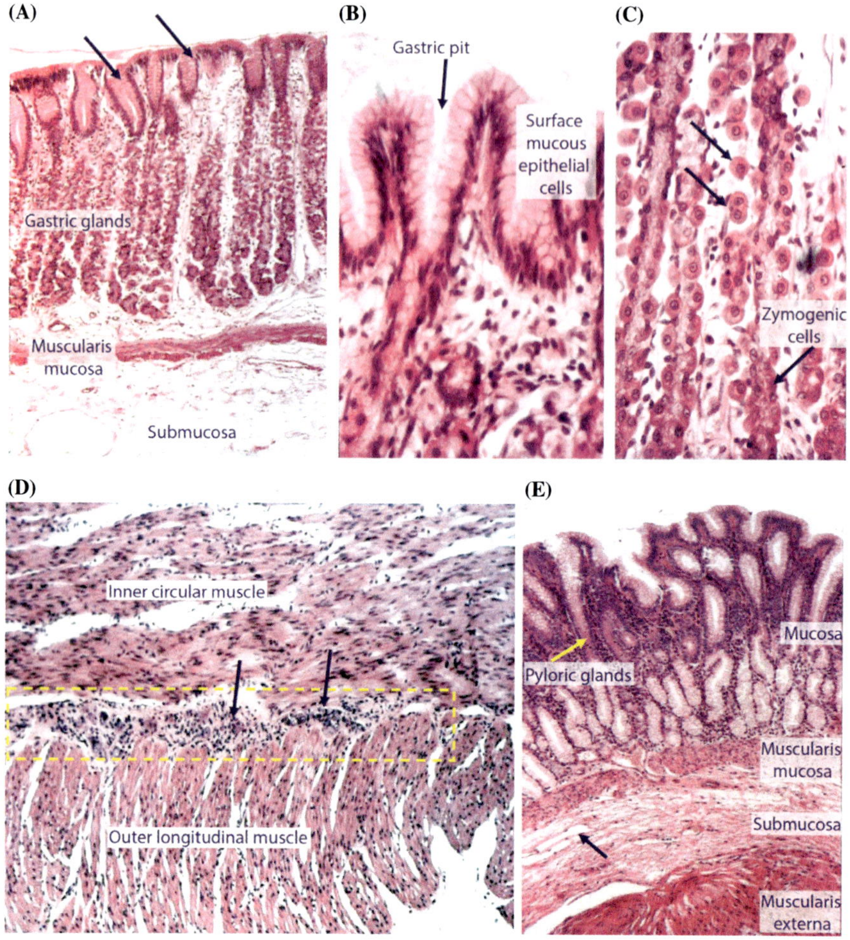

Figure 5.12. Stomach. (A) Stomach — fundus. The gastric mucosa extends from the surface down to the muscularis mucosa, which separates it from the submucosa. The mucosal surface shows many tiny gastric pits (arrows). It is lined by the simple columnar epithelium composed of surface mucous epithelial cells, which secrete mucus, forming a protective layer — mucous theca. **(B)** The theca may be eroded by *Helicobacter pylori*, causing a gastric (peptic) ulcer (which may be treated with a proton pump inhibitor, amoxylin, and erythromycin). Many tubular gastric glands **(A)** open into the base of the gastric pits. Note the lack of villi in the gastric mucosa. (H&E stain.) **(C) Gastric glands (Fundus, body).** The gastric glands are tubular glands that open into the base of gastric pits. The gland is lined by two major cells: parietal (oxyntic) cells (arrows) and zymogenic cells. The eosinophilic parietal cells secrete HCl and intrinsic factor, while the zymogen cells (small basophilic) located nearer to the base secrete pepsinogen (converted to pepsin). (H&E stain.) **(D) Myenteric nerve plexus (Auerbach's plexus).** This is an autonomic nervous plexus (area outlined) that lies between the inner circular muscle and external longitudinal muscle of the muscularis externa to which it innervates. The plexus

artery, a branch of the gastroduodenal artery. The lesser curvature is supplied by the left gastric artery, a direct branch of the coeliac trunk, anastomosing with the right gastric artery, a branch of the proper hepatic artery (variable origin). The fundus of the stomach is supplied by the short gastric arteries, which arise from the splenic artery.

(C) **Innervation (Fig. 5.12; Fig. 5.13):** The stomach is innervated by the parasympathetic component of the right and left vagus nerves, sympathetic nerves, and visceral afferent fibers.

- Parasympathetic innervation: The preganglionic parasympathetic nerve fibers terminate at the post-ganglionic neurons in the intramural ganglia within the myenteric nerve plexus (Auerbach's) innervating the muscularis externa for peristalsis and the submucous plexus (Meissner) innervating the secretory glands. Vagal stimulation increases gastric motility and secretion and relaxes the pyloric sphincter.
- Sympathetic innervation: Preganglionic sympathetic fibers arise from T6–T9 spinal segments and travel via greater splanchnic nerve to synapse in the celiac ganglion. The postganglionic fibers reach the stomach via the celiac plexus along branches of the celiac trunk. Sympathetic stimulation inhibits gastric motility and secretion and causes contraction of the pyloric sphincter.
- Visceral afferent fibers (sensory) convey sensations of hunger and distension from the stomach to the nucleus of the tractus solitarius (NTS) and are involved in the vomiting reflex (via area postrema).
- The visceral pain fibers follow the course of the sympathetic nerves entering the spinal cord at the T7 segment. The pain originating from the stomach is referred to the T7 dermatome at the epigastrium.

Figure 5.12. (*Continued on facing page*) is composed of preganglionic parasympathetic nerve fibers (vagus) and postganglionic parasympathetic ganglion cells (arrows). Contraction of both muscle layers causes peristalsis. (H&E stain.) **(E) Stomach — pylorus.** The mucosa extends from the surface to the muscularis mucosa. Many mucous pyloric glands open into the base of the deep gastric pits (yellow arrow). They secrete gastrin, which is a peptide hormone that stimulates the secretion of HCl by the parietal (oxyntic cells). The submucosa is composed of connective tissue with blood vessels and lacteals (blue arrow). The muscularis externa has two sublayers: inner circular and outer longitudinal. (H&E stain.)

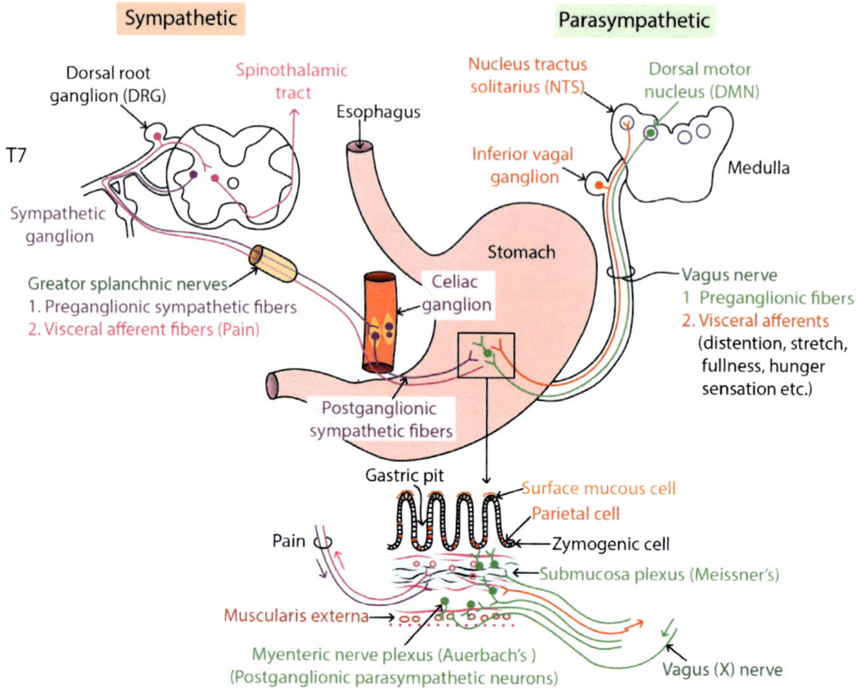

Figure 5.13. Stomach (innervation). The stomach is innervated by both parasympathetic and sympathetic nerves. The parasympathetic supply is by the vagus nerve (X), which originates from the brainstem, medulla. The preganglionic neurons are localized in the dorsal motor nucleus (DMN) of the vagus nerve. They send their long extending axons to synapse with the postganglionic parasympathetic neurons, forming the myenteric nerve plexus (Auerbach's) and the submucous plexus that supply the muscularis externa and gastric gland cells, respectively. The vagus also carries visceral afferent nerve fibers whose sensory neurons are in the inferior vagal ganglion. The afferent fibers mediate different sensations for the physiological reflex project (red arrow) to the nucleus tractus solitarius (NTS). The sympathetic supply is by the preganglionic sympathetic neurons localized in the lateral horn of the spinal cord at the thoracic segment, e.g., T7. The preganglionic sympathetic fibers traverse through the sympathetic ganglion, forming the greater splanchnic nerves. The splanchnic nerves synapse with the postganglionic sympathetic neurons in the celiac ganglia. The postganglionic fibers supply the musculature and glands. The greater splanchnic nerves also carry pain fibers from the stomach to enter the spinal cord at the T7 segment. The neurons for pain sensation are localized in the dorsal root ganglion (DRG). Referred pain from the stomach is, therefore, to the T7 dermatome over the epigastrium.

(D) Histology — cell types and functions: The wall of the stomach has four main layers: mucosa, submucosa, muscularis externa, and serosa (*adventitia is where the surface is devoid of peritoneal covering*).

i. *Mucosa* **(Fig. 5.12A, B)**

It is lined by the simple columnar epithelium composed exclusively of surface mucous epithelial cells. The mucous secretion by the epithelial cells forms a protective "theca" or coating against the acidic medium. The gastric mucosa with gastric pits is thrown into many folds which are known as rugae. In the fundus and body of the stomach, gastric glands open into the base of the gastric pits. The gastric gland is lined by different cell types, as follows:

1. *Parietal (oxyntic) cells* **(Fig. 5.12 C)**

   These are acidophilic cells which produce hydrochloric acid (HCl) in the lumen of stomach using proton pumps (H+/K+-ATPase) to maintain the acidic medium . By electron microscopy, the cells show numerous mitochondria, intracellular canaliculi and microvilli. HCl is essential for the conversion of pepsinogen (inactive) to pepsin (active) for protein digestion **(Fig. 5.10)**. Besides producing HCl, the parietal cells also secrete the intrinsic factor (glycoprotein) for the absorption of vitamin B12.

   A common cause of peptic ulcer is infection with *Helicobacter pylori* flora in the gastric mucosa which may trigger inflammation and destruction of the mucous theca. Once this protective barrier is compromised, the acidic medium may erode the mucosa, leading to ulcer formation. Clinically, proton pump inhibitors are commonly used to inhibit the excess production of HCl.

   Additionally, reflux of acid into the esophagus (gastroesophageal reflux, GERD) may chronically irritate the esophageal lining and cause metaplasia in its lining cells.

2. *Zymogenic (chief) cells* **(Fig. 5.12C)**: These cells are localized near to the base of the gastric glands. They secrete pepsinogen (inactive form) which is activated by HCl to form pepsin for protein digestion in the lumen of the stomach.
3. *Enterochromaffin cells (argentaffin or enteroendocrine cells)*: They secrete serotonin (5-HT) which is involved in peristaltic movement.
4. *Stem cells*: These are undifferentiated cells, giving rise to other cell types.

   The base of the gastric glands lies adjacent to the muscularis mucosae, a thin layer composed of smooth muscle fibers. Contraction of this layer helps move the mucosal layer and facilitates the emptying of glandular secretions into the stomach lumen.

The mucosa of the cardiac and pyloric regions does not contain typical gastric glands. Instead, these regions contain cardiac glands and pyloric glands, **(Fig. 5.12E)**, respectively. Both types of glands primarily secrete mucus, which helps protect the stomach lining from mechanical damage and the acidic gastric environment.

In addition, the pyloric glands contain gastrin-secreting cells (G cells). These cells release gastrin, a hormone that stimulates parietal (oxyntic) cells in the gastric glands of the body and fundus of the stomach to secrete hydrochloric acid (HCl) and intrinsic factor. Intrinsic factor is a glycoprotein that is essential for the absorption of vitamin B12 in the distal ileum.

ii. *Submucosa*

It is composed mainly of dense irregular connective tissue forming bedding for the mucosa. Between the connective tissue fibers are blood vessels and the submucous nerve plexus (Meissner's plexus).

iii. *Muscularis externa*

It is composed mainly of inner circular and outer longitudinal muscle layers (smooth muscle). In some areas, an innermost oblique layer is present.

Contraction of the muscle layers help mixing the food into a semifluid chyme for transportation. Between the inner circular and outer longitudinal muscle layers is the myenteric nerve plexus (Auerbach's nerve plexus) **(Fig. 5.12D)**.

iv. *Serosa/Adventitia*

The stomach surface is covered by a layer of the peritoneum (visceral layer).

Lymphatic drainage

The lymphatic vessels follow the course of arteries supplying the stomach and drain ultimately to the aortic lymph nodes.

5. Liver

The liver, which is the largest glandular organ in the body, lies primarily in the right hypochondrium of the abdomen, and may extend into the epigastrium and left hypochondrium. In normal conditions, the liver is not palpable, but it can be felt in an enlarged liver as seen in hepatomegaly or in newborns. The surface of the liver is covered by a layer of peritoneum, which is absent superiorly where it is in direct contact with the diaphragm, the so-called "bare area of the liver". The liver has a superior diaphragmatic and visceral surface related to different organs, e.g., the right kidney. At the visceral surface is the porta hepatis which contains the hepatic portal vein, hepatic artery, and hepatic ducts **(Fig. 5.14; Fig. 5.15)**.

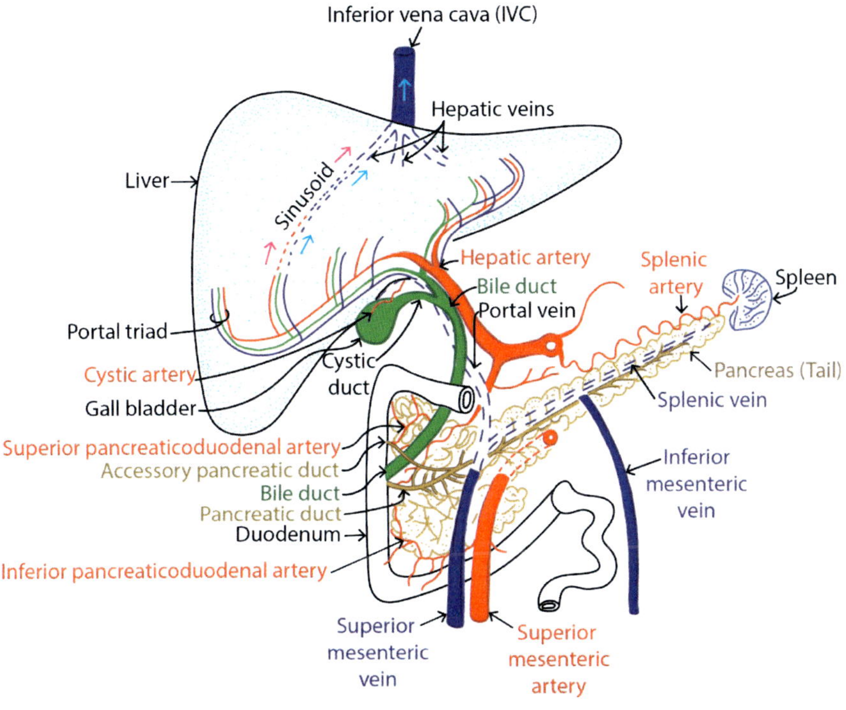

Figure 5.14. Upper gastrointestinal tract: Liver, gall bladder, bile duct, duodenum, and pancreas. The liver receives the blood supply from the hepatic artery and portal vein. After passing through the liver sinusoids, the confluent blood is drained into the inferior vena cava (IVC) via the hepatic veins. Bile secretion is drained by the hepatic ducts via the gall bladder and bile duct and then into the second part of the duodenum. The bile duct grooves the head of the pancreas posteriorly. The pancreas lies in the curvature of the duodenum, whose tail is related to the spleen on the left. It receives arterial supply from the superior and inferior pancreatico-duodenal arteries as well as the splenic artery. The portal vein is formed by the union of the superior mesenteric vein and splenic vein (posterior to the neck of the pancreas), which receives the drainage from the inferior mesenteric vein.

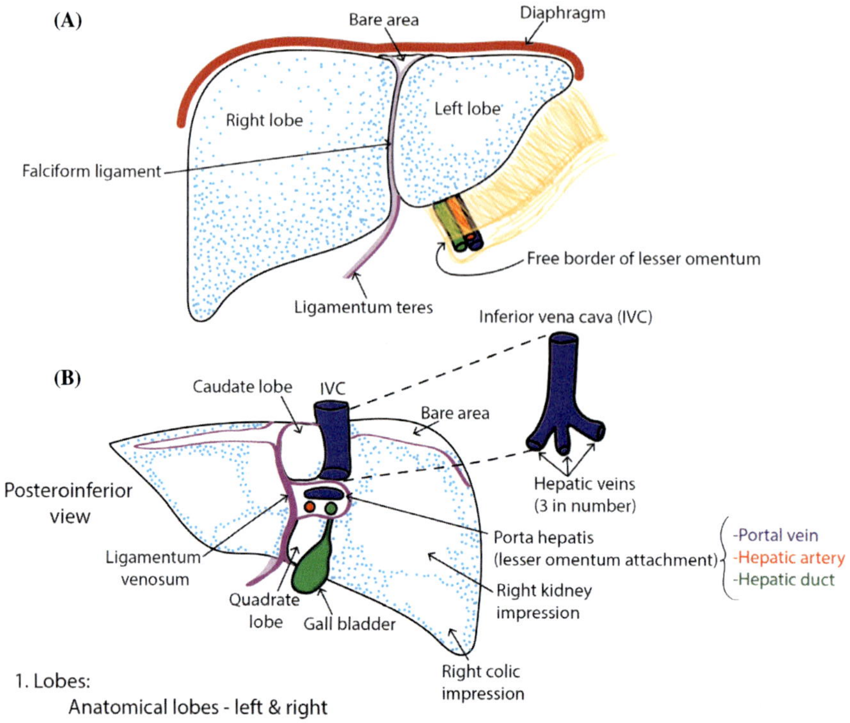

1. Lobes:

Anatomical lobes - left & right
- falciform ligament
- ligament and ligamentum venosum (posterior)

Functional lobes - Based on blood supply and biliary drainage
- Along IVC and gall bladder
- Caudate and Quadrate lobes - Left lobe

2. Functions: Carbohydrate storage (glycogen), production of serum (plasma) proteins e.g. Albumin, Fibrinogen and Prothrombin.
- Bile: Bile salt and Bilirubin; conjugation of free bilirubin → conjugated bilirubin (glucuronide)
- Cholesterol, Lipoprotein (LDL & HDL)
- Hormones: Insulin-like growth factor (IGF-1) and Angiotensinogen

Figure 5.15. Liver. (A) Anterior view of the liver showing the right and left lobes (anatomical division) divided by the falciform ligament. The liver is covered on its surface by the peritoneum except over the bare area beneath the diaphragm. **(B)** Posterior and postero-inferior views of the liver showing the left and right anatomical lobes, which are separated by the ligamentum venosum. The lesser omentum is attached to the margin of the porta hepatis, which shows the openings of the hepatic artery, hepatic duct, and portal vein. Above the porta hepatis is the caudate lobe, and below it is the quadrate lobe. The left functional lobe (based on biliary drainage) includes the caudate and quadrate lobe along an imaginary line extending from the inferior vena cava to the gall bladder. The right functional lobe is to the right of this line. The postero-inferior aspect is related to the right kidney and right colic flexure.

The lesser omentum attaches to the margin of the porta hepatis, connecting the liver to the stomach and duodenum.

Lobes of the liver (Fig. 5.15): Anatomically, the liver is divided into left and right lobes demarcated anteriorly by the falciform ligament and posteriorly by the ligamentum teres and ligamentum venosum. The caudate and quadrate lobes are part of the right anatomical lobe. Functionally, the liver is divided into right and left functional lobes based on blood supply (portal vein and hepatic artery) and biliary drainage. On the liver's surface, this functional division is marked by the inferior vena cava and gallbladder. In this functional classification, the caudate and quadrate lobes are considered part of the left functional lobe.

b. **Functions**: The liver has multiple essential functions, including, the storage of carbohydrates as glycogen, production of serum (plasma) proteins (e.g., albumin) and blood clotting factors (e.g., fibrinogen, prothrombin), bile (bile salt and bilirubin), cholesterol, lipoproteins (LDL, HDL), and some hormones such as insulin-like growth factor (IGF-1), and angiotensinogen. It also functions in detoxification of drugs, toxins, and metabolic byproducts.

c. **Hepatocytes and sinusoids**: The portal vein, hepatic artery, and bile duct are held together by connective tissue in the liver and they ramify into small branches, each forming a "portal triad" **(Fig. 5.16A)**. Six of such triads form a hexagonal hepatic lobule (classic), the center of which is occupied by the central vein. Blood from the hepatic artery and portal vein drains into the central vein via sinusoids **(Fig. 5.16B)**. From the central veins, the blood is drained into the inferior vena cava via the hepatic veins. The main liver cells or hepatocytes are arranged in the form of cell plates. Between them are the blood sinusoids lined by endothelial cells and Kupffer's cells, which are monocyte-derived macrophages **(Fig. 5.16C)**. Deep to the sinusoids is the perisinusoidal space or space of Disse in which hepatic stellate cells (Ito cells) are present. The hepatic stellate cells are for the storage of vitamin A and are implicated in cirrhosis.

The cytoplasm of hepatocytes is rich in smooth endoplasmic reticulum (involved in detoxification) and glycogen (carbohydrate storage). Some hepatocytes are binucleated.

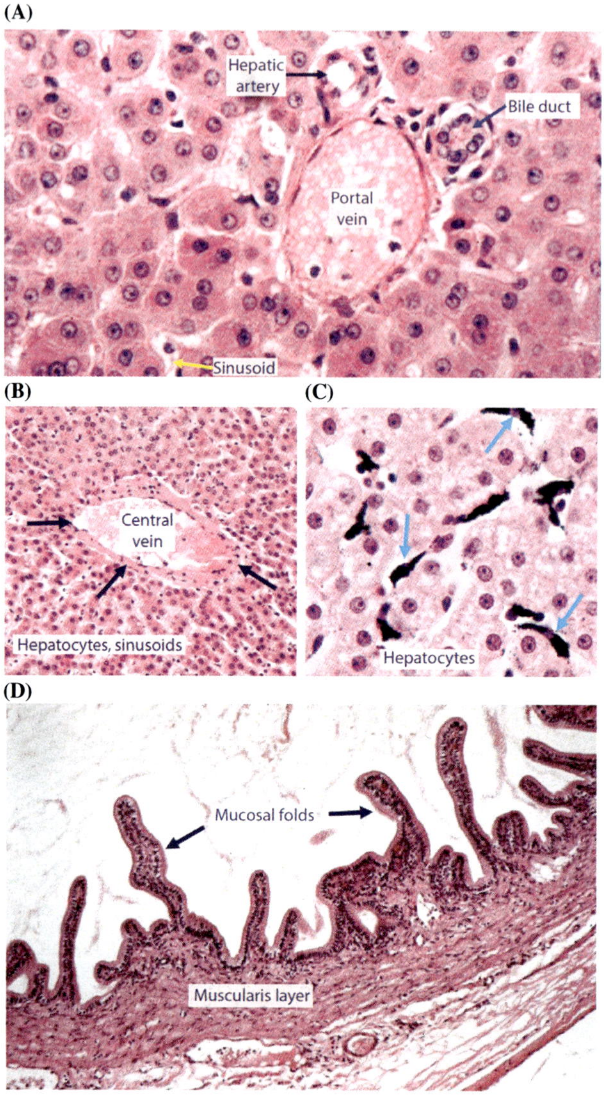

Figure 5.16. Liver. (A) A portal triad: hepatic artery, portal vein, and bile duct. Between the hepatic cells, which are arranged in cords, are the sinusoids (yellow arrow) lined by endothelial cells and Kupffer's cells. (H&E stain.) **(B)** Hepatocytes in columns or cords. Between them are sinusoids (capillaries). Blood from the hepatic artery and portal vein flows through the sinusoids (arrows), draining into the central vein. (H&E stain.) **(C)** Arrows indicate phagocytic Kupffer's cells (nucleus, arrows), which are labeled with carbon particles (black), and injected intravascularly into a rat. The Kupffer's cells had earlier ingested the carbon particles in circulation. (H&E stain.) **(D) Gall bladder.** The wall has a mucosa and muscularis layer. The mucosa is thrown into many folds, lined by the simple columnar epithelium. The epithelial cells show a distinct brush (striated) border formed by a palisade of microvilli that facilitate absorption. Note the lack of goblet cells in the epithelial lining. (H&E stain.)

d. **Gall bladder and biliary drainage (Fig. 5.15; Fig. 5.16)**

On the visceral (inferior) surface of the liver, the pear-shaped gallbladder is located in a fossa related to the quadrate lobe. It is surrounded by a layer of peritoneum except for the area in contact with the liver. It has four parts: fundus, body, neck, and cystic duct. The body of the gallbladder is in contact with the quadrate lobe, and the neck continues into the cystic duct leading to the biliary tree. The cystic duct joins with the common hepatic duct to form the (common) bile duct. The fundus is surface marked at the tip of the right ninth costal cartilage intersecting with the linea semilunaris **(Fig. 5.2)**.

The main function of the gall bladder is to concentrate the bile. Its lumen is lined by the simple columnar epithelium with a distinct striated or brush border (microvilli) that facilitates water absorption **(Fig. 5.16D)**. Its wall consists of smooth muscle fibers and lacks submucosa. The gall bladder is supplied by the cystic artery, which arises from the hepatic artery.

In the liver, hepatocytes secrete bile, which drains into bile canaliculi that merge into bile ductules and then into larger intrahepatic bile ducts. These ducts converge to form the right and left hepatic ducts, which join at the porta hepatis to form the common hepatic duct. Just below this, the common hepatic duct unites with the cystic duct from the gallbladder to form the common bile duct. The common bile duct then passes posterior to the head of the pancreas, where it usually joins the main pancreatic duct. The combined duct which is knowns as hepatopancreatic duct (ampulla of Vater) opens into the second part of the duodenum at the major duodenal papilla **(Fig. 5.14)**.

Applied anatomy

i. Calot's triangle (also called the hepatocystic triangle) is bounded medially by the common hepatic duct, superiorly by the inferior surface of the liver, and inferiorly by the cystic duct. This anatomical triangle is an important surgical landmark used to identify the cystic artery during cholecystectomy **(Fig. 5.14)**.

ii. Obstructive jaundice may occur due to a tumor in the head of the pancreas, which obstructs the common bile duct, preventing bile from reaching the duodenum.

6. Pancreas

a. Location, parts, and relations (Fig. 5.14)

The pancreas is a retroperitoneal gland that lies transversely across the posterior abdominal wall, extending from the duodenum on the right to the hilum of the spleen on the left. The pancreas is lobulated rather than truly encapsulated and is divided into the head, neck, body, tail, and uncinate process. The head of the pancreas lies within the C-shaped curve of the duodenum, while the uncinate process extends posterior to the superior mesenteric vessels. The tail of the pancreas passes within the splenorenal (lienorenal) ligament together with the splenic vessels and reaches the hilum of the spleen. Posterior to the neck of the pancreas, the superior mesenteric vein joins the splenic vein to form the portal vein. The main pancreatic duct runs through the pancreas and usually joins the common bile duct to form the hepatopancreatic ampulla (ampulla of Vater), which opens into the second part of the duodenum at the major duodenal papilla. An accessory pancreatic duct, when present, opens into the second part of the duodenum at the minor duodenal papilla, which lies superior to the opening of the main pancreatic duct.

b. Exocrine and endocrine gland

The pancreas is covered by connective tissue capsule which forms many fibrous septa dividing the parenchyma into numerous lobules. It consists of both exocrine and endocrine components. The exocrine part is a compound acinar gland in which acinar cells **(Fig. 5.17A)** secrete digestive enzymes such as trypsinogen (inactive precurosor of trypsin), lipase, and amylase. Trypsinogen is activated by enterokinase secreted by Brunner's glands of the duodenum to form trypsin. The branching ducts terminate as the intercalated ducts at the serous acinus (acini). Some lining cells of the intercalated duct extend into the lumen of the acinus, forming the centro-acinar cells, which produce bicarbonate ions. The secretions from the acini pass into a system of intercalated ducts, which drain into intralobular and interlobular ducts and eventually into the main pancreatic duct. The secretion of bicarbonate is stimulated by the hormone secretin, released from the duodenal mucosa, which helps neutralize the acidic chyme entering the duodenum from the stomach.

The endocrine part **(Fig. 5.17B)** consists of the islets of Langerhans composed of alpha-, beta-, and delta cells. The alpha cells produce glucagon, the beta cells produce insulin, and the delta cells produce somatostatin. The

(A)

(B)

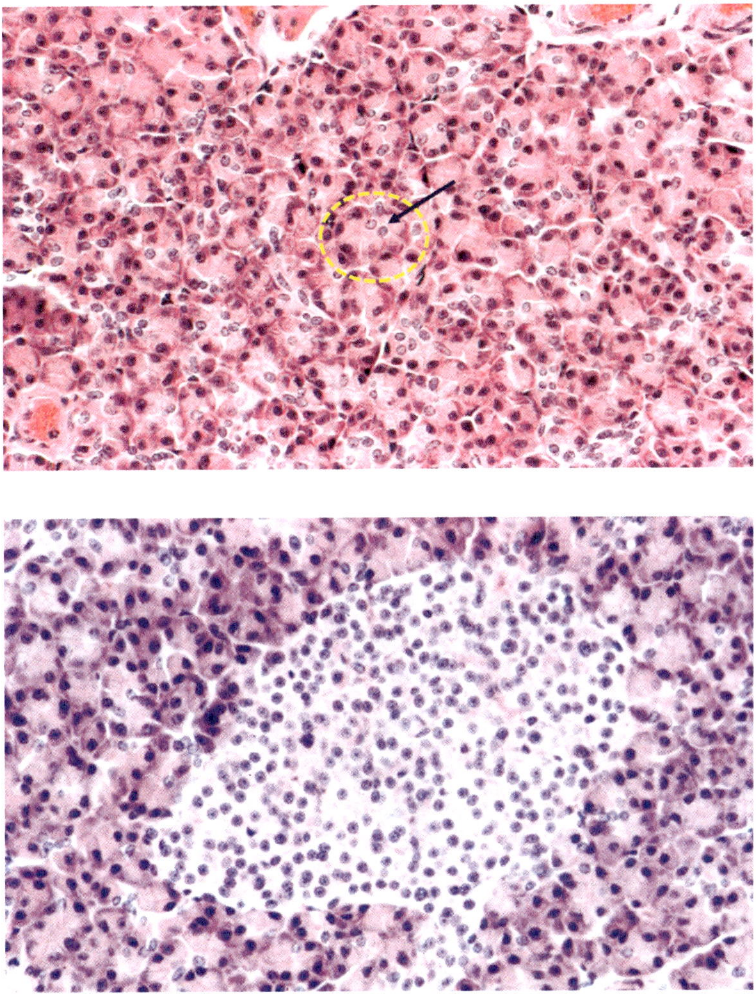

Figure 5.17. Pancreas. **(A)** Showing the exocrine part of the pancreas, which is made up of closely packed serous acini. The acinus (circled) is formed by serous acinar cells that secrete trypsinogen, amylase, etc. In the center of the acinus are the centroacinar cells (arrows, palely stained cells). Under the stimulation of secretin (from the duodenum), the centrocinar cells secrete bicarbonate ions, which help neutralize the acidic chyme from the stomach. The centroacinar cells are lining cells of the intercalated duct. Unlike the salivary glands, striated ducts, as observed in the salivary glands, are absent in the pancreas. (H&E stain.) **(B)** Showing the endocrine part of the pancreas — islet of Langerhans. The islet consists of alpha (glucagon), beta (insulin), and delta (somatostatin) cells, which are palely stained. They are indistinguishable from each other unless immunohistochemical staining using specific antibodies is used. (H&E stain.)

hormones act in concert to maintain an optimal blood glucose level. (*For more details regarding the endocrine part, refer to the chapter on the Endocrine System.*)

b. Arterial supply

The arteries supplying the pancreas are the (a) splenic artery, a branch of the coeliac trunk; (b) superior pancreatico-duodenal artery, a branch of the gastroduodenal artery; and (c) inferior pancreatico-duodenal artery, a branch of the superior mesenteric artery.

c. Embryological development

The pancreas is derived from both the ventral and dorsal pancreatic buds from the foregut. The dorsal pancreatic bud forms the head, body, and tail; the ventral pancreatic bud forms the uncinate process.

A developmental abnormality may result in annular pancreas, in which pancreatic tissue encircles the second part of the duodenum, potentially causing duodenal obstruction.

DIGESTIVE SYSTEM: LOWER GASTROINTESTINAL TRACT

The partially digested semi-fluid food (chyme) from the stomach passes through the pyloric canal, which consists of pyloric sphincter (smooth muscle). Pyloric sphincter is innervated by the vagus nerve which relaxes the sphincter allowing the chyme to enter the small intestine for further digestion and absorption. The chyme first passes through the small intestine, which consists of duodenum, jejunum, and ileum, where most digestion and nutrient absorption occur. It then moves into the large intestine including caecum, ascending colon, transverse colon, descending colon, sigmoid colon, and rectum, before finally reaching the anal canal **(Fig. 5.18)**. Undigested waste products are excreted from the body through the anal canal.

SMALL INTESTINE

The small intestine consists of the duodenum, jejunum, and ileum **(Fig. 5.18)**. Its main functions are the digestion of chyme received from the stomach and the absorption of water and nutrients. To facilitate these functions, the luminal surface of the small intestine is highly modified to increase its absorptive capacity. The mucosal surface possesses numerous finger-like projections known as intestinal villi. The jejunum exhibits mucosa and submucosa features notably prominent circular folds (plicae circulares) that increase the area for absorption. At the cellular level, the surface of the lining epithelial cells has numerous microvilli. Taken together, these structural specializations enhance the surface area for digestion and absorption.

A. **Duodenum:** The first part of the small intestine is the duodenum, which extends from the pyloric sphincter to the duodenojejunal flexure **(Fig. 5.18)**. It presents a C-shaped structure, the curvature of which accommodates the head and uncinate process of the pancreas. It is divided into four parts: the first (superior), second (descending), third (horizontal), and fourth (ascending) parts. Most parts of the duodenum are retroperitoneal except for its proximal segment immediately distal to the pylorus.

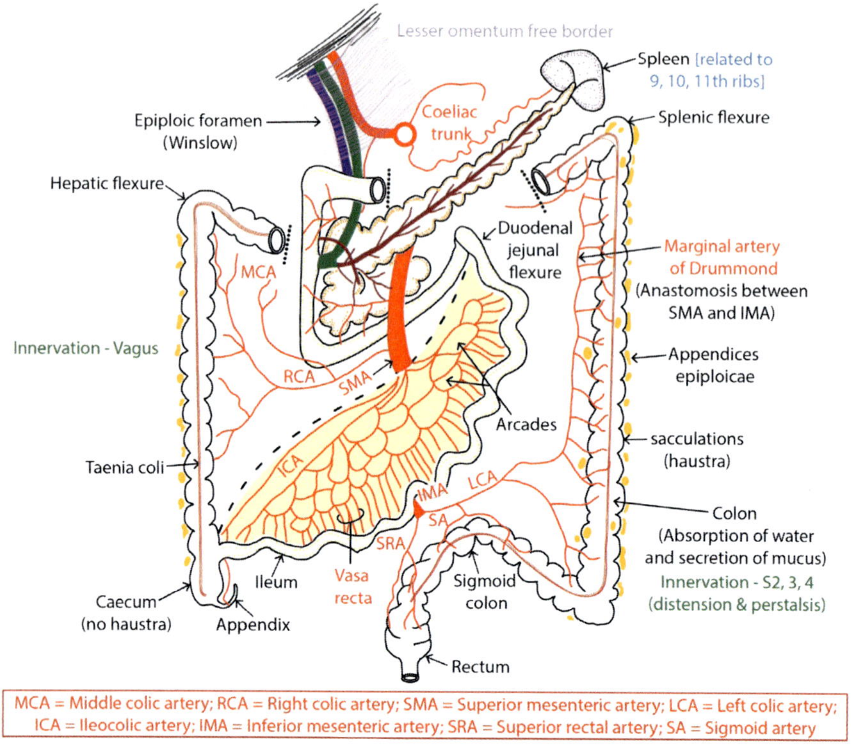

Figure 5.18. Lower gastrointestinal tract — small and large intestines. The small intestine begins at the duodenum. At the duodenojejunal flexure, it continues as the jejunum and ileum, which empties into the caecum at the ileocecal junction. The caecum continues as the ascending colon. At the right colic flexure (hepatic flexure), it turns to the left till the left colic flexure (splenic flexure). The descending colon turns downward to become the sigmoid colon, rectum, and anal canal in succession. Three main arteries supply the lower gastrointestinal tract and associated organs: the coeliac trunk, superior mesenteric artery (SMA), and inferior mesenteric artery (IMA). The coeliac trunk supplies the stomach, pancreas, and spleen. The SMA supplies the duodenum; also, it gives rise to many arterial arcades and vasa recta, supplying the jejunum and ileum. It also gives rise to the ileocolic artery (ICA), right colic artery (RCA), and middle colic artery (MCA), supplying the caecum, appendix, ascending colon, and transverse colon. The inferior mesenteric artery (IMA) gives rise to the left colic artery (LCA), sigmoidal artery (SA), and superior rectal artery (SRA) supplying the descending colon (through the marginal artery of Drummond), sigmoid colon, and rectum, respectively. The colon is characterized by the presence of sacculations (haustra), appendices epiploicae, and taenia coli.

The common bile duct and the main pancreatic duct converge to form the hepatopancreatic ampulla (ampulla of Vater), which opens into the second (descending) part of the duodenum at the major duodenal papilla. The release of bile and pancreatic secretions at this site is regulated by the sphincter of

Oddi (*Refer to the section on Liver & Pancreas*). The duodenum receives its arterial supply from the superior pancreatico-duodenal artery (a branch of the coeliac trunk) and the inferior pancreatico-duodenal artery (a branch of the superior mesenteric artery). Both superior and inferior pancreatico-duodenal arteries anastomose. It is innervated by the parasympathetic component of the vagus nerve, whose preganglionic nerve fibers terminate at the myenteric and submucous nerve plexuses described above (*Refer to the section on stomach innervation*).

Histologically, the duodenal wall comprises four layers: mucosa, submucosa, muscularis externa, and serosa. The mucosa has numerous intestinal villi lined by the simple columnar epithelium, consisting of columnar and goblet cells **(Fig. 5.19 A, B)**. At the base of the intestinal villi lie the intestinal glands (crypts of Lieberkühn) which are invaginations in the intestinal mucosa. These short glands extend down to the muscularis mucosae which separates the intestinal crypts from the submucosa. These crypts comprise enterocytes, stem cells, enteroendocrine cells and Paneth cells **(Fig. 5.19C)**. Paneth cells are filled with acidophilic granules containing lysozyme for bactericidal function. The enterocyte apart from its absorptive function, also produces enterokinase that activates pancreatic trypsinogen (inactive form) to trypsin (active form), facilitating protein digestion.

The duodenum has endocrine function through its enteroendocrine cells. It secretes secretin in response to acidic chyme, inhibiting the parietal (oxyntic) cells of the stomach and stimulating pancreatic centroacinar cells to release fluid rich in bicarbonate ions, helping maintain duodenal pH homeostasis. The duodenum also secretes cholecystokinin (CCK) in response to fats and amino acids, stimulating the contraction of the gall bladder musculature to release bile, relaxing the sphincter of Oddi, and promoting pancreatic enzyme secretion.

A distinctive histological feature of the duodenum is the presence of Brunner's glands **(Fig. 5.19A, C, D)** in the submucosa, secreting alkaline mucus to neutralize the acidic medium from the stomach. The muscularis externa is composed of inner circular and outer longitudinal muscle layers, which are involved in peristalsis of the gut **(Fig. 5.19A)**. The peristaltic movement is regulated by myenteric nerve plexus. The serosa covers the surface of the duodenum except the region where it is retroperitoneal.

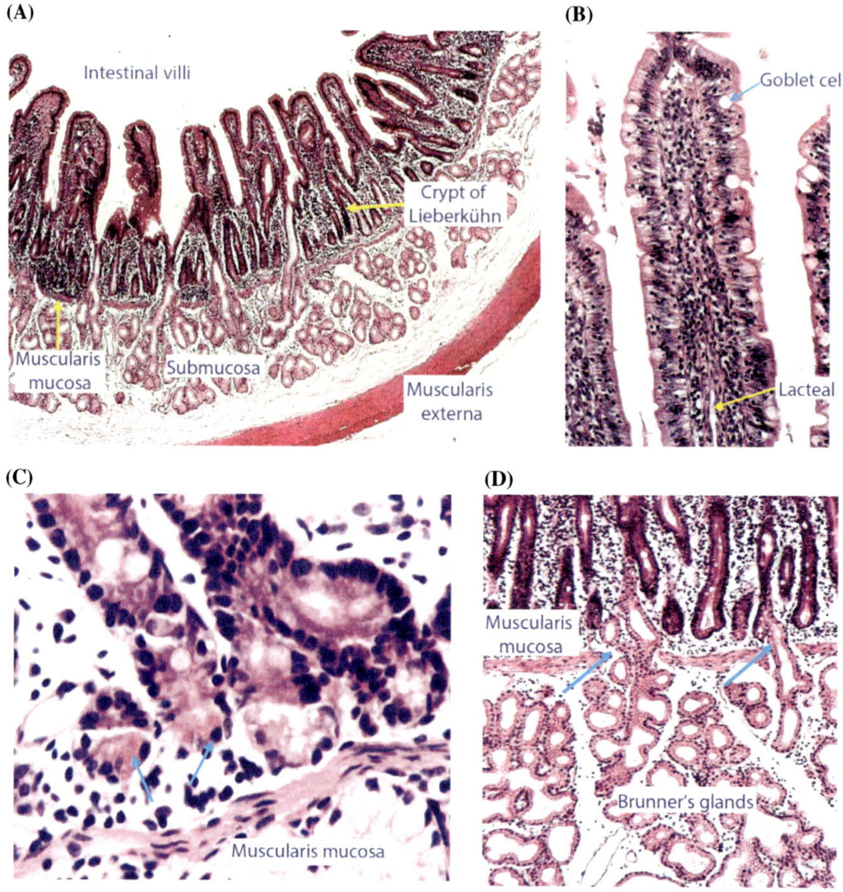

Figure 5.19. Duodenum. (A) The mucosa shows many finger-like projections — intestinal villi. Opening between the intestinal villi at the base are crypts of Lieberkuhn, which lie above the muscularis mucosa. The submucosa is occupied by Brunner's glands, which secrete alkaline mucus into the crypt of Liberkuhn to neutralize the acidic medium from the stomach. The muscularis externa is made up of inner circular and outer longitudinal muscles. **(B)** An intestinal villus is lined by the simple columnar epithelium bearing a prominent brush border (microvilli). Blue arrow indicates a goblet cell. The core of the villus contains connective tissues, lacteals, lymphocytes (dense dots). **(C)** Crypt of Lieberkuhn (enlarged view). Note the acidophilic Paneth cells (arrows), which secrete lysozyme that is bactericidal. **(D)** Brunner's glands discharge their secretions into the crypts of Lieberkuhn. Note that their ducts pass through the muscularis mucosa. (H&E stain.)

B. Jejunum (Fig. 5.20): The second part of the small intestine is the jejunum, which lies mainly in the upper left of the abdomen. It extends from the duodenojejunal junction to the ileum which is located predominantly in the lower right abdomen. The jejunum and ileum are suspended from the

(A)

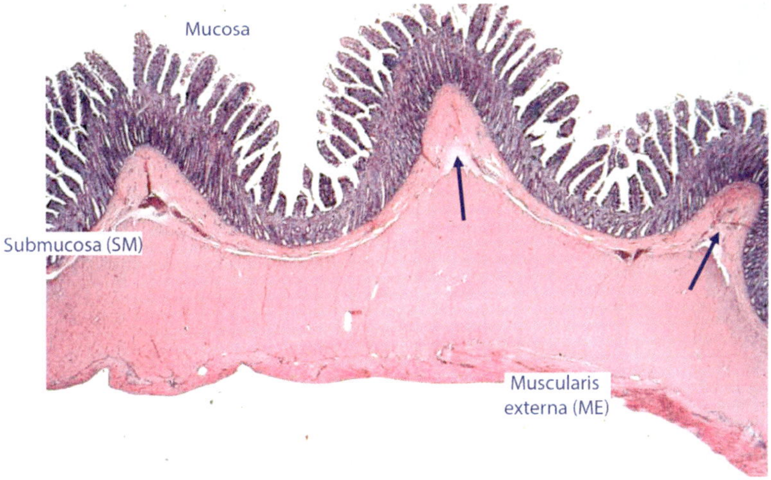

(B)

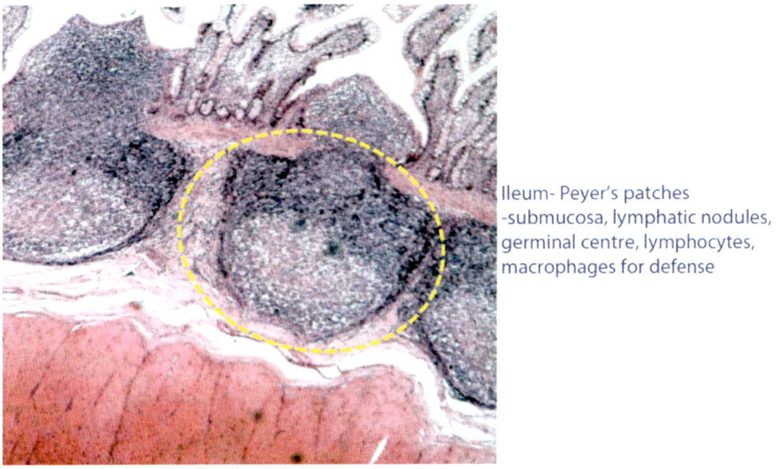

Figure 5.20. **(A) Jejunum.** The mucosa shows many villi longer than those in the duodenum and ileum. The submucosa (SM) projects into the lumen as circular folds (plica circularis) (arrows); both are to increase the surface area for absorption. The muscularis externa (ME) has inner circular and outer longitudinal layers involved in peristalsis. **(B) Ileum.** It is characterized by the presence of lymphatic nodules (follicles) (circled area) in the submucosa. They are collectively referred to as the Peyer's patches. Each lymphatic nodule has a pale germinal center. It contains B and T lymphocytes and macrophages for defense. (H&E stain.)

posterior abdominal wall by the mesentery which provides support and transmit blood vessels and nerves. The jejunum is supplied by branches of the superior mesenteric artery, forming arterial arcades and long vasa recta **(Fig. 5.18)**. Compared to the ileum, the jejunum has a thicker wall, more prominent circular folds (plicae circulares), and taller intestinal villi **(Fig. 5.20A)**.

C. **Ileum:** It is the terminal part of the small intestine, located mainly in the lower right abdomen and it terminates at the ileocecal junction **(Fig. 5.18)**. It receives its blood supply from branches of the superior mesenteric artery forming more arterial arcades and shorter vasa recta compared to the jejunum **(Fig. 5.18)**.

Histologically, like the duodenum and the jejunum, the ileum also consists of mucosa, submucosa, muscularis externa, and serosa and is lined by the simple columnar epithelium. The mucosa and submucosa contain many lymphoid aggregations, including nodules or follicles and prominent Peyer's patches, which play an important role in gut immunity **(Fig. 5.20B)**. Intestinal glands are present, while Brunner's glands are absent. The ileum is involved in both absorption and immune defense. The distal ileum is particularly important for the absorption of vitamin B12 which is bound to intrinsic factor and reabsorption of bile salts.

A clinically relevant feature is Meckel's diverticulum, a congenital remnant of the vitelline duct and its inflammation can lead to Meckel's diverticulitis.

LARGE INTESTINE (Fig. 5.18)

It extends from the caecum, which is located in the right iliac region and continues as the ascending colon from the right lumbar region up to the right colic flexure (hepatic flexure) in the right hypochondrium. From there, it extends as the transverse colon with its mesocolon (mesentery) to the left colic flexure (splenic flexure) in the left hypochondrium. The descending colon from the splenic flexure extends up to the left iliac region and continues as the sigmoid colon (with the sigmoid mesocolon). The rectum begins at the rectosigmoid junction and terminates at the anal canal.

A. **Colon:** The ascending and descending colons are retroperitoneal, while the transverse colon has a transverse mesocolon (a mesentery), which is attached to the posterior abdominal wall. The proximal two-thirds and distal one-third of the transverse colon mark the junction between the midgut and hindgut. The sigmoid colon has a similar mesentery, which is sigmoid mesocolon, that appears like an inverted "V".

The main functions of the colon are the absorption of water and secretion of mucus. It is lined by the simple columnar with goblet cells **(Fig. 5.21B, C)**. Intestinal villi are absent in the large intestine, including all parts of the colon, cecum, appendix, and rectum.

The colon exhibits segmental sacculations (haustra) **(Fig. 5.18)**, which slow down the transport of chyme to facilitate water absorption. The outer surface of the colon presents three longitudinal muscular bands which are taenia coli aiding in peristaltic movement. Appendices epiploicae which are pockets of subserosal fat are found in the outer walls, but their function is unclear. These unique features are absent in the vermiform appendix, caecum, and rectum.

The superior and inferior mesenteric arteries supply the large intestine. The superior mesenteric artery gives rise to the ileocolic artery, right colic artery, and middle colic artery, which supply the colon till the proximal two-thirds of the transverse colon. The distal one-third of the transverse colon, along with the descending colon and the rectum, is supplied by the inferior mesenteric artery. Branches of the inferior mesenteric artery include the left colic artery, sigmoidal arteries, and superior rectal artery. The marginal artery of Drummond and vasa recta provide collateral arterial circulation between the superior and inferior mesentery arteries along the margin of the colon **(Fig. 5.18)**. The marginal artery is clinically important in the event of mesentery ischemia.

In all parts of the colon, the mucosa is lined by simple columnar epithelium with numerous goblet cells. Intestinal villi and crypts of Lieberkuhn are absent. The intestinal glands open directly on the mucosal surface **(Fig. 5.21B, C)**.

As seen in the small intestine, the colon has four main layers: mucosa, submucosa, muscularis externa, and serosa. As mentioned above, the colon has three bands of taenia coli and appendices epiploicae, which are absent in the small intestine.

B. **Caecum:** The caecum receives contents from the ileum at the ileocaecal junction and resembles the colon histologically. Caecum has taenia coli while sacculations and appendices epiploicae are absent. It is supplied by the ileocaecal artery. The function of cecum is unclear.

C. **Appendix (Fig. 5.21A):** This “worm-like” tubular structure is attached to the caecum, which is often in a retrocaecal position. It has a layer of

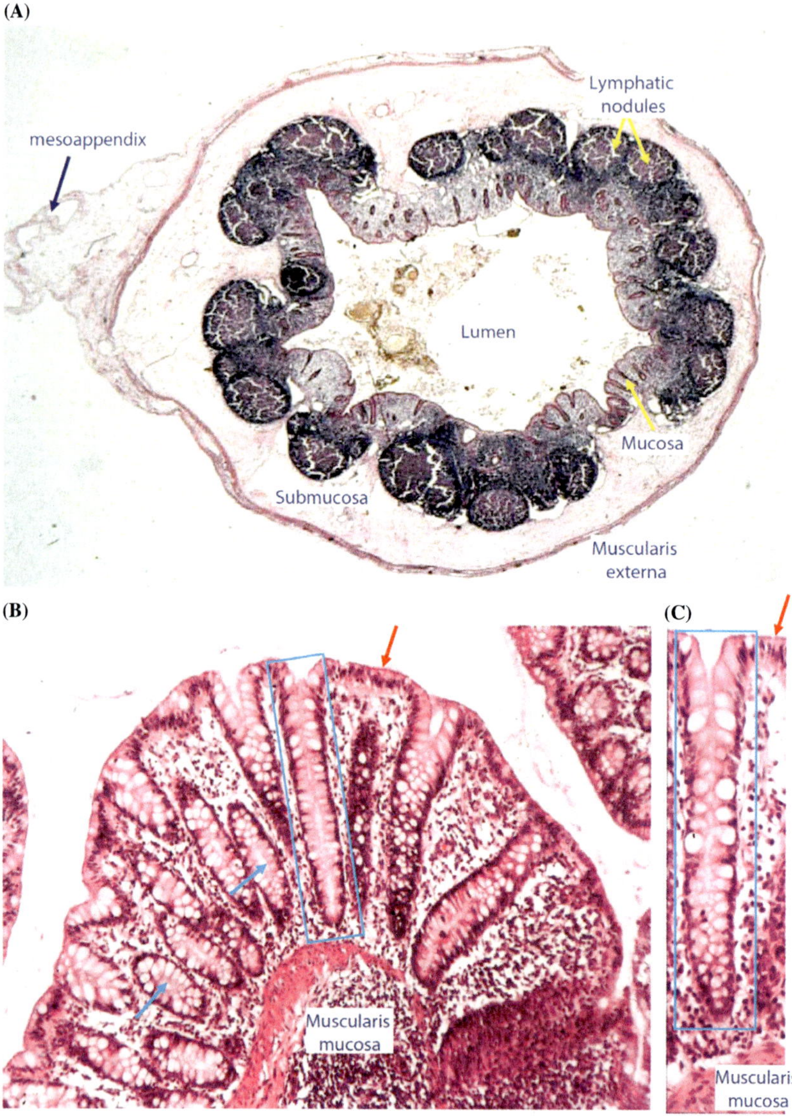

Figure 5.21. **(A) Appendix.** The mucosa, which appears smooth, shows many tubular intestinal glands lined by goblet and simple columnar cells. Note the lack of intestinal villi. The submucosa is occupied by many lymphatic nodules. A thin layer of muscularis externa is seen. The mesoappendix (mesentery) conveys the artery and nerves supplying the organ. Pain caused by inflammation of the appendix (appendicitis) is referred to the T10 dermatome at the umbilical region. (H&E stain.) **(B) Colon.** The mucosa is devoid of intestinal villi. The surface is relatively smooth, lined by simple columnar cells **(red arrow in B and C)** and goblet cells. Many intestinal glands (boxed area) open into the lumen. Blue arrows indicate oblique profiles of intestinal glands. **(C) Intestinal gland (boxed area).** Note the plentiful of goblet cells. The columnar cells are for the absorption of water, while the goblet cells secrete mucus. (H&E stain.)

mesentery, mesoappendix, carrying the appendicular artery that arises from the posterior caecal artery. The mucosa and submucosa have numerous lymphoid follicles **(Fig. 5.21A)**. The function of the appendix is not clear, although they may be involved in immune functions. The inflammation of the appendix (appendicitis) may occurr due to a viral infection or chyme obstruction.

D. Rectum (Fig. 5.22A, B):

1. It begins at the level of S3 vertebral segment and ends opposite to the coccyx **(Fig. 5.22A)**. It is about 12.5 cm in length. The rectum presents two curvatures: sacral and lateral flexures. The lower part of the rectum is enlarged, called the ampulla **(Fig. 5.22B)**. Circular valves (one on the right and two on the left) project into the lumen.
2. **Peritoneal relations:** Peritoneum covers the anterior and sides of the upper one-third of the rectum and the anterior surface of the middle one-third of the rectum. However, the lower one-third of the rectum is devoid of peritoneal covering **(Fig. 5.22A)**.
3. **Relations:** In the male, the rectum is related to the prostate gland anteriorly and the rectovesical septum (Denovillier's fascia or septum) **(Fig. 5.22A)**. In the female, it is related to the vagina anteriorly. Posteriorly, it is related to the anococcygeal body, piriformis muscle, and sacral plexus.
4. **Innervation**: The muscles and the glands in the rectum receive their parasympathetic innervation from the pelvic splanchnic nerves (S2, 3, 4), **(Fig. 5.22B)**. The visceral afferents arise from the stretch receptors for the detection of fullness sensation (able to differentiate between feces and flatus).
5. **Arterial supply**: The rectum is supplied by the superior, middle, and inferior rectal arteries **(Fig. 5.22B)**. The superior rectal artery is a branch of inferior mesenteric artery.
6. **Venous drainage**: The rectum drains via the superior rectal vein, inferior mesenteric vein, and portal vein **(Fig. 5.22B)**.
7. It does not have taenia coli or haustra (sacculations).
8. It is lined by the simple columnar epithelium with numerous goblet cells.
9. Its main function is the absorption of water and secretion of mucus.

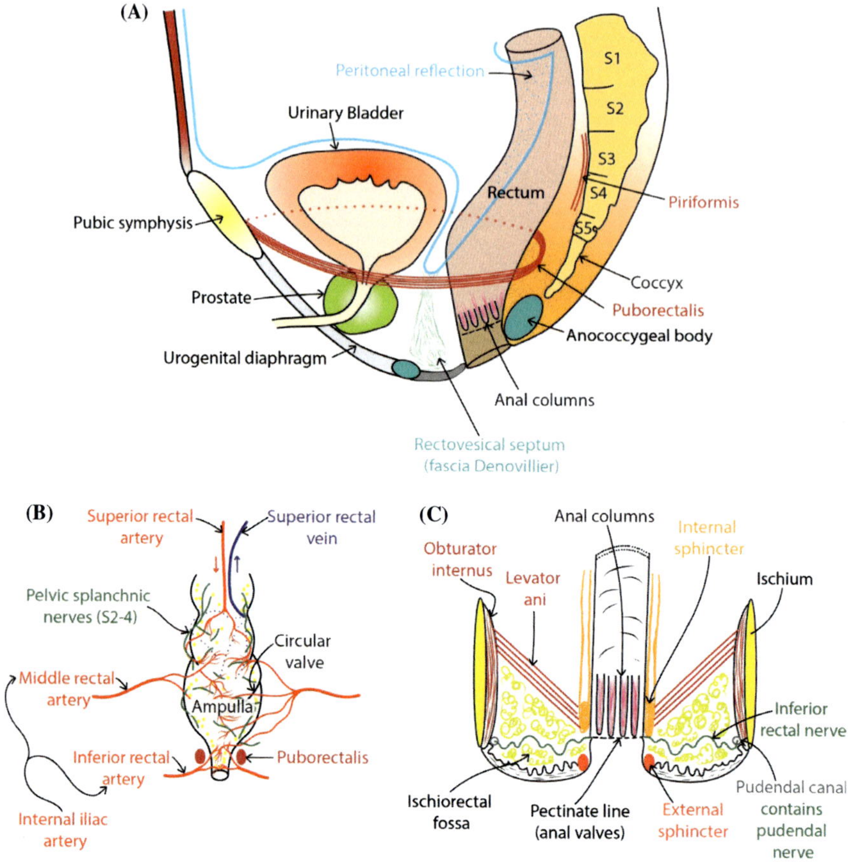

Figure 5.22. **(A) Rectum.** A sagittal section through the male pelvis showing the rectum and the urinary bladder. The rectum begins at the level of S3. It terminates at the puborectalis sling. It lies posterior to the urinary bladder, separated by the recto-vesical pouch. (In the female, it lies posterior to the pouch of Douglas). It is related to the peritoneum anteriorly in its upper part (see text). **(B) Rectum.** It presents one right and two left lateral flexures. Inferiorly, the dilated lower part is the ampulla. The rectum ends at the level of the puborectalis. It receives its arterial supply from the superior rectal artery. The lower part of the rectum is supplied by the middle and inferior rectal arteries. The venous drainage is by the superior rectal vein. It is innervated by the pelvic splanchnic nerves (S2, 3, 4). **(C) Anal canal.** A frontal section through the anal canal. The upper part of the canal shows the vertical anal columns. The lower ends of the anal columns form the anal valve (pectinate line). It is related laterally to the ischiorectal fossa containing adipose tissue. The upper part of the anal canal is lined by the simple columnar epithelium, whereas the lower is lined by the stratified squamous epithelium. The pectinate line forms the "watershed" for this. In the lateral wall of the ischiorectal fossa is the pudendal canal, which encloses the pudendal nerve. The inferior rectal nerve, a branch of the pudendal nerve, supplies the lower part of the anal canal. The upper part of the canal is supplied by the pelvic splanchnic nerves (S2, 3, 4).

a. Applied anatomy

i. Rectal polyps are precancerous growths in the mucosa.

ii. Hemorrhoids are dilated submucous veins in the rectal and anal region, which may be internal or external.

b. Innervation of the large intestine

i. *Parasympathetic innervation*: Parasympathetic component of the vagus innervates the large intestine up to the proximal two-thirds of the transverse colon (midgut derivative). Distal to this (hindgut derivatives), the parasympathetic innervation is provided the pelvic splanchnic nerves (S2, 3, 4).

ii. *Sympathetic innervation*: Sympathetic fibers arise from the thoracolumbar segments (T10–L2) and reach the large intestine via the superior mesenteric plexus and inferior mesenteric plexus.

iii. *Sensory*: Visceral afferent fibers carrying sensations of distension (e.g., due to gas) generally follow parasympathetic pathways, whereas pain fibers typically follow sympathetic pathways.

ANAL CANAL (Fig. 5.22A, C)

A. Anal canal, which is the terminal part of the gastrointestinal tract (digestive tube) extends from the rectum and runs downward and backward. The junction of the rectum and anal canal is marked by the presence of anorectal ring which is formed by the internal sphincter, puborectalis (levator ani), and deep part of the external sphincter.

B. **Relations:** It is related to ischiorectal fossa laterally, prostate gland in male and vagina in female anteriorly and anococcygeal body posteriorly.

C. **Internal Features (Fig. 5.22C):**

1. Its mucosa has vertical anal columns whose lower ends are joined by anal valves, forming the pectinate line which marks the lower end of the hindgut developmentally.
2. The pectinate line divides the anal canal into the upper two-thirds which is lined by the simple columnar epithelium and lower one-third which is lined by the stratified squamous epithelium **(Fig. 5.23)**. Some circumanal glands are present deep to the epithelium **(Fig. 5.23)**.

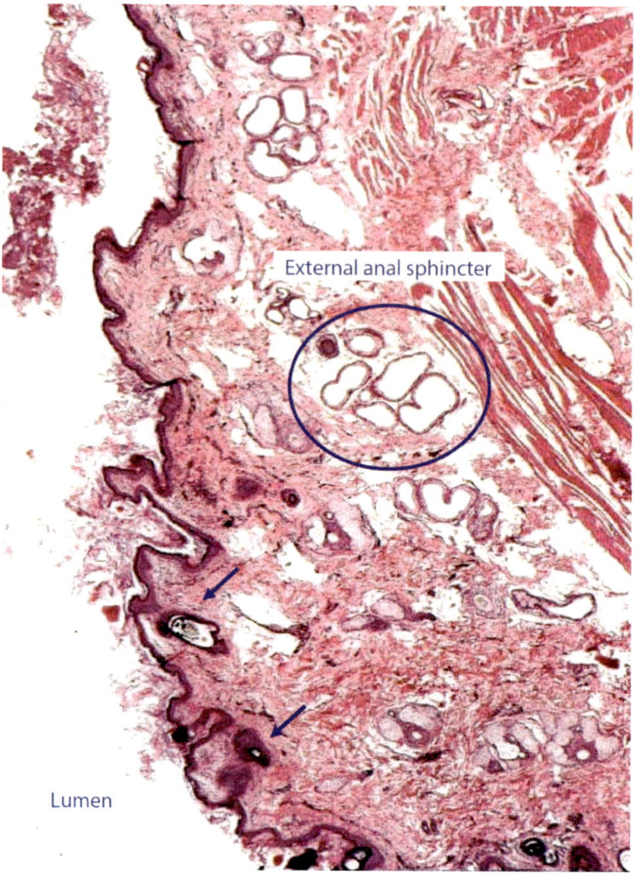

Figure 5.23. Anal canal. The lumen is lined by the stratified squamous epithelium; at its lower part, the epithelium is keratinized, bearing hair follicles (arrows). Some circumanal glands (circled area) lie deep to the epithelium. Bundles of skeletal muscles form the external anal sphincter (supplied by the inferior rectal nerve). (H&E stain.)

3. **Arterial supply:** The upper part of the anal canal is supplied by the superior rectal artery (a branch of the inferior mesentery artery), while the lower part of the anal canal is supplied by the inferior rectal artery (a branch of the internal iliac artery). Middle rectal artery from the internal iliac artery supplies mainly the musculature.
4. **Innervation:** The upper part of the anal canal is innervated by the pelvic splanchnic nerves (S2–4) and visceral afferents (insensitive to pain, sensitive to stretch). The lower part of the anal canal is innervated

by the inferior rectal nerve (a branch of the pudendal nerve), which is sensitive to somatic pain.

5. **Internal anal sphincter:** It is formed by a thickening of the inner circular muscle (smooth) which is surrounded by skeletal muscle (levator ani puborectalis) and the deep part of the external anal sphincter **(Fig. 5.23)**. If it is weakened, it may result in fecal incontinence.
6. **Clinical considerations:**
   - Anal abscess arises due to perianal abrasions, boils and infection of anal glands.
   - Hemorrhoids: It can be internal or external based on pectinate line.

ISCHIORECTAL FOSSA (Fig. 5.22C)

The ischioanal fossae are wedge-shaped fat-filled spaces located on either side of the anal canal, between the anal canal and the lateral pelvic wall, inferior to the pelvic diaphragm. The ischiorectal fossa allows anal canal to expand during defecation.

It is bounded laterally by the obturator internus muscle and the obturator fascia containing pudendal canal. Superiorly, it is bounded by the pelvic diaphragm while the inferior boundary is formed by the skin. Anteriorly, it extends into the anterior recess above the perineal membrane (urogenital region) while it is bounded by the gluteus maximus muscle and sacrotuberous ligament posteriorly. The ischiorectal fossae contain fat and connective tissues and communicate with each other. The inferior rectal nerve from the pudendal nerve traverses through the fossa to supply the external sphincters and the perianal skin. Anal abscess (infections) is relatively common and may spread from one side of the fossa to the other.

PORTAL SYSTEMIC ANASTOMOSIS (Fig. 5.24)

The portal vein carries blood rich in nutrients (except most lipids) which are absorbed from the small intestine and transported to the liver for storage, detoxification, and metabolism. The portal vein is formed by the union of the superior mesenteric vein and splenic vein, posterior to the neck of the pancreas. It ascends posterior to the first part of the duodenum, and then runs within free border of the lesser omentum to enter the liver at the porta hepatis. The

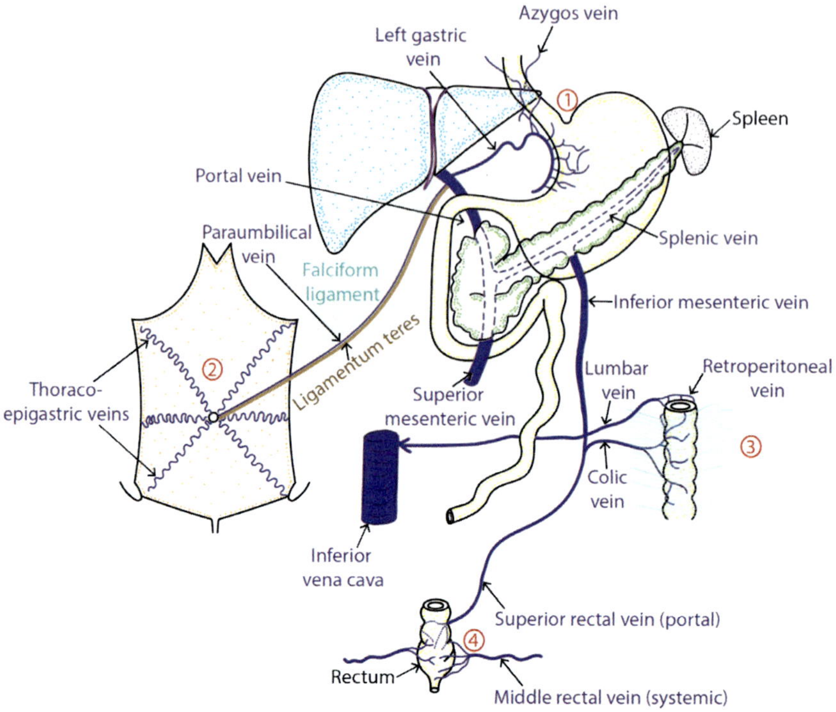

1. Portal vein - Left gastric vein - esophageal vein - Azygos vein
(Esophageal varices)

2. Portal vein - Paraumbilical vein - Thoracoepigastric veins
(Caput medusae)

3. Inferior mesenteric vein - Colic veins - Retroperitoneal veins - Inferior vena cava
(Portal vein) (Splenic vein)

4. Inferior mesenteric vein - Superior rectal vein - Middle rectal vein
(Portal vein) (Splenic vein) - Inferior rectal vein
(Hemorrhoids)

Figure 5.24. Porto-systemic anastomosis. The portal vein is formed by the union of the superior mesenteric vein (SMV) and the splenic vein posterior to the neck of the pancreas. It then ascends to enter the liver. Sites of porto-systemic anastomosis:

1. The left gastric vein, which drains into the portal vein, has connections with the tributaries of the azygos vein in the walls of the lower esophagus.
2. The paraumbilical vein in the falciform ligament connects the portal vein with the thoracoepigastric veins.
3. The inferior mesenteric vein, which drains into the splenic vein, has connections with the colic veins, lumbar veins, and inferior vena cava.
4. The inferior mesenteric vein drains the superior rectal vein, which has connections with the middle and inferior rectal veins in the rectum.

inferior mesenteric vein draining the descending colon and rectum joins with the splenic vein. The portal vein has many tributaries, which form anastomosis with the systemic veins at different sites; hence, in the event of cirrhosis or liver diseases (caused by portal hypertension), the drainage of portal circulation may be impeded. Thus, the anastomotic veins may become dilated (varicosed) or ruptured.

The following are sites of portal systemic anastomosis:

1. Portal vein receives drainage from the left gastric vein, which communicates with the esophageal vein and the azygos vein (systemic). Dilation of anastomotic veins at the lower part of the esophagus may result in esophageal varices (dilated veins) or their rupture.
2. Portal vein connects with the paraumbilical veins in the falciform ligament. The paraumbilical veins connect with the thoracoepigastric veins (systemic) through the umbilicus in the anterior abdominal wall. Enlarged veins in the anterior abdominal wall ("caput medusae") are indicative of liver pathology.
3. Portal vein drains the inferior mesenteric vein via the splenic vein. The inferior mesenteric vein has connections with the colic veins (descending colon) and retroperitoneal veins (systemic) that drain into the inferior vena cava.
4. Portal vein drains the superior rectal vein via the inferior mesenteric vein. The superior rectal vein has connections with the middle and inferior rectal veins (systemic). Dilation of these anastomotic veins in the submucosa of the rectum may result in hemorrhoids.

Chapter 6

ENDOCRINE SYSTEM

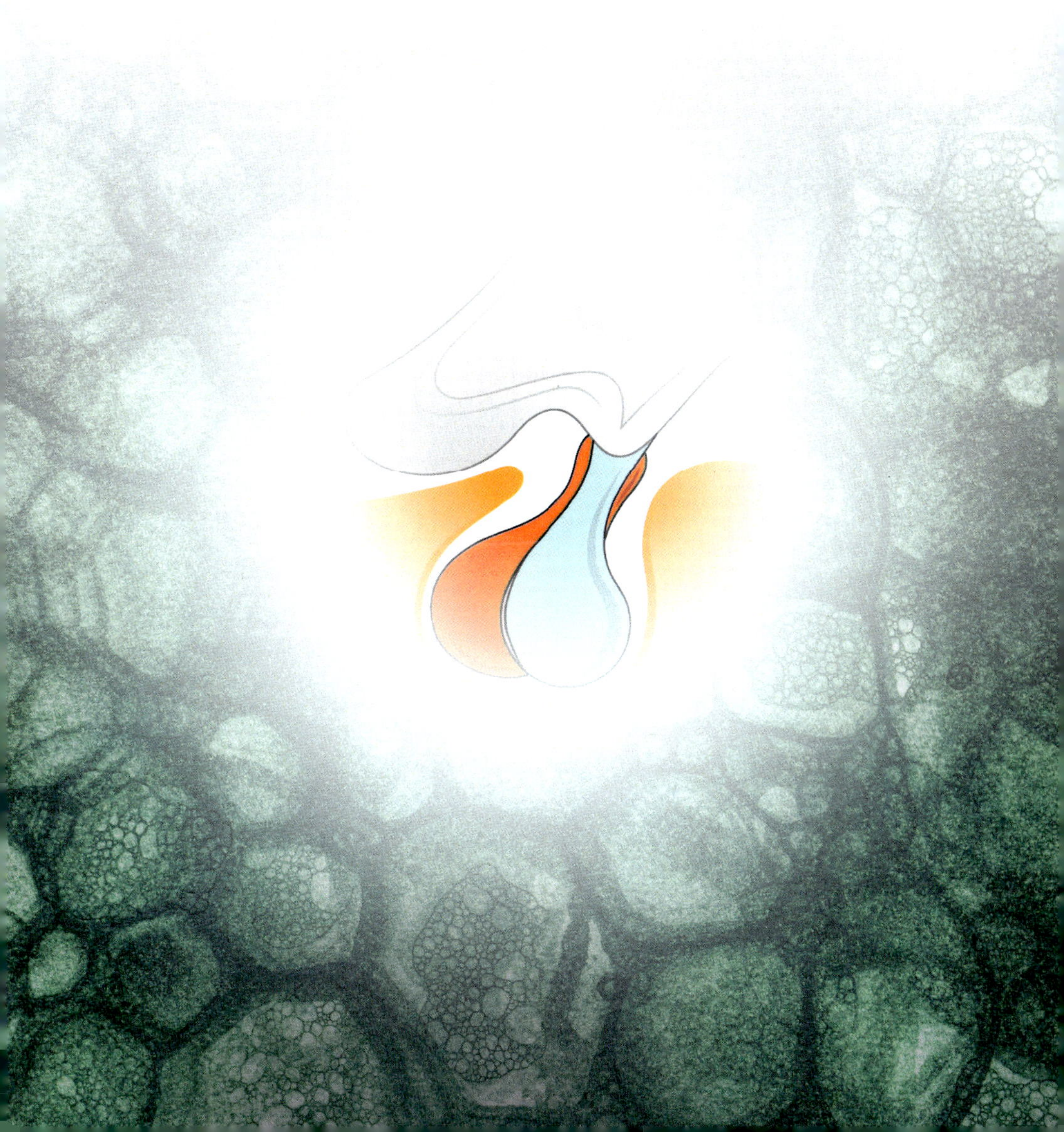

ENDOCRINE SYSTEM

Endocrine glands are defined as the "ductless glands" because they release their secretory products directly into the blood circulation. Hormones from the endocrine glands act on target tissues or organs away from the site of their synthesis. A common feature of the endocrine glands is the presence of fenestrated capillaries or sinusoids, which receive the hormone secretions for circulation to the target site. Hormones are divided into three classes: steroid hormones (i.e., testosterone and estradiol), peptide hormones (i.e., insulin and prolactin), and amino acid-derivatives (i.e., catecholamines and thyroxine).

The endocrine glands comprise the following: the pituitary gland (hypophysis), hypothalamus, pineal gland, thyroid, parathyroid, suprarenal (adrenal) gland, islets of Langerhans in pancreas, gonads (testis in males & ovaries in females), and enteroendocrine cells along the gastrointestinal tract.

PITUITARY GLAND (HYPOPHYSIS)

The pituitary gland produces several hormones that influence the activity of other endocrine glands. This gland lies in a depression of the sphenoid bone, the sella turcica, at the base of the skull. It is connected to the hypothalamus by a slender stalk, the infundibulum **(Fig. 6.1)**. The pituitary can be divided into an anterior lobe, the adenohypophysis, and a posterior lobe, the neurohypophysis, on anatomical and developmental grounds. During embryogenesis, adenohypophysis is derived from an out pocketing of the oral ectoderm (Rathke's pouch); the neurohypophysis as an evagination from the neuroectoderm (presumptive diencephalon). The adenohypophysis is further subdivided into a pars distalis, a pars tuberalis and a pars intermedia. The neurohypophysis consists of pars nervosa and the infundibulum **(Fig. 6.1)**.

A. Adenohypophysis (Anterior Pituitary)

Pars distalis accounts for 75 % of the mass of the adenohypophysis, is highly cellular, and comprises two main cell types based on the staining affinity of their cytoplasm: chromophils and chromophobes. The chromophils stain

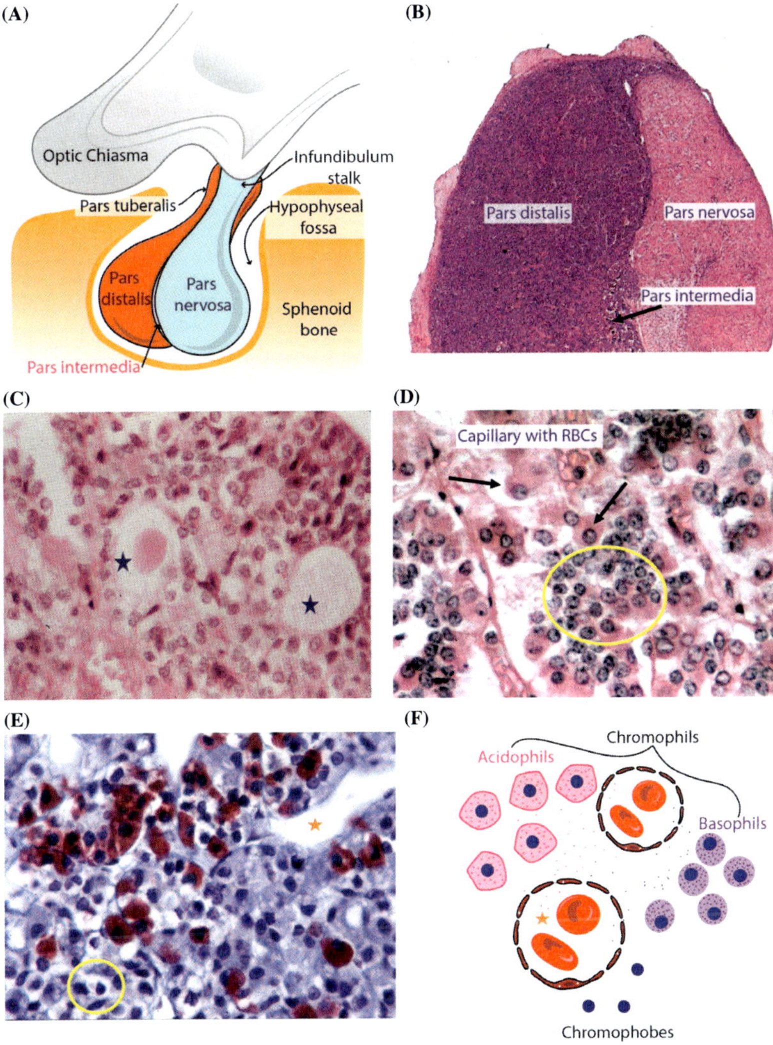

Figure 6.1. Pituitary gland (hypophysis). (A) Diagrammatic picture showing the three parts of the gland: pars distalis, pars intermedia, and pars nervosa. Adenohypophysis = pars distalis + pars tuberalis + pars intermedia. Neurohypophysis = pars nervosa + infundibulum + infundibulum stalk. Note that the gland lies in the hypophyseal fossa at the body of the sphenoid. Note the pars nervosa is connected to the hypothalamus (III ventricle) via the infundibulum stalk. **(B)** A horizontal section through the three main parts of the gland: pars distalis, pars intermedia, and pars nervosa. (Hematoxylin and eosin (H&E) stain.) **(C) Pars intermedia.** It contains closely packed cells, with some of them forming small follicles (asterisk) containing colloids. Pars intermedia secretes melanocyte-stimulating hormone and endorphins. (H&E stain.) **(D) Pars distalis.** Showing chromophils (arrows), chromophobes (circled), and fenestrated capillary containing red blood cells. (H&E stain.) **(E) Pars distalis.** Showing acidophils (red cytoplasm) and basophils (blue cytoplasm), chromophobes (circled), and fenestrated capillary (asterisk) (Azan stain) **(F)** A semi-diagrammatic picture showing the three constituent cell types in the pars distalis.

either acidic or basic dye and they are named acidophils (pink) and basophils (blue), respectively (**Fig. 6.1**). Chromophobes do not stain intensely and chromophils stain strongly. Both acidophils and basophils are rich in cytoplasm (**Fig. 6.1**) which contains numerous secretory granules. With recent advances in immunohistochemistry, the cell types in the pars distalis can be identified on the basis of hormones they produce. The hormones produced by the cell types in pars distalis include somatotropin (GH), corticotropin (ACTH), thyrotropin (TSH), gonadotropins (FSH, LH), and lactotropin (prolactin).

Hormones of the adenohypophysis:

1. **Growth hormone (GH):** stimulates cell growth, particularly, skeletal muscle cells and chondrocytes (cartilage cells). Overproduction of GH causes pituitary gigantism and GH deficiency causes pituitary dwarfism.
2. **Prolactin (PRL):** promotes milk secretion from the mammary gland.
3. **Thyroid-stimulating hormone (TSH):** stimulates thyroid hormone synthesis from the thyroid gland.
4. **Adrenocorticotropic hormone (ACTH):** stimulates the secretion of steroid hormones by adrenal gland.
5. **Follicle stimulating hormone (FSH):** promotes ovarian follicle development and estrogen secretion in women and stimulates spermatogenesis in men.
6. **Luteinizing hormone (LH):** induces ovulation and secretion of progesterone (that prepares the body for possible pregnancy) in women and androgen (male sex hormone) secretion in men.

Pars tuberalis forms a sleeve around the infundibulum of neurohypophysis. Pars intermedia is located just posterior to a cleft or series of small cystic cavities that represent the residual lumen of Rathke's pouch. The cells present in the pars intermedia secrete melanocyte-stimulating hormone (MSH) for the dispersion of melanin granules. It is reported that they also secrete an endorphin-like substance.

B. Hypothalamo-hypophyseal Portal System (Fig. 6.2)

The secretion of hormones from the pars distalis is regulated by neurohormones released from the hypothalamus through the hypothalamo-hypophyseal portal

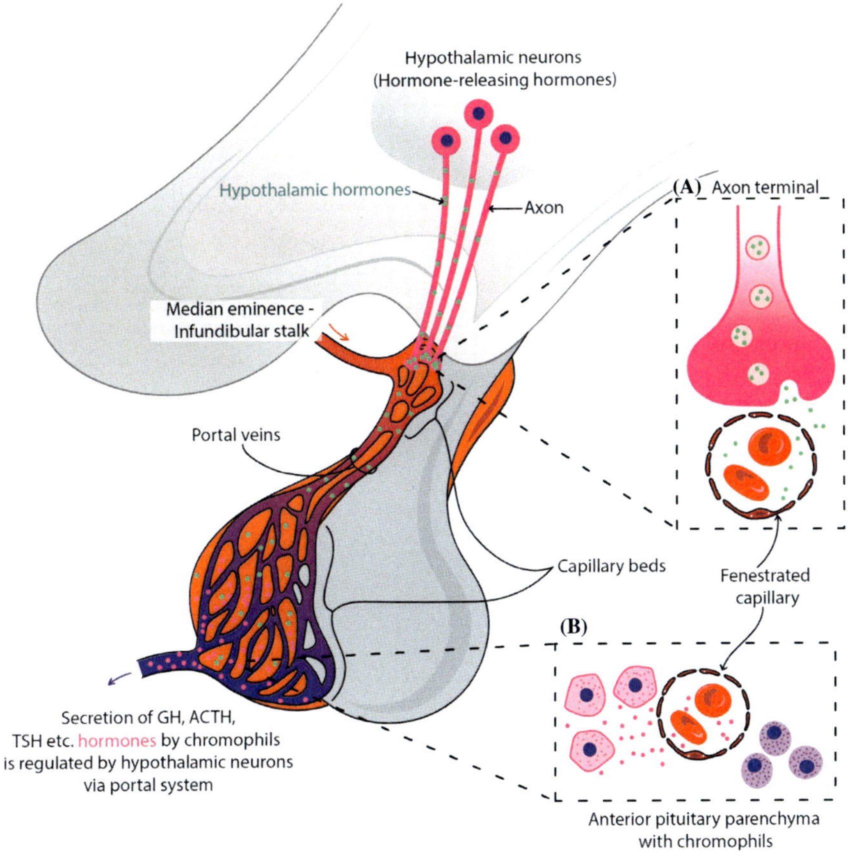

Figure 6.2. Hypothalamo-hypophyseal portal system. Hypothalamic neurons secrete specific hormone-releasing factors, which are transported via their axons to be released into the blood capillaries **(A)** in the median eminence/infundibular stalk. The hormone-releasing factors are then transported by the portal veins to the blood capillaries in the pars distalis. By this, they regulate the secretion of different hormones by the chromophils in the pars distalis **(B)**.

system. Hypothalamic neurons secrete specific releasing and inhibitory hormones into the primary capillary plexus located in the median eminence.

The hypothalamic releasing hormones include:

- Thyrotropin-releasing hormone (TRH): stimulates release of TSH
- Corticotropin-releasing hormone (CRH): stimulates release of ACTH
- Gonadotropin-releasing hormone (GnRH): stimulates release of FSH and LH
- Growth hormone–releasing hormone (GHRH): stimulates release of GH

The hypothalamic inhibitory hormones include:

- Growth hormone–inhibiting hormone (GHIH, Somatostatin): inhibits GH
- Prolactin-inhibiting hormone (PIH, Dopamine): inhibits prolactin (PRL)

These hormones are then transported via the portal veins to the secondary capillary plexus in the pars distalis. There, they regulate the secretion of specific hormones by the various cell types in the adenohypophysis **(Fig. 6.2)**.

C. Neurohypophysis (Posterior Pituitary)

The pars nervosa of the neurohypophysis **(Fig. 6.1)** is connected to the hypothalamus via the infundibulum. It mainly consists of unmyelinated axons of hypothalamic neurons and a specific type of glial cells called pituicytes, which constitute approximately 25% of its volume. Pituicytes do not possess secretory activity and function as supporting cells, similar to neuroglia in the central nervous system.

Neurosecretory cells located in the supraoptic nucleus (SON) and paraventricular nucleus (PVN) of the hypothalamus synthesize the neurohormones vasopressin (antidiuretic hormone, ADH) and oxytocin. These hormones are transported along unmyelinated axons through the infundibular stalk to the pars nervosa **(Fig. 6.3)**.

The axon terminals in the pars nervosa contain accumulations of neurosecretory granules known as Herring's bodies **(Fig. 6.4)**, which appear as eosinophilic (pink-staining) dilations in H&E sections. The neurohypophysis does not synthesize hormones; rather, it stores and releases ADH and oxytocin produced in the hypothalamus. These hormones are released from the axon terminals into the surrounding capillary network for systemic circulation.

ADH promotes water reabsorption in the kidneys, thereby reducing urine output. Its deficiency results in diabetes insipidus, a condition characterized by the inability to concentrate urine, leading to excessive urination and persistent thirst.

In women, oxytocin stimulates contraction of uterine smooth muscle during labor and parturition and induces contraction of myoepithelial cells surrounding the alveoli and ducts of the mammary glands during milk ejection.

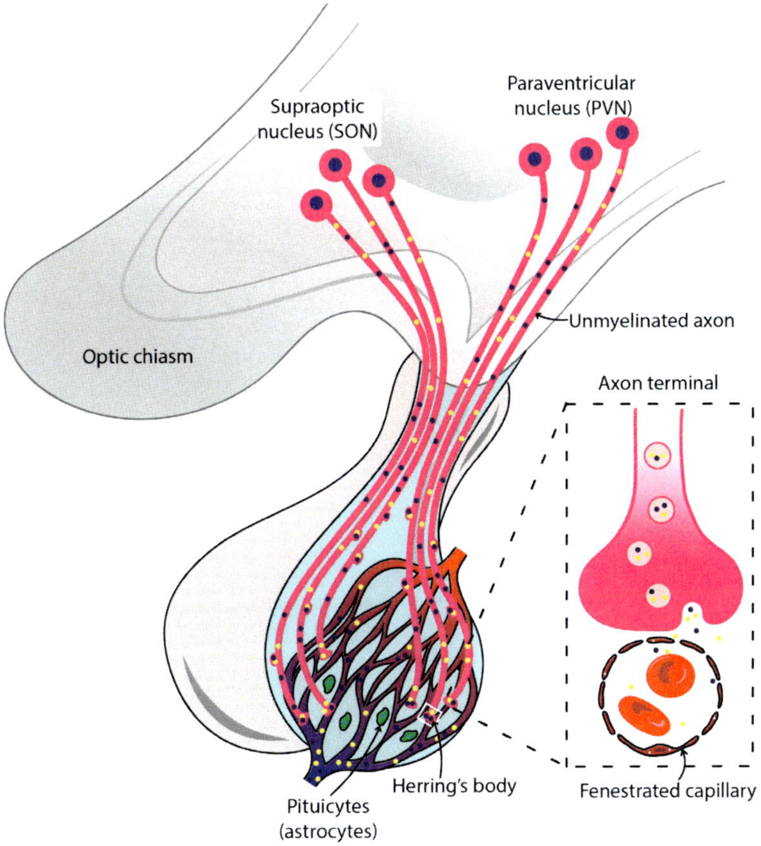

Figure 6.3. Neurohypophysis and hypothalamo-hypophysial tract. The neurohypophysis lies posterior to the adenohypophysis. It consists of the pars nervosa and infundibulum/stalk. It is connected to the median eminence of the hypothalamus below the III ventricle. The neurons in the supraoptic optic nucleus (SON) and paraventricular nucleus (PVN) are modified to become neurosecretory cells. The long extending non-myelinated axons descend through the infundibulum (stalk) to terminate in the pars nervosa. By axonal flow, the neurosecretions are transported to the pars nervosa. The axon terminals with the neurosecretions impinge on the capillary walls. The neurosecretions (vasopressin ADH and oxytocin) are released into the circulation. Herring's bodies are dilated axon terminals laden with neurosecretions. Pituicytes are modified astrocytes in the pars nervosa.

PINEAL GLAND

The pineal gland which is an endocrine gland located at the roof of the III cerebral ventricle (epithalamus). It is composed primarily of pinealocytes, along with interstitial (glial) cells, and a small number of astrocytes and microglia. The gland

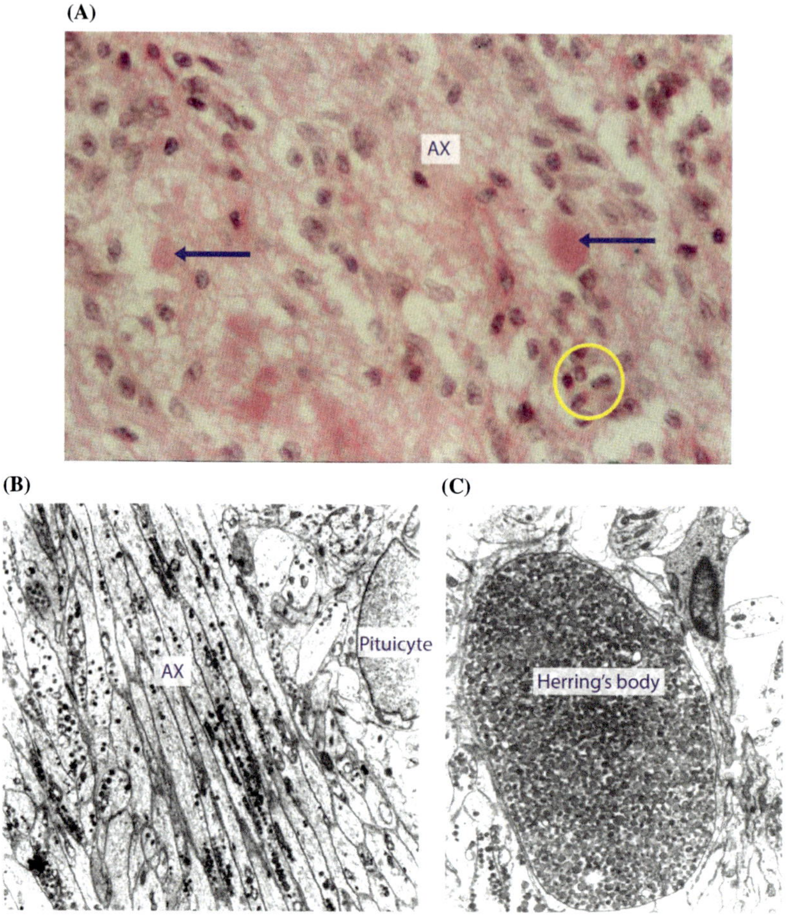

Figure 6.4. Pars nervosa. **(A)** It contains closely packed unmyelinated axons (AX). Dilated axons laden with neurosecretions (pinkish in staining) are Herring's bodies (arrows). Between the unmyelinated axons are many pituicytes (modified astrocytes) (circled area). (H&E stain.) **(B)** Electron micrograph showing closely packed unmyelinated axons (AX) filled with electron dense neurosecretory granules. On the right is a portion of a pituicyte. **(C)** Electron micrograph of a Herring's body laden with neurosecretory granules. The neurosecretory granules are rich in oxytocin and vasopressin (ADH).

is highly vascular, containing numerous capillaries. The pinealocytes synthesize and secrete melatonin involved in regulating circadian rhythms.

Melatonin is commercially available for the management of mild sleep disturbances, such as jet lag. It also exhibits antioxidant and anti-inflammatory properties as a neurohormone. With age, calcification of the pineal gland may occur, forming structures known as corpora arenacea (brain sand).

THYROID GLAND

The thyroid gland consists of two lobes, right and left, anterolateral to the larynx (thyroid and cricoid cartilages) and trachea in the neck. These lobes are united by the isthmus that overlies the tracheal rings **(Fig. 6.5)**.

The relations, arterial supply, and venous drainage of the thyroid gland are described in the chapter 10 titled the Head and Neck.

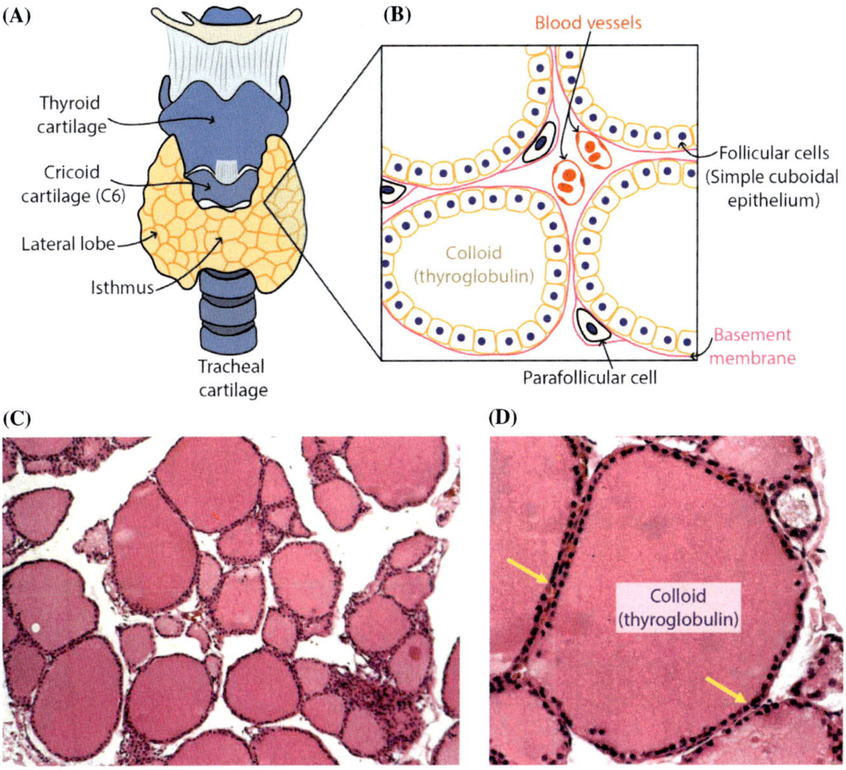

Figure 6.5. Thyroid gland. **(A)** It is closely associated with the trachea. It has two lateral lobes extending from the thyroid cartilage to the 6th tracheal ring. The two lateral lobes are interconnected by the isthmus overlying the 2nd to 4th tracheal rings. The pyramidal lobe extends upward from the isthmus. **(B)** In a tissue section, the gland is composed of many thyroid follicles filled with colloid (thyroglobulin) secreted by the follicular cells. The follicular cells are the simple cuboid epithelium. Between the follicles are loose connective tissue and fenestrated blood capillaries where thyroid hormones are released. **(C)** Showing many thyroid follicles of different sizes. **(D)** The follicle is lined by the simple cuboidal epithelium composed of the follicular cells (arrows). Note that all follicles are filled with thyroglobulin (pinkish) colloid, which appears homogeneous. (H&E stain.)

In a histological section, the thyroid gland is composed of numerous follicles of varying sizes and is covered by a thin, connective tissue capsule from which septa extend into the gland **(Fig. 6.5)**. Each follicle is lined by a simple cuboidal epithelium **(Fig. 6.5)**, consisting of follicular cells resting on a thin layer of basement membrane. The follicular lumen contains colloid, a gelatinous material rich in thyroglobulin. The height of the epithelium is indicative of the functional activity of the thyroid gland. When the follicular cells are stimulated, the cuboidal cells become columnar.

In general, follicle cells are divided into two types: 1. principal or follicular cells and 2. parafollicular cells (calcitonin-secreting cells or C cells). Most of the follicular epithelial cells are principal cells. These cells synthesize thyroglobulin which is stored in the lumen and subsequently release into the capillaries. TSH secreted by adenohypophysis stimulates the follicular cells to synthesize thyroid hormones (T3 and T4). These are structural derivatives of tyrosine to which 3/4 iodine atoms have been attached. T4 roughly accounts for 90% of all thyroid secretions. T3 is secreted in small amounts **(Fig. 6.6)**.

By electron microscopy, it has been shown that the thyroglobulin is synthesized in the rough endoplasmic reticulum and processed in the Golgi apparatus before being secreted into the follicular lumen by exocytosis. At the apical membrane, it undergoes iodination. When needed, iodinated thyroglobulin is reabsorbed by endocytosis and enzymatically cleaved to release triiodothyronine (T3) and thyroxine (T4), which are then secreted into the bloodstream from the basal surface. **(Fig. 6.6)**.

The parafollicular or C cells lie between the cuboidal follicles and the basement membrane **(Fig. 6.6)**. These cells are larger than those of the follicular epithelial cells and stain less intensely. The most characteristic feature of these cells is the presence of numerous dense secretory granules. These cells produce a hormone called the calcitonin which regulates calcium ion concentrations in body fluids and inhibits the osteoclasts and decreases bone resorption, thus lowering the blood calcium level.

Thyroid disorders:

- ***Hypothyroidism*:** Goiter (due to iodine deficiency), Myxedema (adults) and Cretinism (children)
- ***Hyperthyroidism*:** Graves' disease

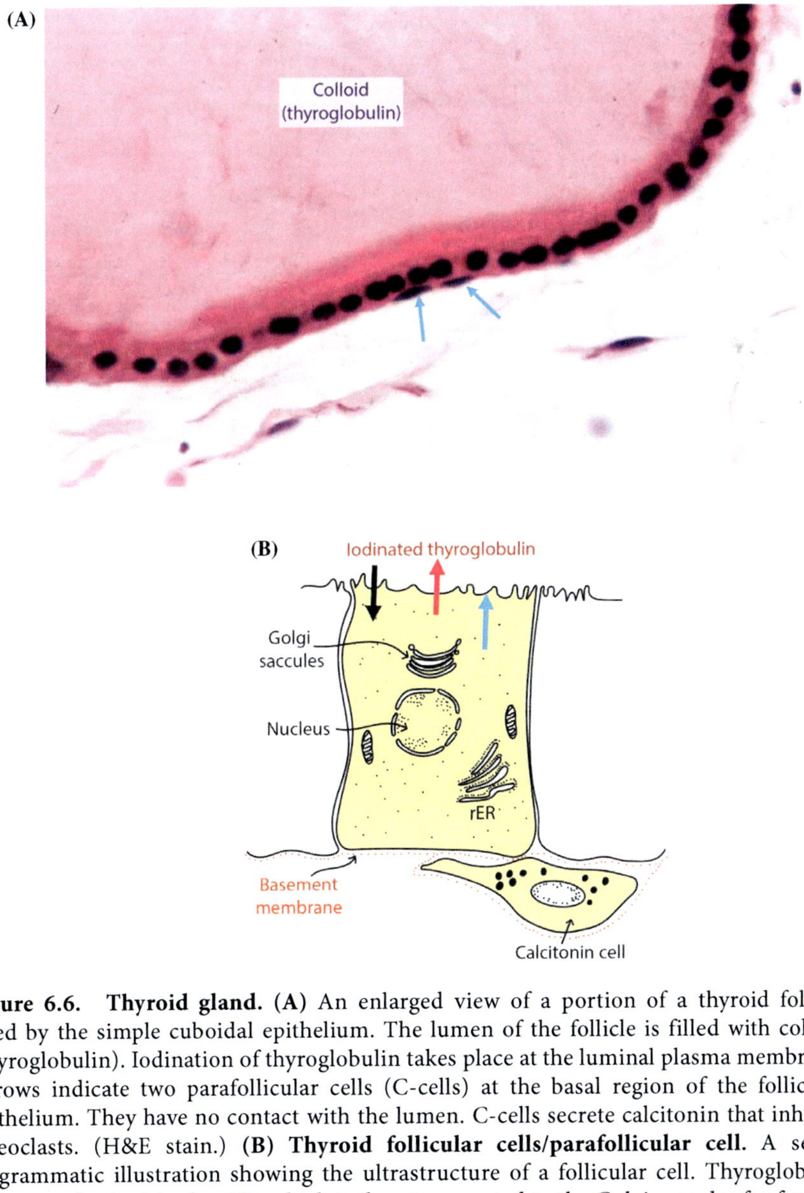

Figure 6.6. Thyroid gland. (A) An enlarged view of a portion of a thyroid follicle lined by the simple cuboidal epithelium. The lumen of the follicle is filled with colloid (thyroglobulin). Iodination of thyroglobulin takes place at the luminal plasma membrane. Arrows indicate two parafollicular cells (C-cells) at the basal region of the follicular epithelium. They have no contact with the lumen. C-cells secrete calcitonin that inhibits osteoclasts. (H&E stain.) **(B) Thyroid follicular cells/parafollicular cell.** A semi-diagrammatic illustration showing the ultrastructure of a follicular cell. Thyroglobulin is first synthesized in the rER, which is then transported to the Golgi saccules for further packaging (glycosylation). Thyroglobulin is iodinated at the apical plasma membrane (blue arrow) and released into the lumen (red arrow). Iodinated thyroglobulin is internalized by the cell (black arrow) by endocytosis. It is hydrolyzed to give rise to tri-iodothyronine (T3) and thyroxine (T4). T3/T4 is discharged into the blood circulation in the interfollicular region. A calcitonin cell is closely associated with the follicle. Its secretion (calcitonin) is released directly into the blood circulation.

PARATHYROID GLANDS

Two pairs of parathyroid glands (a superior and inferior on either side) are found embedded in the connective tissue capsule on the posterior surface of the thyroid gland. They are derived embryologically from the 3rd and 4th pharyngeal pouches. There are two basic cell types, chief (principal) cells and oxyphil cells, identified in the glandular epithelium. The main cellular constituent is the chief cells **(Fig. 6.7)**, which secrete parathyroid hormone (PTH). The PTH stimulates

(A)

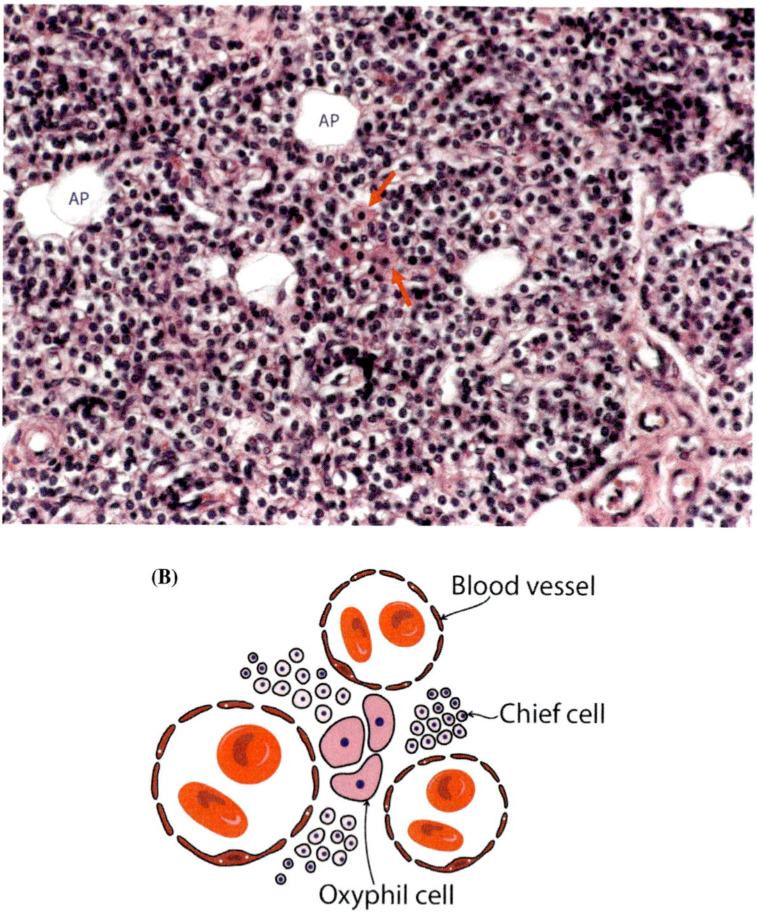

(B)

Figure 6.7. Parathyroid gland. (A) It is composed mainly of chief cells, along with some oxyphil cells and adipocytes. The chief cells secrete a parathyroid hormone that stimulates the osteoclasts. The oxyphil cells show pinkish cytoplasm (arrows) whose function is unclear. Occasional adipocytes (AP) are present. (H&E stain.) **(B)** Semi-diagrammatic illustration showing chief cells and oxyphil cells.

osteoclasts involved in bone resorption, which, therefore, raises the blood calcium level. The oxyphil cells constitute a minor portion of the parenchymal cells **(Fig. 6.7)**, and their function is uncertain. They are distinctly larger than the chief cells.

***Hyperparathyroidism*:** Serum calcium levels are increased. This condition frequently produces pathologic deposits of calcium in kidneys and arteries.

***Hypoparathyroidism*:** Serum calcium levels are decreased. This condition causes spastic contractions of the skeletal muscles and generalized convulsions called tetany.

SUPRARENAL (ADRENAL) GLAND

Adrenal glands are a pair of flattened, triangular organs that sit on the superior poles of the kidneys. Hence, they are also called the suprarenal glands. Each gland is enclosed in a thick, connective tissue capsule. The gland consists of two parts, a central medulla and an outer cortex **(Fig. 6.8)**.

The adrenal cortex is composed of zona glomerulosa (outer layer adjacent to the capsule), zona fasciculata (middle layer), and zona reticularis (inner layer adjacent to the medulla) **(Fig. 6.8)**. The cortex is derived embryologically from the mesoderm, whereas the medulla is derived from the ectoderm specifically from neural crest cells and shares a developmental origin with the sympathetic neurons.

A. **Zona Glomerulosa (Fig. 6.8):** The zona glomerulosa consists of columnar or pyramidal cells arranged in rounded clusters surrounded by capillaries. They secrete mineralocorticoids (e.g., aldosterone, a steroid hormone that acts on the principal cells of the distal convoluted tubule and collecting tubule/duct) for maintaining electrolytes ($Na+/K+$) and water balance in the body.
B. **Zona Fasciculata (Fig. 6.8):** The zona fasciculata consists of cells which are arranged in parallel columns separated by sinusoids. The cells have a lightly stained spherical nucleus and acidophilic cytoplasm with numerous lipid droplets. The lipid is extracted during histological procedures, thus giving the cells a vacuolated (foamy) appearance. This zone produces steroids collectively known as glucocorticoids (Cortisol, Corticosterone and

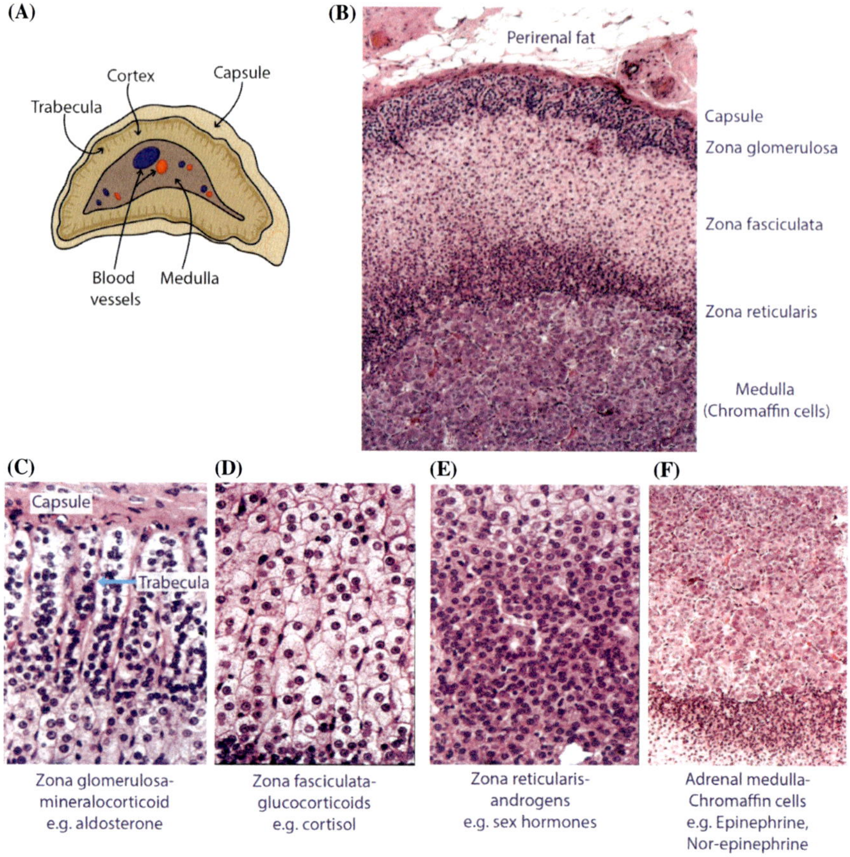

Figure 6.8. Adrenal (suprarenal) gland. (A) A semi-diagrammatic illustration showing a section through the gland. The surface is covered by a layer of capsule. Extending from the capsule into the parenchyma are finger-like projections, trabeculae. The cortex is developmentally derived from the mesoderm, whereas the medulla is from the neural crest cells (neuroectoderm). **(B)** The surface is covered by a layer of fibrous capsule. It has two parts: cortex and medulla. The cortex is composed of zona glomerulosa, zona fasciculata, and zona reticularis. The cortex is derived embryonically from the mesoderm, while the medulla is derived embryonically from the neural crest shared by the sympathetic neurons. (H&E stain.) Hormonal secretions from different layers of the cortex **(C–E)** and medulla **(F)**. (H&E stain.)

Cortisone). These hormones accelerate the rates of glucose synthesis and glycogen formation (Carbohydrate metabolism). Synthesis and secretion of glucocorticoids is stimulated by ACTH from the adenohypophysis.

C. **Zona Reticularis (Fig. 6.8):** The zona reticularis consists of small, rounded cells arranged in branching and anastomosing cords. The cells are smaller than those of the other two zones and possess intensely stained nuclei and lipofuscin granules in their cytoplasm. This zone secretes small amounts of sex hormones, mainly androgens, and to a lesser extent, estrogens.

D. **Medulla:** The adrenal medulla is composed of endocrine parenchymal cells (called chromaffin cells) arranged in cords **(Fig. 6.8)** and supported by a reticular fiber network, numerous blood vessels and a few parasympathetic ganglion cells. The medulla contains two populations of secretory cells, which produce epinephrine (adrenaline) and norepinephrine (noradrenaline), like sympathetic neurons. These hormones are collectively called the catecholamines. Epinephrine makes up 80% of the secretions from the medulla, the rest being norepinephrine. The secretion of catecholamines is initiated by impulses conveyed in the preganglionic sympathetic fibers that end on the chromaffin cells. These are secreted in large quantities in response to intense emotional reactions (fight, fright, and flight).

Cushing syndrome is caused by excessive production of glucocorticoids.
Conn syndrome is produced by excessive production of aldosterone.
Addison disease is caused by autoimmune destruction of the adrenal cortex.

ISLETS OF LANGERHANS IN PANCREAS

The islets of Langerhans represent the endocrine part of the pancreas. They are widely distributed in the pancreas among the exocrine acini **(Fig. 6.9)**. Each islet is composed of alpha cells, beta cells, and delta cells, which secrete glucagon (raises blood glucose level), insulin (lowers blood glucose level), and somatostatin (inhibits secretion by other cells), respectively. There cells can be identified immunohistochemically with specific antibodies.

Quiz: *What are Type 1 and Type 2 diabetes?*

GONADS

Ovary: The ovarian follicular cells secrete progesterone and estrogen. (*Refer to the chapter on the Female Reproductive System.*).
Quiz: *What are the roles of progesterone and estrogen during the menstrual cycle?*

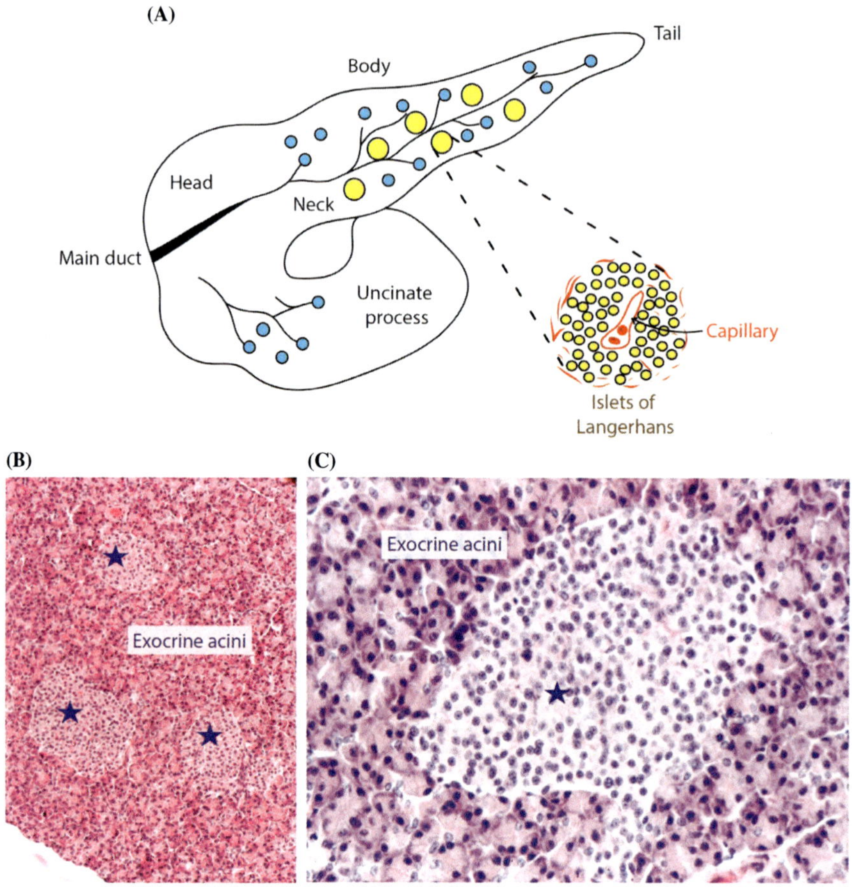

Figure 6.9. Pancreas. (A) It has different parts: uncinate process, head, neck, body, and tail. It has both an exocrine gland and an endocrine gland. The exocrine part is made up of a compound alveolar gland, which secretes trypsin, amylase, lipase, bicarbonate ions, etc. The main duct opens into the second part of the duodenum. The endocrine part is made up of islets of Langerhans (yellow), which secrets glucagon, insulin, and somatostatin into the blood capillaries. **(B) Pancreas — islets of Langerhans (asterisk).** The islets are embedded between the exocrine acini or alveoli. It is composed of alpha cells, which secrete glucagon, beta cells, which secrete insulin, and delta cells, somatostatin. It is not possible to differentiate them by the H&E stain (only by an immunohistochemical method using specific antibodies).

Testis: Leydig's (interstitial) cells secrete testosterone. (*Refer to the chapter on the Male Reproductive System.*)

Quiz: *Which cell organelle is very well developed in steroid hormone-synthesizing cells?*

OTHERS

Some cells lining the digestive tract also function as endocrine cells and secrete hormones. For example, the enteroendocrine cells (including argentaffin cells) secrete hormones such as serotonin, which plays an important role in regulating gut motility. Other endocrine cell types in the gastrointestinal tract include gastrin-secreting cells and secretin-secreting cells, which help regulate digestive processes.

Chapter 7

MALE REPRODUCTIVE SYSTEM

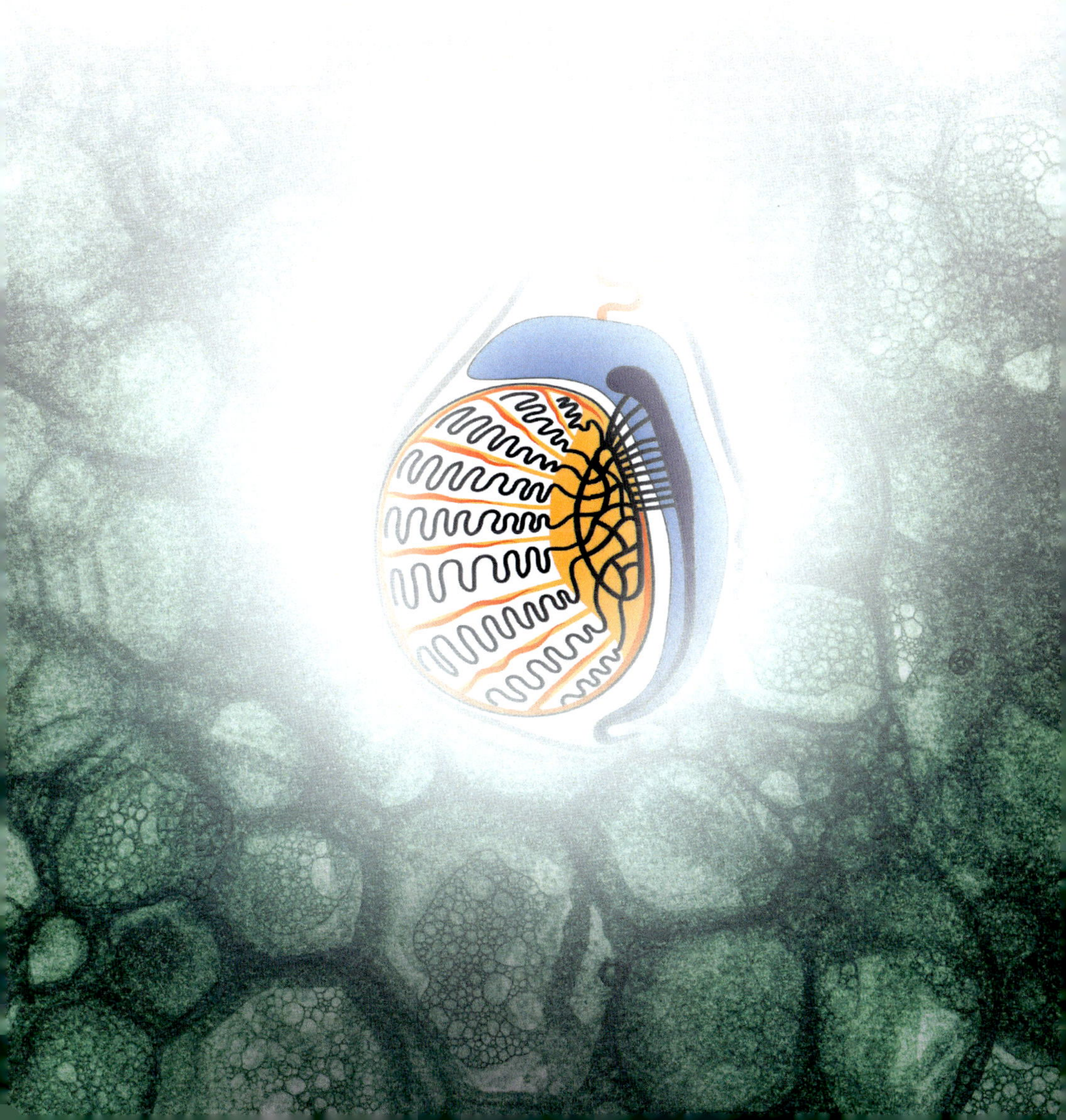

MALE REPRODUCTIVE SYSTEM

The male reproductive system located mainly in the perineum below the pelvic diaphragm. The perineum contains the reproductive organs and their parts as well as the urethra and anal canal. When viewed from below, the perineum is a diamond-shaped area bounded by the pubic symphysis anteriorly, the ischiopubic rami anterolaterally, the sacrotuberous ligaments posterolaterally, and the coccyx posteriorly **(Fig. 7.1)**. An imaginary line drawn between the two ischial tuberosities divides the perineum into two triangular areas: the urogenital (UG) triangle anteriorly and the anal triangle posteriorly **(Fig. 7.1)**. The urogenital triangle contains the external genitalia both in the male and in the female. (*For illustrations, refer to the chapter on the Female Reproductive System.*) The anal triangle contains the terminal part of the gastrointestinal tract, the anal canal.

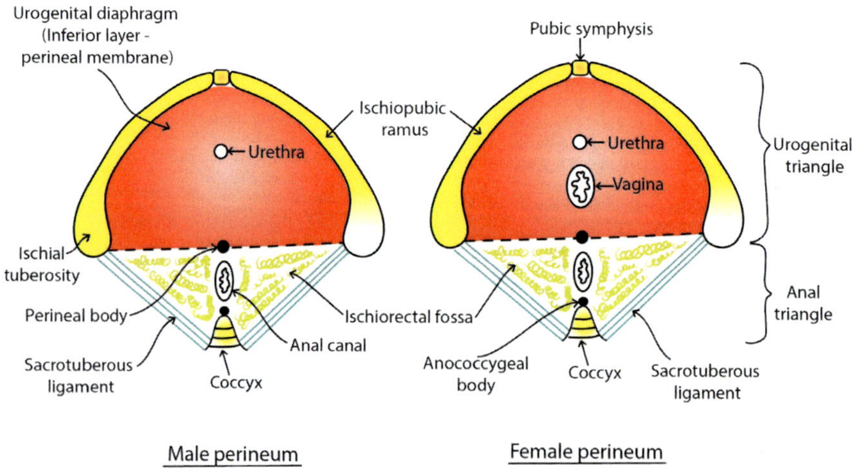

Figure 7.1. Perineum. A. Male perineum. B. Female perineum. Note the perineum is bounded by the ischiopubic rami, ischial tuberosities, sacrotuberous ligament, and coccyx. The diamond-shaped perineum is divided into the urogenital triangle and anal triangle. In the male, the urogenital diaphragm that bridges the ischiopubic rami (urogenital triangle) is pierced by the urethra (membranous urethra); in the female, it is pierced by the urethra and vagina.

UROGENITAL TRIANGLE

Bridging the two-ischiopubic rami in the urogenital triangle is the urogenital (UG) diaphragm (whose inferior fascial layer that spans the pubic arch is the perineal membrane) **(Fig. 7.1)**. In the male, the membranous urethra passes through the UG diaphragm, whereas in the female, both the urethra and vaginal canal pass through the UG diaphragm **(Fig. 7.1)**. At the center of the diamond-shaped perineum lies the perineal body, a fibromuscular structure that serves as a site for muscle attachment. (*Refer to the chapter on the Female Reproductive System for illustrations*)

MALE REPRODUCTIVE SYSTEM

The male reproductive system consists of a pair of testes, epididymis, vas deferens, seminal vesicles, prostate gland, and associated ducts, as well as the penis and urethra **(Fig. 7.2)**. The system is responsible for the production of spermatozoa

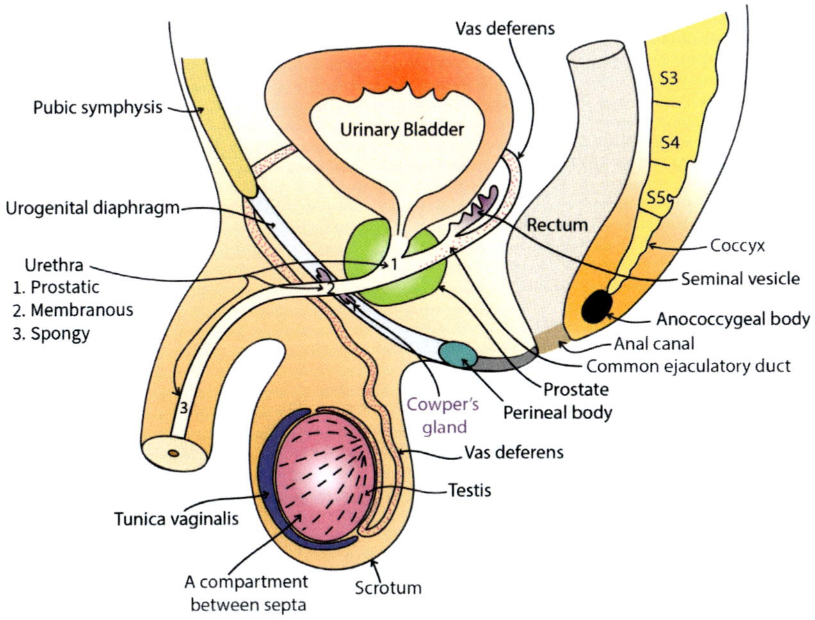

Figure 7.2. Testis and the duct system. The testis lies in the scrotum. It is capped by the tunica vaginalis anteriorly as well as its sides. The testis is divided into many compartments by fibrous septa, and each compartment contains extremely coiled seminiferous tubules. Posteriorly, it is capped by the epididymis, which leads to the vas deferens that is joined by the seminal vesicle to form the common ejaculatory duct. The ejaculatory duct opens into the prostate urethra, which leads into the membranous urethra through the urogenital (UG) diaphragm and ultimately into the penile urethra.

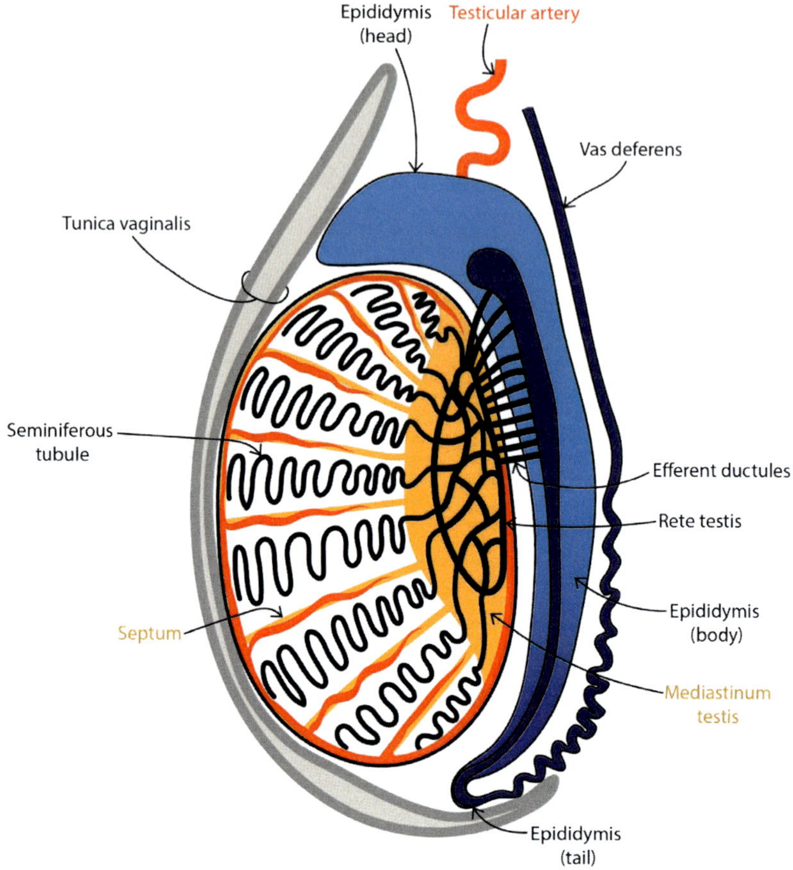

Figure 7.3. Duct system of the male reproductive system. It begins from the seminiferous tubules, through the rete testis, efferent ductules, epididymis, vas deferens, and common ejaculatory duct. By this route, the spermatozoa are transported ultimately to the penile urethra (see **Fig. 7.2**). The testis is supplied by the testicular artery, which arises from the abdominal aorta.

and their transport to the exterior **(Fig. 7.3)**. The external genitalia include the penis and scrotum (which contains the testes, epididymis and a part of vas deferens). The internal genital organs include the vas deferens, seminal vesicles, ejaculatory ducts, and prostate gland, which are located within the pelvis.

Testis

1. **General features:** The testis which is covered anteriorly and on sides by tunica vaginalis as a blind sac **(Fig. 7.2)**, is enclosed in the scrotal sac,

which has a slightly lower body temperature compared with the rest of the body.

The scrotum has several layers: skin (outermost), dartos fascia (with some smooth muscle fibers), external spermatic fascia, cremaster fascia/muscle, and internal spermatic fascia.

Quiz: *What causes the wrinkling of scrotal skin in cold weather? What is the purpose of this?*

2. **Histology** In a histological section, the testis has a dense fibrous capsule, tunica albuginea. From the tunica albuginea, fibrous septa extend inward and divide the testicular parenchyma into many lobules **(Fig. 7.4)**. Each lobule contains extremely coiled seminiferous tubules. The seminiferous tubules converge to form straight tubules (tubuli recti), which drain into the rete testis **(Fig. 7.3)**. The seminiferous tubules are lined by multi-layered germ cells at different stages of spermatogenesis. These differentiate in sequence as follows **(Fig. 7.4)**: spermatogonia (2N) → primary spermatocytes (2N) → secondary spermatocytes (2N) → spermatids (1N) → spermatozoa (1N). After release into the lumen, spermatozoa pass through the following pathway: seminiferous tubules → rete testis → efferent ductules → epididymis → vas

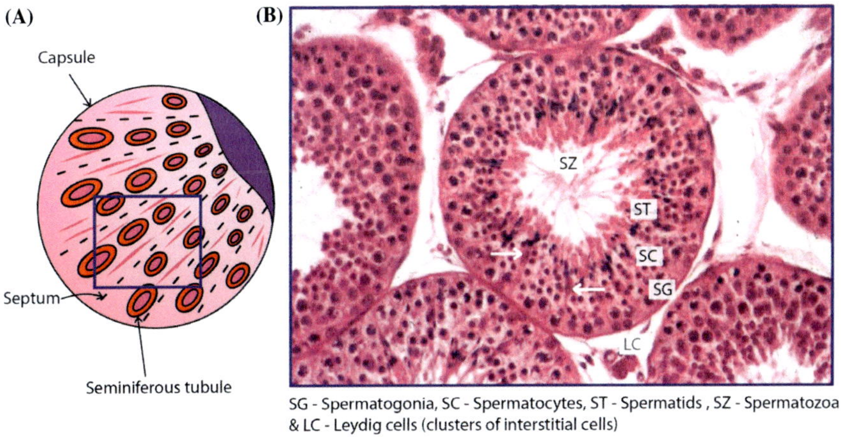

Figure 7.4. Testis — seminiferous tubules. (A) Transverse section through the testis showing different compartments of its parenchyma. Many seminiferous tubules are in cross-sectional profiles. **(B)** Boxed area in (A). The tubules show different associations of germ cells undergoing different stages of spermatogenesis: spermatogonia (SG), spermatocytes (SC), spermatids (ST), and spermatozoa (SZ). Between the germ cells are the Sertoli cells (white arrows). Clusters of interstitial cells (cells of Leydig, LC) may be seen between the tubules. They secrete testosterone. (Hematoxylin and eosin (H&E) stain.)

deferens → common ejaculatory duct → urethra (prostatic, membranous, and penile) **(Fig. 7.3)**.

Between the germs cells are the Sertoli cells, which are supporting cells that provide a proper environment for spermatogenesis and form the blood-testis barrier via tight junctions. At the base of the seminiferous tubules, myoepithelial cells are located **(Fig. 7.5)**. In the interstitial spaces between seminiferous tubules are blood vessels and clusters of interstitial (Leydig) cells, which secrete testosterone **(Fig. 7.5; Fig. 7.6)**.

3. **Arterial supply and venous drainage of the testis.** It is supplied by the testicular artery which is a branch from the abdominal aorta **(Fig. 7.3)**.

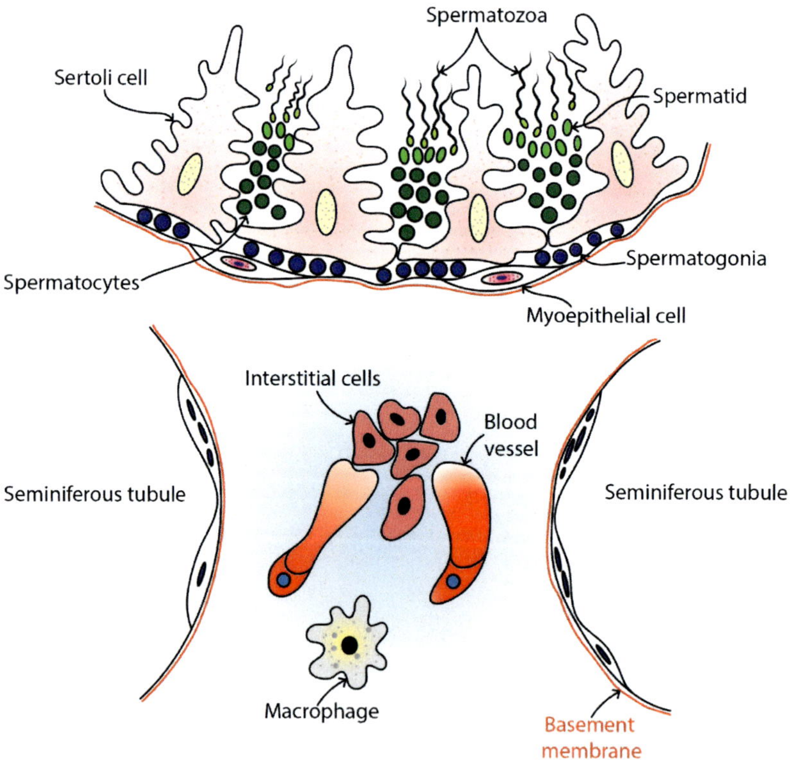

Figure 7.5. Germ cells, Sertoli cells, and interstitial cells in the testis. The germ cells comprise the spermatogonia (2N), spermatocytes (2N), spermatids (1N), and spermatozoa (1N). The Sertoli cells are supporting cells that create a proper environment for spermatogenesis. They are held together at the base by tight junctions. Myoepithelial cells are located at the base invested by a layer of basement membrane. Between the seminiferous tubules are the interstitial cells, phagocytes, and blood vessels (BV).

Quiz: *What is the blood-testis barrier? What other "blood–tissue" barriers have you learned?*

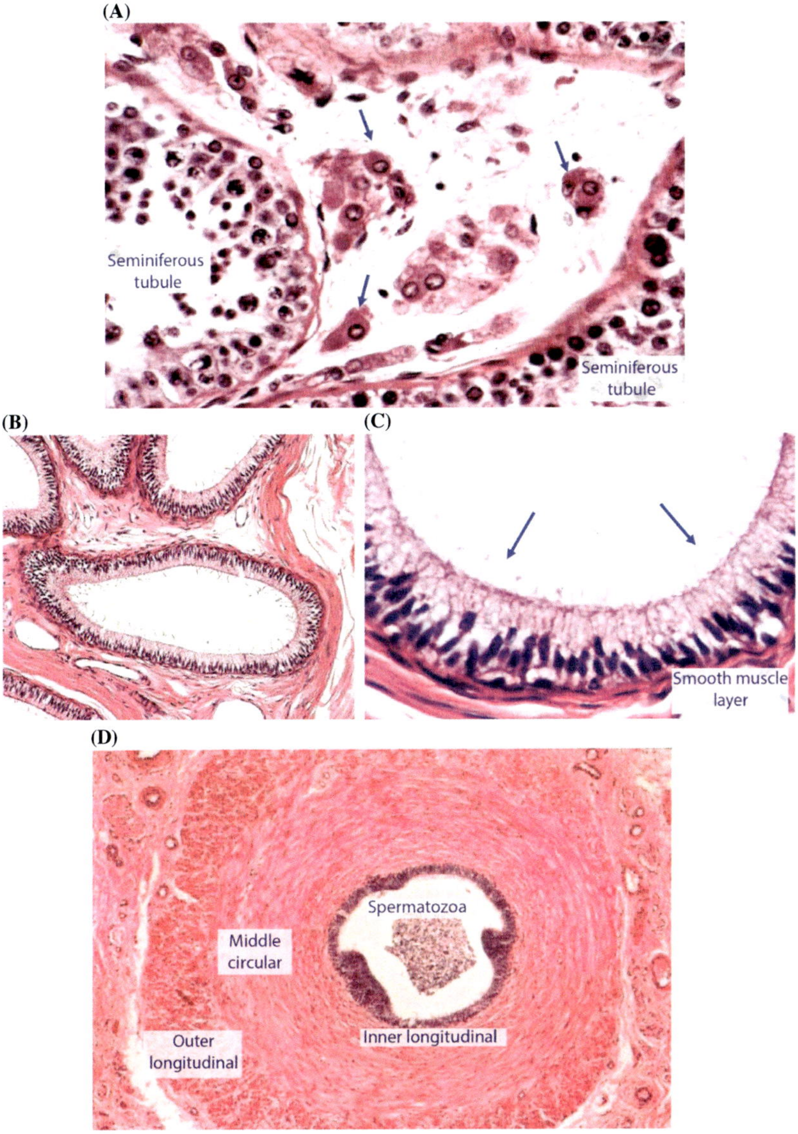

Figure 7.6. **(A) Testis — interstitial cells (Leydig cells).** The cells (arrows) are distributed between the seminiferous tubules. They secrete testosterone. (H&E stain.) **(B) Epididymis.** The lumen is lined by the pseudostratified columnar epithelium. **(C) Epididymis.** The epithelial cells show long stereocilia. They represent branched microvilli (arrows) that facilitate secretion. The wall has a thin layer of smooth muscle. (H&E stain.) **(D) Vas deferens.** It is a muscular tube lined by the pseudostratified columnar epithelium. The thick muscular wall consists of three layers: inner longitudinal, middle circular, and outer longitudinal. (H&E stain.)

Quiz: *What cell organelle is well developed in the interstitial cells?*

Venous drainage occurs via the pampiniform plexus, a network of veins that surrounds the testicular artery in the spermatic cord and functions as a countercurrent heat exchange system, helping to cool arterial blood before it reaches the testis.

Efferent Ductules (Fig. 7.3)

These are small tubules lined by the simple cuboidal epithelium. They connect the rete testis with the epididymis.

Epididymis (Fig. 7.3; Fig. 7.7)

It is a tubular structure consisting of the head, body, and tail, and is continuous with the vas deferens. The head receives spermatozoa from the efferent ductules. The epididymis is the site of sperm maturation, storage, and transport. It is lined by the pseudostratified columnar epithelium with basal cells. The lining cells possess long, non-motile, branched projections called stereocilia (modified microvilli), which are involved in absorption and secretion, helping in sperm maturation (**Fig. 7.6**). The wall also contains connective tissue and some smooth muscle cells.

Vas Deferens

The vas deferens is a long, thick-walled muscular tube measuring approximately 30 cm in length. It ascends within the spermatic cord through the inguinal canal to reach the posterior surface of the urinary bladder (**Fig. 7.2**). Near its termination, it crosses superior to the ureter and joins the duct of the seminal vesicle to form the ejaculatory duct. The ejaculatory ducts from both sides open into the prostatic urethra on either side of the seminal colliculus (verumontanum) within the prostate gland. Histologically, the vas deferens is lined by the pseudostratified columnar epithelium with basal cells (**Fig. 7.6D**). Its lumen appears star-shaped, due to mucosal folds and contraction of the thick smooth muscle coat, which consists of inner longitudinal, middle circular, and outer longitudinal layers.

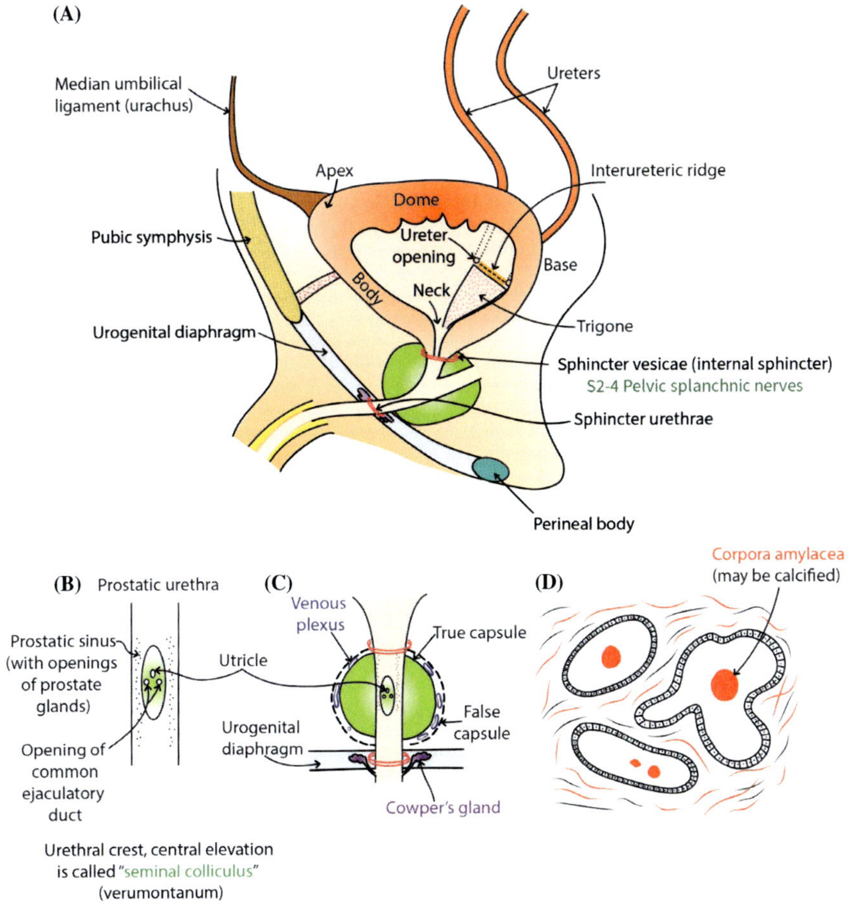

Figure 7.7. Prostate gland and prostatic urethra. (A) The prostate lies below the bladder neck, guarded by the sphincter vesicae (smooth muscle). It rests on the urogenital (UG) diaphragm. **(B)** The gland surrounds the prostatic urethra, which passes through the UG diaphragm as the membranous urethra. **(C)** The gland is covered by a layer of true capsule, and further exteriorly is a layer of false capsule. Between the two layers of the capsule, the venous plexuses are present. On the posterior wall of the prostatic urethra is the urethral crest, whose central elevation is the seminal colliculus "verumontanum." The prostatic sinus lateral to the urethral crest receives minute openings of the prostate gland. The openings of the common ejaculatory ducts lie on the sides of the urethral crest. The utricle is a blind opening on the urethral crest. **(D)** In a histological section, the prostate gland is composed of a compound tubulo-alveolar gland. The alveoli show the presence of corpora amylacea (prostatic concretions).

Ejaculatory Duct

This is formed by the union of vas deferens and duct of the seminal vesicle **(Fig. 7.2)**.

Prostate Gland

1. It is a chestnut-sized gland, located inferior to the neck of the urinary bladder.
2. It lies on the UG diaphragm **(Fig. 7.7; Fig. 7.8)**.
3. It can be palpated on digital rectal examination as it is closely related to the anterior wall of the rectum **(Fig. 7.2)**.
4. It is covered by a layer of true fibrous capsule and outer false fibrous capsule (prostatic sheath). Between these lies the prostatic venous plexus, which communicates with the vertebral venous plexus (Batson's plexus) **(Fig. 7.7)**.

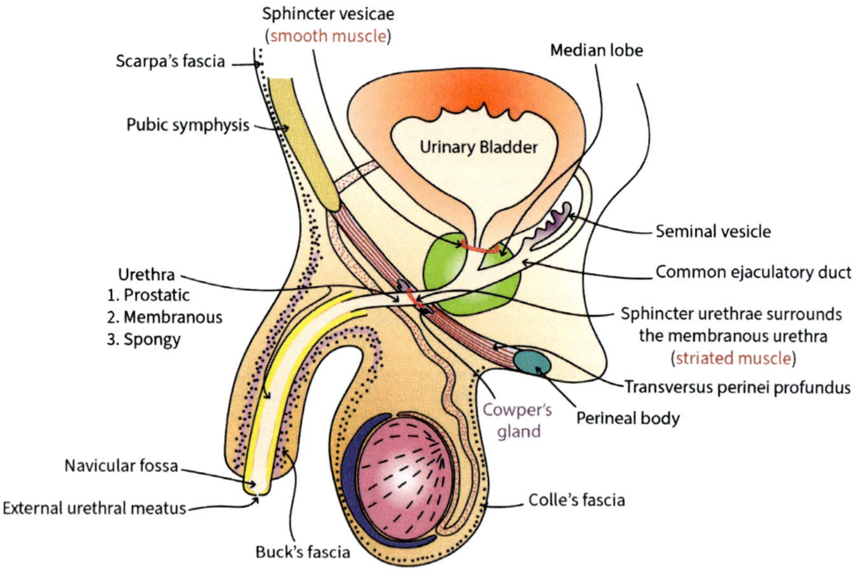

Figure 7.8. Prostate and male urethra. The prostate lies beneath the bladder neck, surrounded by the sphincter vesicae. It rests on the urogenital (UG) diaphragm containing the sphincter urethrae, transversus perinei profundus, and Cowper's gland. The prostate has different lobes: median, anterior, lateral, and posterior. The median lobe lies between the common ejaculatory ducts and the prostatic urethra. It may be enlarged in the elderly, causing obstruction to the flow of urine. The urethra in the male has different parts: (1) prostatic urethra (surrounded by the prostate), (2) membranous urethra (in the UG diaphragm), and (3) penile or spongy urethra (in the penis).

This provides a pathway for metastasis of prostatic carcinoma to the vertebral column.

5. Classically, the prostate is described as having anterior, posterior, median, and two lateral lobes. The median (middle) lobe is clinically significant **(Fig. 7.8)**, as enlargement in benign prostatic hyperplasia (BPH) may compress the prostatic urethra and obstruct urine flow, leading to difficulty in micturition.
6. **Histology (Fig. 7.9):** It is a compound tubulo-alveolar gland lined by the pseudostratified columnar epithelium. The lumina of the glands often contain prostatic concretions (corpora amylacea), which may become calcified with age.
7. The prostate gland secretes prostatic fluid, which includes acid phosphatase, prostate-specific antigen (PSA), fibrinolysin, citric acid, and prostaglandins. These components help in liquefaction of semen and enhance sperm motility.
8. The prostatic ducts open into the prostatic sinus, located on both sides of the seminalis colliculus **(Fig. 7.7)**.
9. Prostate-specific antigen (PSA) levels in the blood are used as a clinical marker for assessing prostate abnormalities, including benign prostatic hyperplasia and carcinoma.

Seminal Vesicle (Fig. 7.2; Fig. 7.9)

It is a highly coiled tubular gland that appears irregular and folded due to compression. In a histology section, the lumen is thrown into many folds, giving it a honeycomb-like appearance. The mucosa is lined by the pseudostratified columnar epithelium. The gland secretes viscous, alkaline fluid rich in fructose, prostaglandins, and seminal vesicle proteins, which provide energy for sperm and contribute to semen coagulation. Secretions from both the seminal vesicle and prostate gland contribute to the seminal fluid.

Male Urethra

The male urethra is divided into three parts: prostatic urethra, membranous urethra, and spongy (penile) urethra **(Fig. 7.2; Fig. 7.8)**.

1. Prostatic urethra

This part of the urethra passes through the prostate gland. It is the most dilatable part of the urethra and is lined by a transitional epithelium

(A)

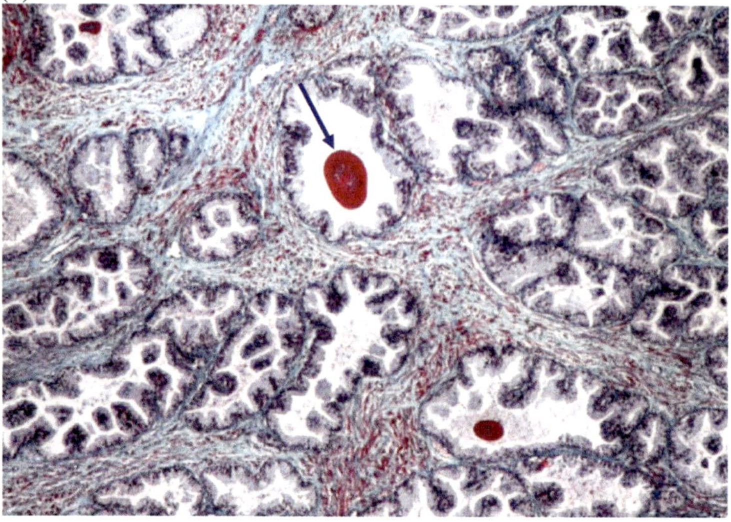

(B)

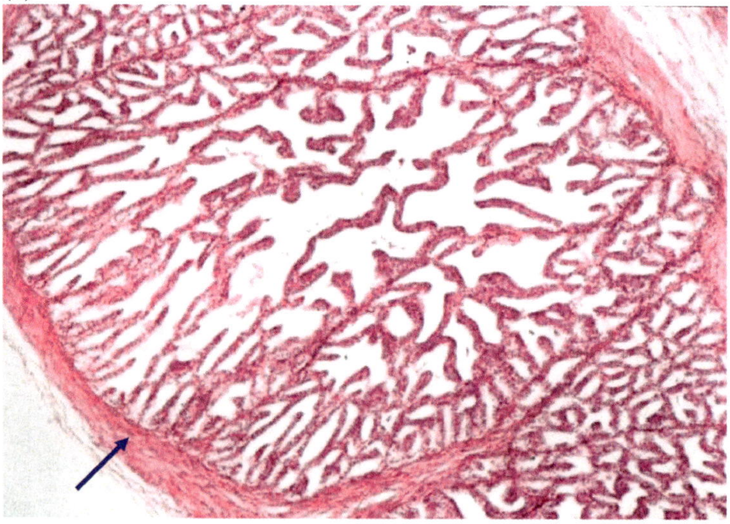

Figure 7.9. **(A) Prostate gland.** It is a compound tubulo-alveolar gland. The alveolus is lined by the pseudostratified columnar epithelium. The lumen contains occasional prostatic concretions (corpora amylacea) (arrow), which may be calcified. It secretes fibrinolysin, acid phosphatase, PSA (prostate-specific antigen), etc. Between the alveoli are collagen bundles (green) and muscles (red). (Masson trichrome stain.) **(B) Seminal vesicle.** It is a long tubular organ that compresses upon itself. The mucosa appears honeycomb-like. It is lined by the pseudostratified columnar epithelium, which produces fructose, vitamin C, etc. Arrow indicates muscular coat. (H&E stain.)

(urothelium). Its posterior wall has the urethral crest with a central elevation, seminalis colliculus (verumontanum) **(Fig. 7.7)**. At the summit of the seminal colliculus is a small blind pouch called the prostatic utricle. On either side of the seminal colliculus open the ejaculatory ducts. On both sides of the urethral crest are grooves called the prostatic sinuses, which receive the openings of the prostatic glands **(Fig. 7.7)**.

2. **Membranous urethra**
   This is the shortest and most fixed part of the urethra. It passes through the UG diaphragm. The deep perineal pouch enclosed by the UG diaphragm contains the Cowper's (bulbourethral) glands. These glands open via ducts into the proximal part of the spongy (penile) urethra, not the membranous urethra. Surrounding the membranous urethra is the external urethral sphincter (sphincter urethrae) which is innervated by the pudendal nerve **(Fig. 7.8)**.
3. **Spongy (penile) urethra**
   This is the longest part of the urethra. It is lined by the stratified columnar epithelium, which undergoes transitional changes to the stratified squamous epithelium nearer to the navicular fossa (dilated part) and the external urethral orifice, the narrowest part of the urethra. Sensory innervation to the urethra is by the perineal branch of the pudendal nerve (S2–4) **(Fig. 7.8)**.

Male External Genitalia — Penis (Fig. 7.10)

The penis has two main parts: the root and the body (shaft).

1. **Root of the penis** — This consists of the bulb of the penis (corpus spongiosum) that is attached to the perineal membrane (inferior layer of the UG diaphragm) and the crura of the penis (corpora cavernosum), which are attached to the ischiopubic rami. Associated with the root of the penis in the superficial perineal pouch are three pairs of perineal muscles: ischiocavernosus which helps maintain erection, bulbospongiosus assists in erection and expels semen during ejaculation, and superficial transverse perineal muscle stabilizes the perineal body. These muscles are innervated by the perineal branches of pudendal nerve.

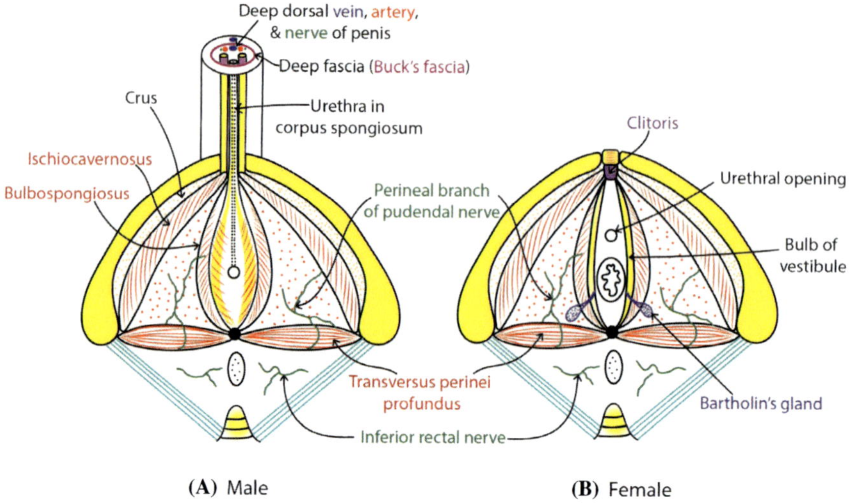

Figure 7.10. Male (A) and female (B) external genitalia. (A) The penis has two parts: the root of the penis and the body of the penis. The root has three pairs of perineal muscles: bulbospongiosus, ischiocavernosus, and transversus perinei superficialis. They are supplied by the perineal branch of the pudendal nerve. The body of the penis has three columns of erectile tissue: corpus cavernosum (paired) and corpus spongiosum, which transmits the urethra. **(B)** The female external genitalia have the same three pairs of perinei muscles.

2. **Body (shaft) of the penis (Fig. 7.10)** — This is made up of three longitudinal columns of erectile tissue: paired corpus cavernosum and a single corpus spongiosum that transmits the urethra. Each tissue column is enclosed by a layer of connective tissue, tunica albuginea. All three tissue columns are enclosed by a common layer of deep fascia, Buck's fascia. Dorsally deep to the skin in the midline are the single dorsal vein of the penis and the paired dorsal artery, and the dorsal nerve of the penis (see below) on both sides.

The penile erection is mediated by the pelvic splanchnic nerves (S2–4) which are called the nervi erigentes. Ejaculation is mediated by the sympathetic nerves.

CLINICAL CONSIDERATIONS

Sildenafil (viagra) is used clinically for the treatment of erectile dysfunction. It acts by inhibiting phosphodiesterase type 5 (PDE5), the enzyme responsible for the breakdown of cyclic guanosine monophosphate (cGMP). An increased level of cGMP causes relaxation of smooth muscles in the corpus cavernosum, thereby resulting in increase in blood flow and erection.

INNERVATION

The main nerves innervating the male and female reproductive systems in the perineum are the pudendal nerve (S2–S4) and the pelvic splanchnic nerves (S2–S4). Both originate from the sacral nerve plexus (L4–S4). For comparison, the illustrations of female external genitalia are shown in **Fig. 7.10**.

Chapter 8

FEMALE REPRODUCTIVE SYSTEM

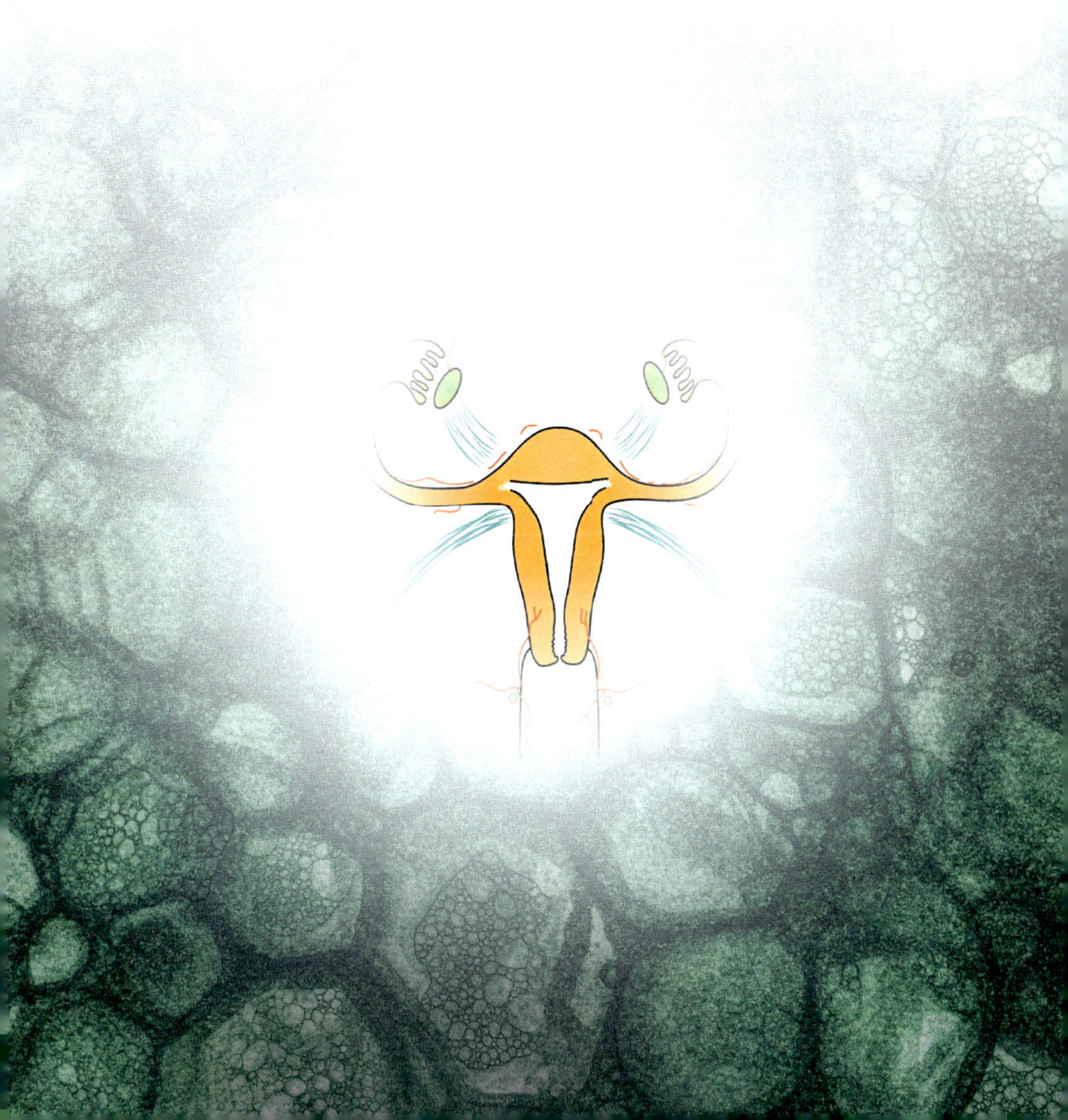

FEMALE REPRODUCTIVE SYSTEM

The upper part of the female reproductive system is housed in the pelvic cavity **(Fig. 8.1)**, whereas the lower part lies in the perineum (urogenital triangle) **(Fig. 8.2)** inferior to the pelvic diaphragm **(Fig. 8.3)**. The pelvic diaphragm provides structural support to the pelvic organs but also acts as a sphincter for the urogenital outlet (urethra and vagina) as well as rectum/anal canal (Digestive tract) **(Fig. 8.4)**.

PELVIC CAVITY AND BONY PELVIS

The pelvic cavity is the space within the pelvis, which is made up of two hip bones. Each hip bone is formed by fusion of the ilium, ischium, and pubis **(Fig. 8.3)**. Posteriorly, the two hipbones articulate with the sacrum at the sacroiliac joint. Anteriorly, they join at the pubic symphysis **(Fig. 8.3)**. In a sagittal section of the male pelvis, the urinary bladder lies most anteriorly, whereas the rectum lies in the curvature of the sacrum posteriorly. Between the bladder and the rectum lies rectovesical pouch which is a downward extension of the peritoneal cavity (greater sac). In the female pelvis, the uterus lies between the bladder and the rectum. Between the bladder and the uterus lies the uterovesical pouch, whereas between the uterus and the rectum lies the rectouterine pouch or pouch of Douglas **(Fig. 8.1)**.

The pelvic cavity has four walls. The anterior wall is related to the body of the pubis; the lateral wall on both sides is formed by the obturator foramen (covered by the obturator membrane and obturator internus muscle) **(Fig. 8.3)**; posteriorly, the cavity is related to the piriformis muscle and the sacral nerve plexus on the sacrum.

Comparison of Male and Female Bony Pelvis

In both male and female, bony pelvis is involved in protection of pelvic organs and locomotion while the female bony pelvis also serves as the birth canal. The pelvic brim or inlet is formed by the sacral promontory posteriorly, ala of sacrum,

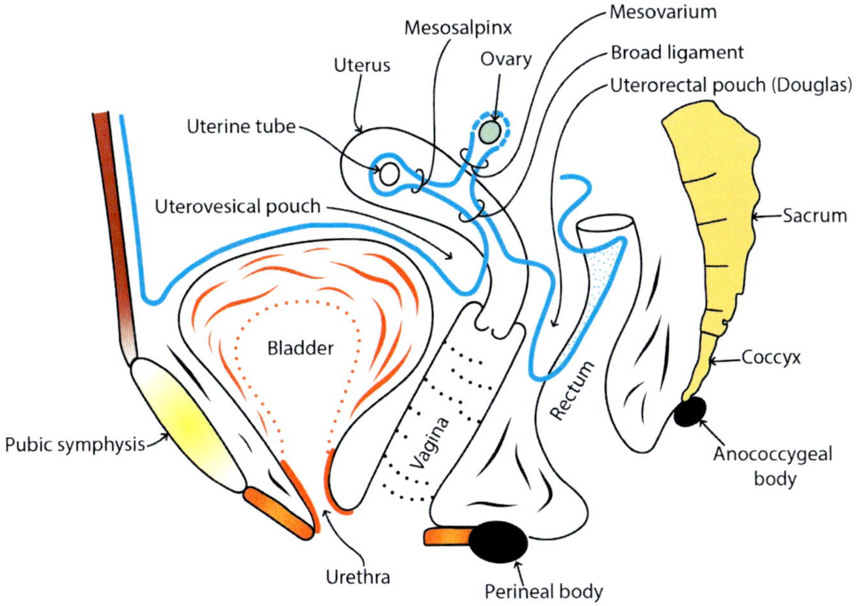

Figure 8.1. Female reproductive system. A sagittal section view through the pelvic cavity showing the female reproductive organs: uterus, uterine tube, and ovary are housed in the pelvic cavity, whereas the lower part of it, the vagina, lies below the pelvic diaphragm in the perineum. Note that the uterus, uterine tube, and ovary are lined by the peritoneum (light blue line). The broad ligament is formed by a double-layered peritoneum; so are the mesosalpinx and mesovarium. The uterovesical pouch and uterorectal pouch are the downward extension of the peritoneal cavity separating the uterus from the urinary bladder and the rectum, respectively.

arcuate line, and iliopectineal line on both sides, and pubic crest anteriorly. It is more rounded in female bony pelvis when compared with male. Also, in the female pelvis, the pubic arch (subpubic angle) is wider (between the thumb and index fingers) than the male (between the index and middle fingers).

Pelvic Diaphragm (Fig. 8.3; Fig. 8.4)

a. This forms the muscular floor of the lower limit of the pelvic cavity. The perineum lies inferior to this.
b. The pelvic diaphragm is composed of muscles attached laterally to a thickened fascia of the obturator internus muscle, known as the tendinous arch (arcus tendinous of levator ani).

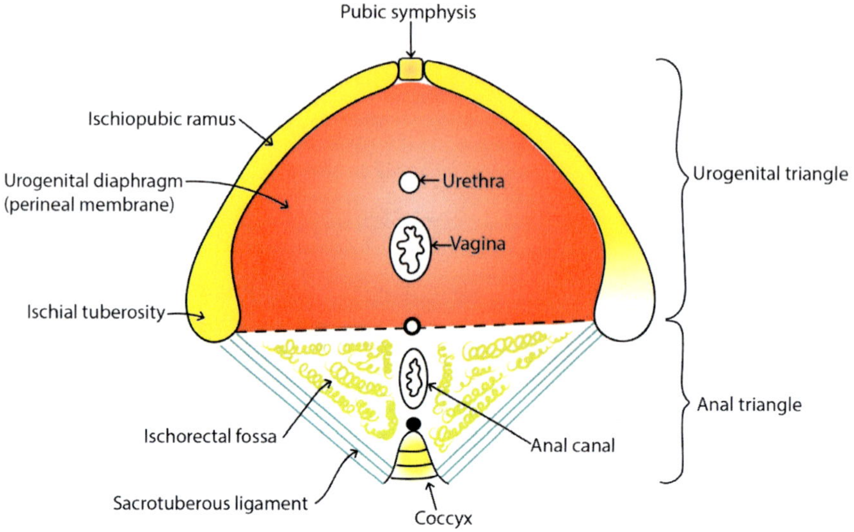

Figure 8.2. Perineum (female as viewed from below). The perineum is a diamond-shaped area bounded by the ischiopubic rami, which articulates anteriorly at the public symphysis, sacrotuberous ligaments, and coccyx. It is divided into two triangles by a line joining the two ischial tuberosities across the perineal body: the urogenital triangle and the anal triangle. In the female, the urogenital triangle forms the outlet of the urethra and vagina. The triangle is bridged by the urogenital diaphragm. The anal triangle is for the outlet of the anal canal flanked by the ischiorectal fossae.

Male: Levator ani (levator prostate, puborectalis, pubococcygeus, iliococcygeus) + ischioccoygeus.

Female: Levator ani (sphincter vaginae, puborectalis, pubococcygeus, iliococcygeus) + ischiococcygeus.

c. The pelvic diaphragm acts like a muscular hammock. Its fibers slope downward and medially toward the midline.
d. It supports the pelvic viscera, including the bladder, rectum and uterus in females, helping maintain continence and organ position.
e. It contributes to sphincteric control of pelvic outlets, supporting urethra, anal canal and vagina (in females).
f. It plays an important role during childbirth by resisting and guiding the descending fetal head, assisting in its rotation in the final stage of delivery.
g. It is innervated by the nerve to levator ani (S3-S4) and the inferior rectal branch of the pudendal nerve (S2-S4).

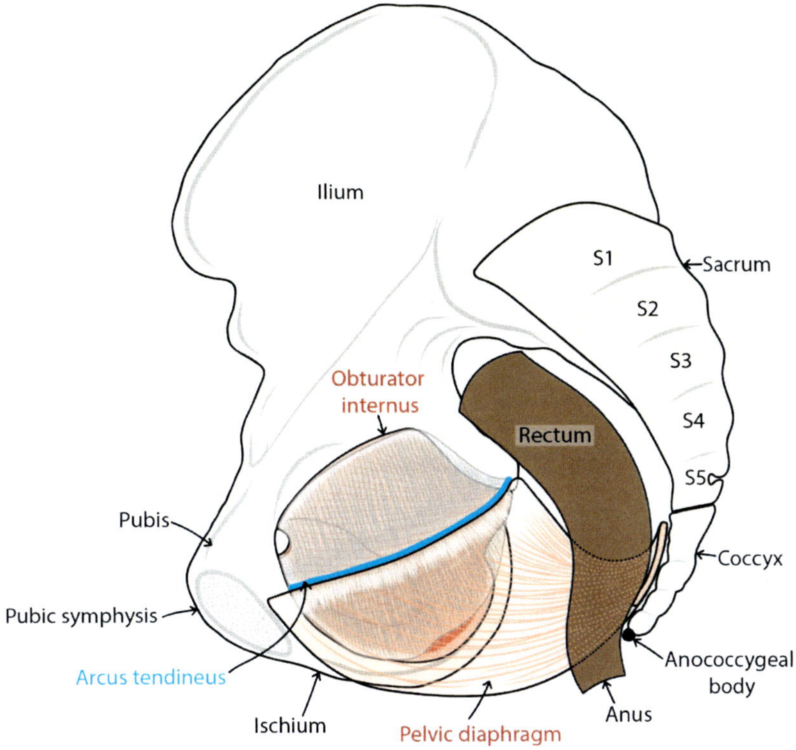

Figure 8.3. Pelvic diaphragm. The muscular pelvic diaphragm is attached to the arcus tendineus across the obturator internus fascia, covering the obturator internus muscle on the medial side of the right hip bone. The pelvic diaphragm from both sides is sloping downward medially to the pelvic organs and posteriorly to the anococcygeal body. It forms the sphincters for the rectum/anal canal and the vagina.

FEMALE REPRODUCTIVE SYSTEM

The female reproductive system comprises a pair of ovaries and uterine tubes (fallopian tubes, oviduct), uterus, vagina **(Fig. 8.5; Fig. 8.6)**, and external genitalia (vulva). The vagina and external genitalia are located in the perineum.

Ovary

a. The organ is an oval and flattened organ. It is attached to the posterior layer of the broad ligament by a peritoneal fold called the mesovarium **(Fig. 8.7)**.

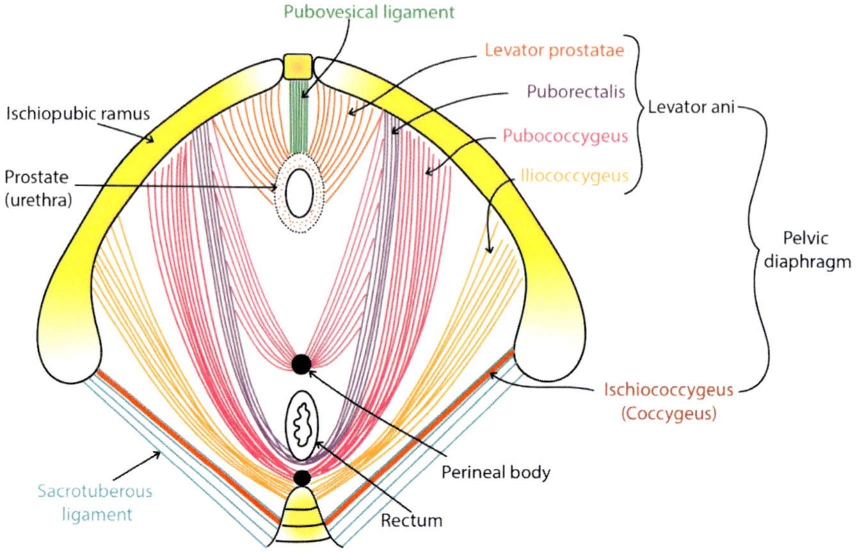

Figure 8.4. Pelvic diaphragm. The muscular pelvic diaphragm forms the floor of the pelvic cavity. Its lateral attachment to the arcus tendineus is shown in **Fig. 8.3**. As viewed from below, the pelvic diaphragm is composed of different parts that differ between male and female pelvis in relation to the visceral organs (prostate, vagina, and rectum). They are involved primarily in sphincteric actions. Details of each part are given in the text.
N.B. It is not necessary to remember all the parts.

b. It is connected to the lateral pelvic wall by the infundibulo-pelvic ligament (suspensory ligament of ovary) and to the lateral wall of the uterus at the junction of the fundus and uterine tube by the ligament of ovary **(Fig. 8.5)**.
c. **Arterial supply:** The ovary is supplied by the ovarian artery, a branch of the abdominal aorta arising at the level of L1–L2. It reaches the ovary through the infundibulo-pelvic ligament **(Fig. 8.5)**.
d. Lymphatics follow the ovarian vessels and drain into the para-aortic (lumbar) lymph nodes.
e. **Histology:** The ovary is covered by a geminal epithelium **(Fig. 8.8; Fig. 8.9)**, which does not generate the ovum. The outer cortex contains many ovarian follicles at various stages of maturation under the influence of follicle-stimulating hormone (FSH): primordial follicle, primary follicle, secondary (growing) follicle, and Graafian follicle (mature) **(Fig. 8.10; Fig. 8.11)**. In a developing follicle, the oocyte is surrounded by multiple layers of granulosa cells, and externally by theca interna and theca externa layers. Following ovulation, the ruptured follicle becomes the corpus luteum and the follicle

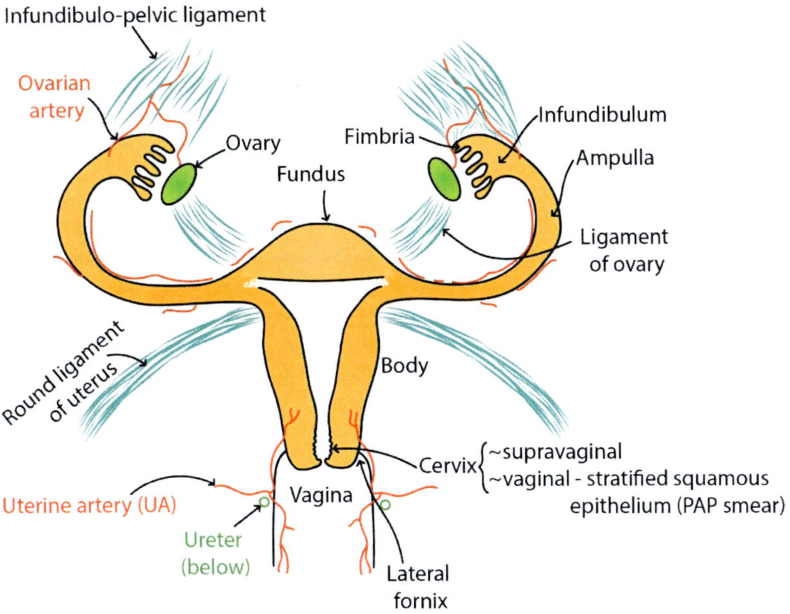

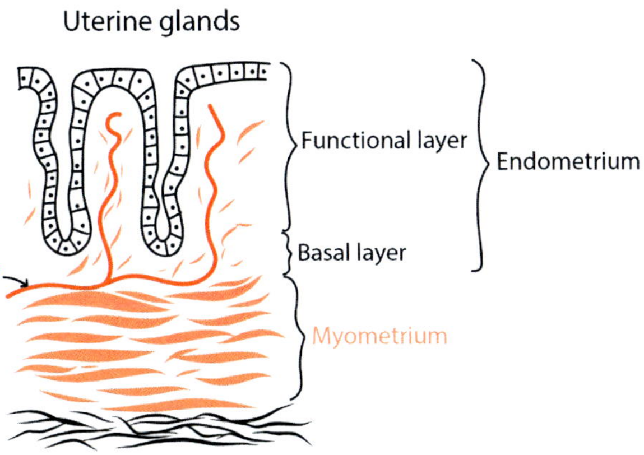

Figure 8.5. Female reproductive system. It consists of the paired ovaries, uterine tubes (fimbria, infundibulum, ampulla, and isthmus), uterus (fundus, body, cervix), and vagina. The uterus wall is made up of endometrium, myometrium, and parametrium. The endometrium shows many simple tubular glands (uterine glands). The endometrium is divided into the superficial functional layer and the deeper basal layer. Arterial supplies are by the ovarian artery via the infundibulo-pelvic ligament and uterine artery (UA), which is closely related to the lateral fornix and the ureter. The cervix has a supravaginal part (lined by the simple columnar epithelium) and vaginal part (lined by the stratified squamous epithelium used for a PAP smear for the screening of cervical cancer).

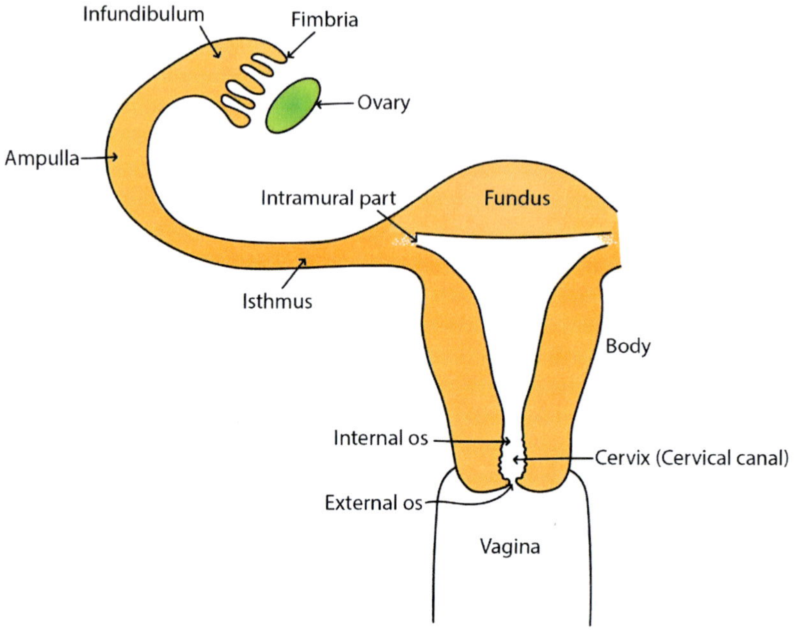

Figure 8.6. Uterus, uterine (fallopian) tube, and ovary. The uterus has the fundus forming the dome, body, and lower part, the cervix. The cervical canal has the internal os and external os that opens into the vagina. The uterine tube begins at the funnel-shaped infundibulum bearing finger-like processes, the fimbriae that are closely associated with the ovary. The ampulla is the longest and most dilated part, while the isthmus is the narrowest part.

cells differentiate into the granulosa lutein cells that secrete progesterone **(Fig. 8.12)**. The outer layer thecal cells become the thecal lutein cells, which secrete estrogens. These hormones regulate the menstrual cycle, particularly the preparation and maintenance of the endometrium in the uterus. Many follicles undergo degeneration, forming atretic follicles **(Fig. 8.13)**. The released oocyte is covered by a layer of zona pellucida (external to the plasma membrane) **(Fig. 8.14)**. Exterior to the zona pellucida lies the corona radiata which is formed by granulosa cells. The inner medulla consists of loose connective tissue containing numerous blood vessels, lymphatics, and nerves.

Uterine (Fallopian) Tube (Fig. 8.6)

The uterine tube, which is also known as the fallopian tube or oviduct, consists of the infundibulum with fimbria (finger-like projections), ampulla (dilated part,

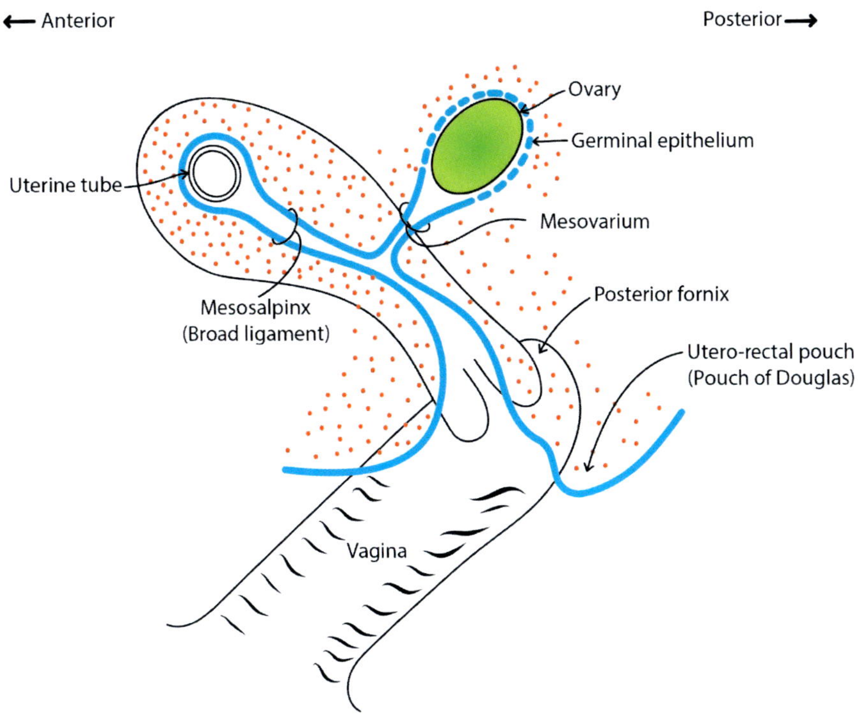

Figure 8.7. Uterus and ovary — peritoneal relations. The uterus is invested by the overlying peritoneum forming a double-layered structure termed the broad ligament consisting of the mesosalpinx (between the uterine tube and mesovarium) and mesovarium that suspends the ovary. The posterior layer of the broad ligament lines the posterior fornix. It is then reflected over the rectum, forming the utero-rectal pouch (pouch of Douglas).

Quiz: *What is the clinical significance of the pouch of Douglas?*

common site of fertilization), isthmus, and intramural part (within the uterus wall). The wall of the uterine tube has three main layers: mucosa, muscularis layer, and serosa **(Fig. 8.15)**. The mucosa is highly folded and lined by the simple columnar epithelium composed of ciliated columnar cells which help propel the oocyte toward the uterus and non-ciliated secretory cells (peg cells), which provide nutrient-rich secretions that support the oocyte and spermatozoa. The muscle layer is composed of inner circular and outer longitudinal layers (smooth muscle) producing peristaltic contraction to help transport the ovum towards the uterus.

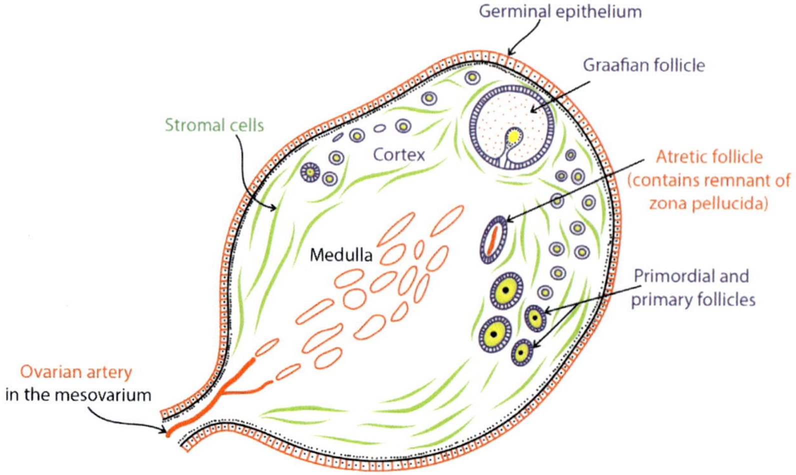

Figure 8.8. Ovary. It is a flattened organ. The surface is lined by a layer of germinal epithelium, which is NOT concerned with germ cell formation. The cortex shows many ovarian follicles at different stages of development (primordial, primary follicles). Also present in it are many spindle-shaped stromal cells (They appear like fibroblasts; some of them may secrete estrogen). Atretic follicles are common. The medulla shows sectional profiles of the ovarian artery that passes through the mesovarium.

Quiz: *Where does the ovarian artery originate?*

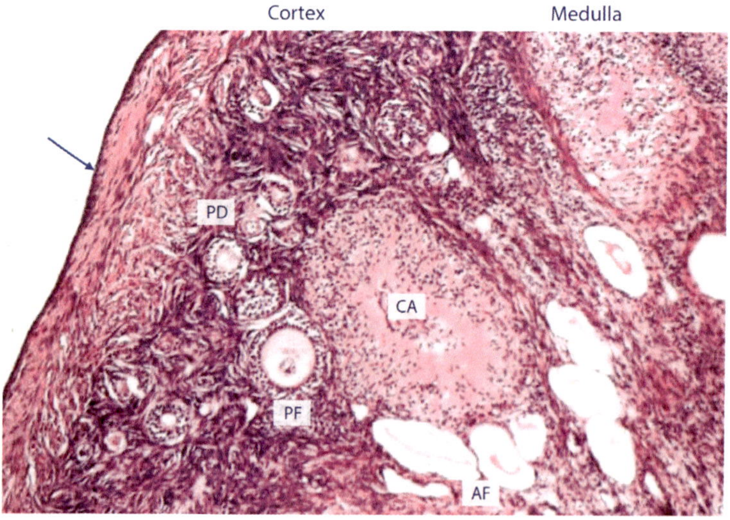

Figure 8.9. Ovary. The surface of the ovary is covered by a layer of germinal epithelium (arrow). The cortex shows primordial follicles (PD), primary follicles (PF), corpus albicans (CA), and atretic follicles (AF). (Hematoxylin and eosin (H&E) stain.)

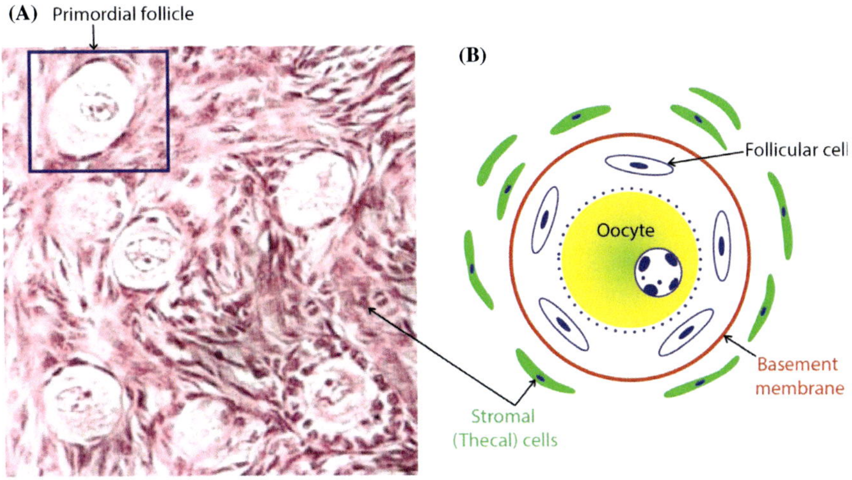

Figure 8.10. Ovary — primordial follicles. (A, B) (boxed area in **A**). Each follicle contains an oocyte that is frozen at the dictyotene stage (meiosis). The follicular cells are flattened cells. Each follicle is delineated by a layer of basement membrane. In response to follicle-stimulating hormone (FSH), the follicular cells start to proliferate. Zona pellucida is formed (dotted blue line). The stromal cells become the thecal cells (secrete estrogen). **(A)** H&E stain. **(B)** Semi-diagrammatic picture.

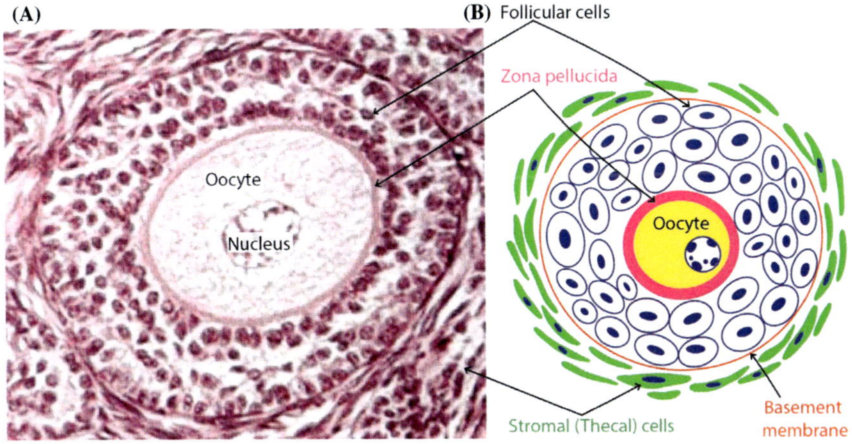

Figure 8.11. Ovary — primary (growing) follicle. (A, B) A primary follicle. Note that it contains an oocyte with a nucleus. The oocyte is invested by a layer of zona pellucida. The follicular cells are multi-layered. Between the follicles are the stromal (thecal) cells. **(A)** (H&E stain).

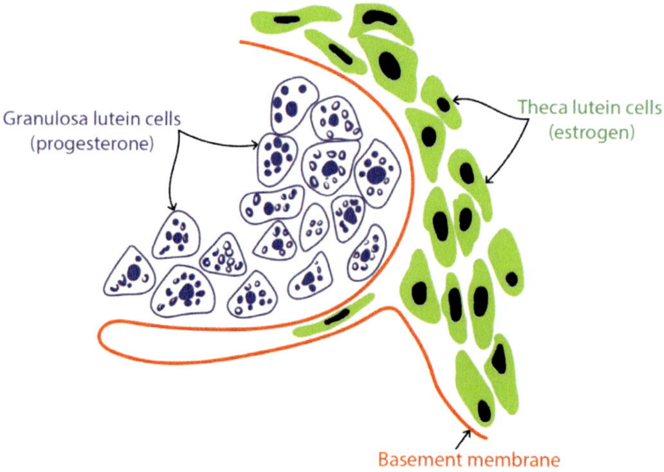

Figure 8.12. Showing a portion of the corpus luteum (yellow body). The granulosa lutein cells are derived from the follicular cells and secrete progesterone; the theca lutein cells are derived from the stromal cells, and they secrete estrogen.

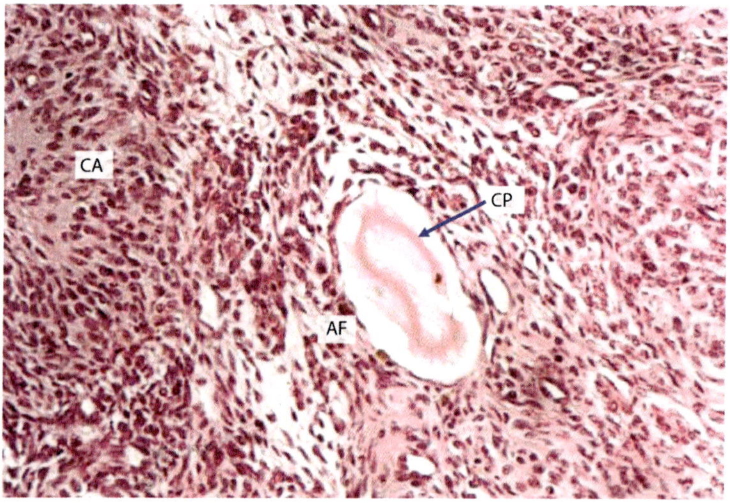

Figure 8.13. Ovary. Showing in the medulla a corpus albicans (CA) (white body) and an atretic follicle (AF). Note the remnant of zona pellucida (CP) in an atretic follicle (AF). (H&E stain).

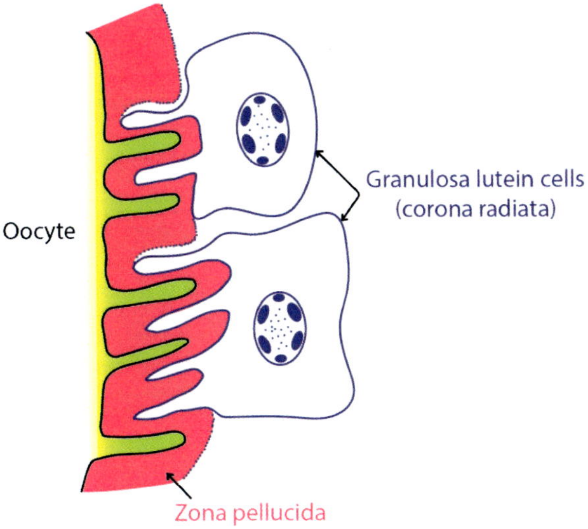

Figure 8.14. Portion of a released oocyte. It is covered by a layer of zona pellucida (external to the plasma membrane). Further exterior to this are the covering granulosa cells forming the corona radiata.

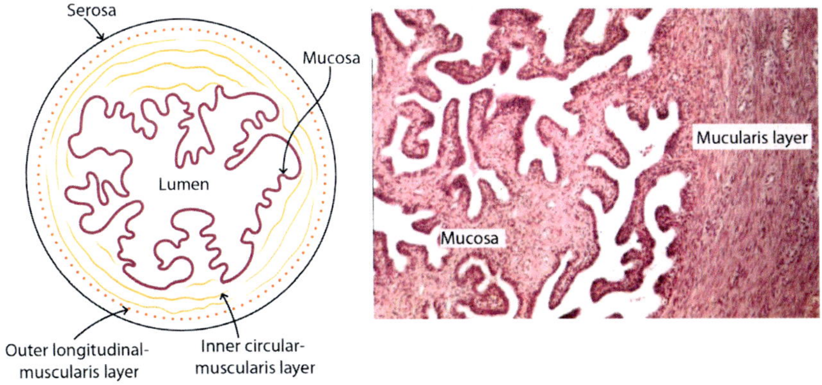

Figure 8.15. Fallopian (uterine) tube. The wall has three layers: mucosa, muscular layer, and serosa. The mucosa, with many folds, is lined by the simple columnar epithelium, composed of ciliated cells and non-ciliated secretory cells (Peg cells). **(A)** Diagrammatic picture. **(B)** (H&E stain).

Uterus

a. **Parts of the uterus (Fig. 8.5; Fig. 8.6):** The uterus has three main parts: the dome-shaped fundus (superior to the level of the openings of the two uterine tubes), body (main central part), and cervix (lower narrow part). The cervix is further divided into:
   - the supravaginal part, a portion above the vagina which communicates with the uterine cavity via internal os and
   - the vaginal part, which projects and opens into the vagina through the external os of the cervical canal.

   The recess formed between the vaginal cervix and the vaginal walls are known as the fornices. These are divided into anterior, posterior and two lateral fornices.

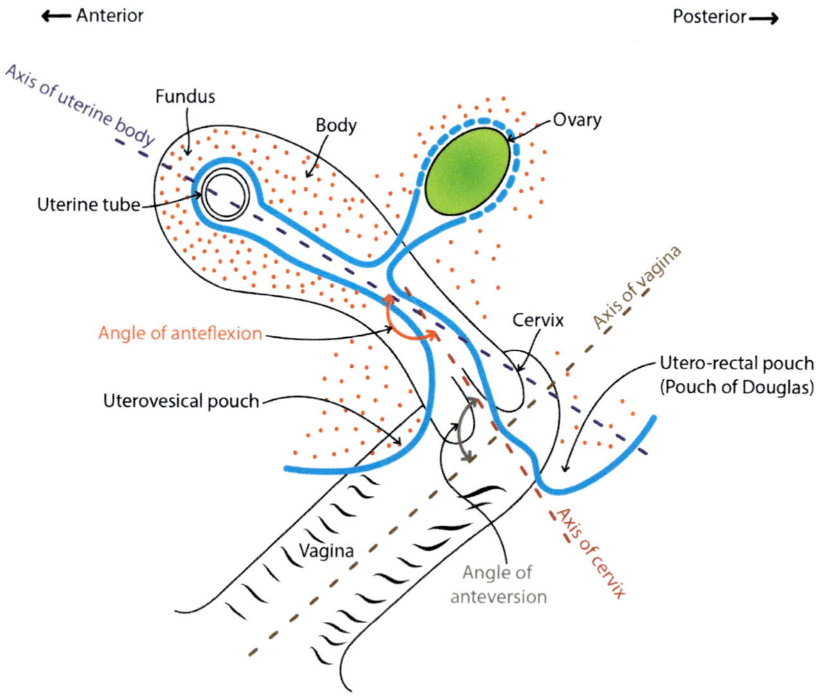

Figure 8.16. Uterus — normal position. Anteflexion is the angulation (dotted lines) between the body of the uterus and cervix. Anteversion refers to the angulation (dotted lines) between the cervix and the vagina. The light blue line represents the peritoneal reflection. Red dotted areas are lined by the peritoneum.

***Quiz:** Describe the support of the uterus.*

b. **Normal position (Fig. 8.16):** The normal position of the uterus is anteflexion (angulation between the body of the uterus and the cervix) and anteversion (angulation between cervix and the vagina). Anteriorly, the peritoneum is reflected from the urinary bladder onto the uterus (fundus), forming the vesicouterine (uterovesical) pouch. Posteriorly, the peritoneum lines the posterior fornix of the vagina and reflects onto the rectum, forming the rectouterine pouch (pouch of Douglas) **(Fig. 8.16)**.

c. **Histology:** The uterine wall consists of three layers: endometrium, myometrium, and perimetrium. The endometrium contains numerous coiled tubular uterine glands lined by simple columnar epithelium. It has two layers: functional and basal layers **(Fig. 8.17)**. The functional layer is sloughed off during menstruation, while the basal layer regenerates the functional layer. Estrogen promotes regeneration and repair of the endometrium during the estrogenic (proliferative) phase. The progesterone supports the growth and maintenance of the endometrium during the luteal phase. The myometrium

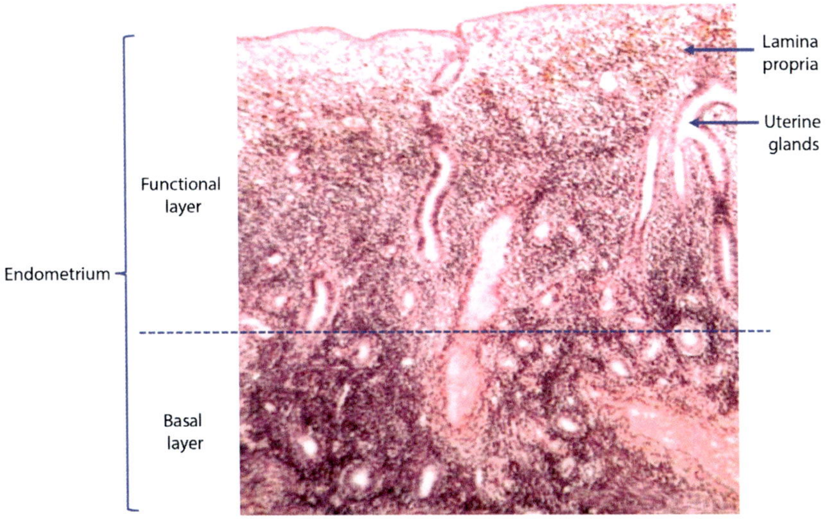

Figure 8.17. Uterus — endometrium. The endometrium has the functional layer and the basal layer. It is lined by the simple columnar epithelium. The superficial functional layer is sloughed off monthly during menstruation, while the basal layer with its stem cells can regenerate. Note the tubular and coiled uterine glands. Between them is the lamina propria containing stromal cells. (H&E stain.)

Quiz: *Which hormone helps the regeneration of endometrium, and which hormone promotes and maintains its growth?*

is composed of smooth muscle responsible for uterine contraction which is stimulated by oxytocin released from the posterior pituitary (pars nervosa) during labor.

d. Arterial supply

The uterus is supplied by the ovarian artery (arising from the abdominal aorta) and the uterine artery (arising from the internal iliac) **(Fig. 8.5; Fig. 8.18)**. The uterine artery crosses over the ureter at the lateral fornix of the vagina ("water under the bridge" relationship). Therefore, during a surgical procedure of the uterus (e.g., hysterectomy) care should be taken to avoid injury or accidental ligation of the ureter.

e. Support of the uterus

- **Muscular support:** Pelvic diaphragm (levator ani)
- **Ligamentous support: (Fig. 8.19)** Pubocervical ligament, cardinal ligament (transverse cervical ligament), uterosacral ligament, broad ligament, and round ligament of the ovary.

Quiz: *What may result to the uterus if its support is weakened or compromised?*

Cervix

The cervix is the lower part of the uterus. It is divided into two parts: supravaginal and vaginal parts **(Fig. 8.5; Fig. 8.6)**. The cervical canal has two openings: internal os and external os. The external os opens into the vagina. The vaginal part of the cervix projects into the vagina and is surrounded by the vaginal fornix **(Fig. 8.5)**. The cervical canal contains numerous branched cervical glands that open into it **(Fig. 8.20)**. The lining epithelium of the cervix (cervical canal) undergoes transitional changes from the simple columnar epithelium in the endocervical canal to the stratified squamous epithelium near the external os. This region of epithelial transition is important clinically, as cervical smears (Papanicolaou or Pap smear) are taken from this region to screen for premalignant or malignant changes.

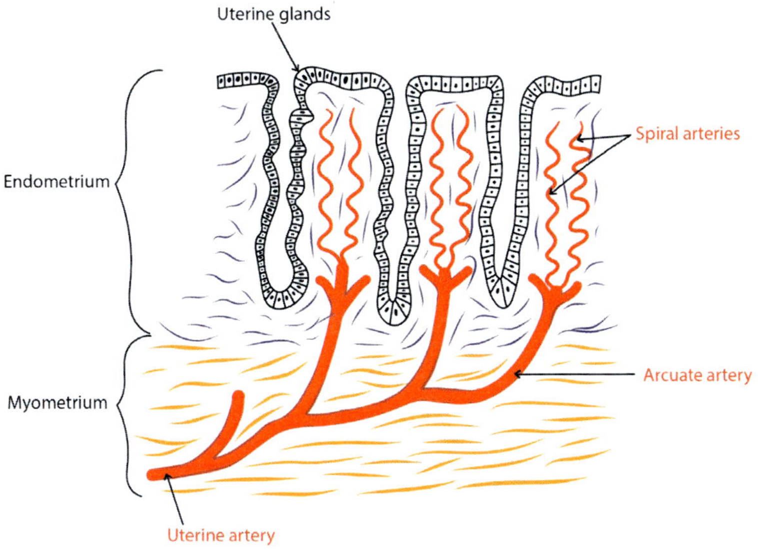

Figure 8.18. Uterus — arterial supply. The uterus is supplied by the uterine artery. It gives off the basal artery, arcuate artery, and then the spiral arteries. During monthly menstruation, the smooth muscles in the spiral arteries undergo spasms; as such, the ischaemic functional layer of the endometrium degenerates and is sloughed off.

Quiz: *Where does the uterine artery originate? What is the other artery that supplies the uterus?*

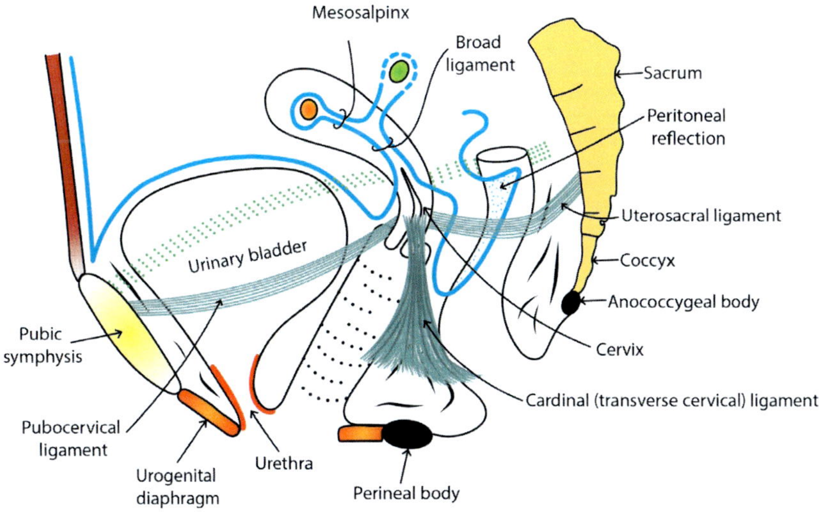

Figure 8.19. Support of the uterus. Showing the ligamentous support of the uterus. (1) Pubocervical ligament. (2) Cardinal ligament (transverse cervical ligament). (3) Uterosacral ligament. The broad ligament may also contribute to its support. Muscular support is by the pelvic diaphragm.

(A)

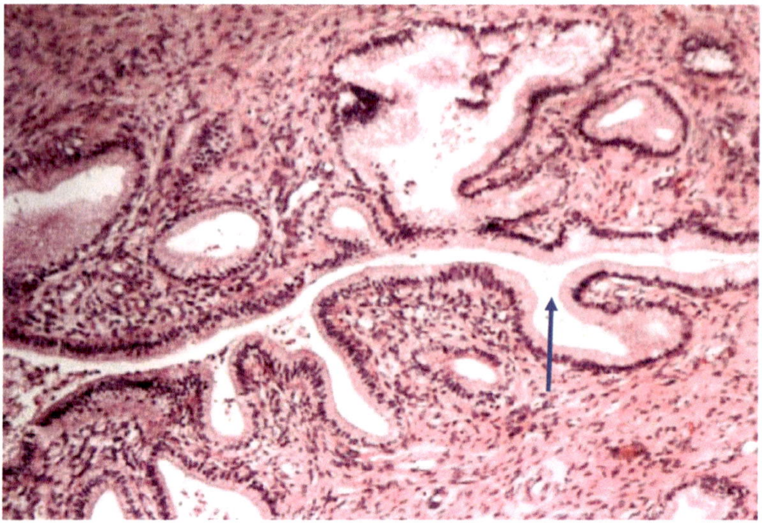

(B)

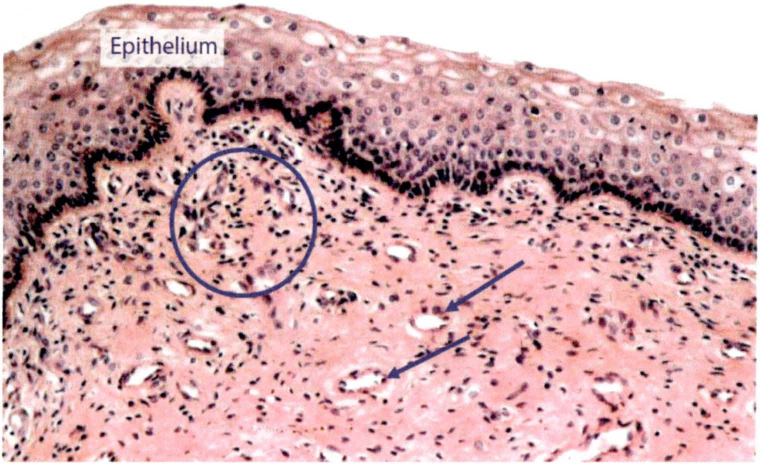

Figure 8.20. **(A) Cervix** — Cervical glands (arrow) are branched tubular glands that secrete mucus that helps protect against invading pathogens. Blockage of the glands may result in the formation of fluid-filled nabothian cysts (benign). (H&E stain.) **(B) Vagina** — The mucous membrane is lined by the stratified squamous epithelium (non-keratinized). The epithelial cells appear empty-looking because the rich glycogen in the cytoplasm was washed off during tissue preparation. The rich glycogen is for the production of lactic acid and maintenance of a low pH of the medium that may help prevent bacterial growth. Note the accumulation of lymphocytes (circled area) in the lamina propria beneath the epithelium. Arrows indicate sinus venosus. (H&E stain.)

Vagina

This is lined by the non-keratinized stratified squamous epithelium **(Fig. 8.20)**. The epithelial cells contain abundant glycogen, which is metabolized by normal vaginal flora to produce lactic acid. This maintains an acidic environment that helps prevent bacterial overgrowth. Deep to the epithelium is a layer of lamina propria with many lymphocytes. The vaginal wall consists of an inner circular and outer longitudinal layer of smooth muscle. Externally, there is a layer of skeletal muscle forming the sphincter vaginae.

Vulva (Fig. 8.21)

The vulva constitutes the external genitalia of the female. It is bounded laterally by the labia majora and labia minora with the clitoris located anteriorly. The urethral and vaginal openings open into the vestibule of the vulva. A pair of greater vestibular glands (Bartholin's glands) is located in the vestibule. The glands open on either side of the vaginal orifice and help in lubrication.

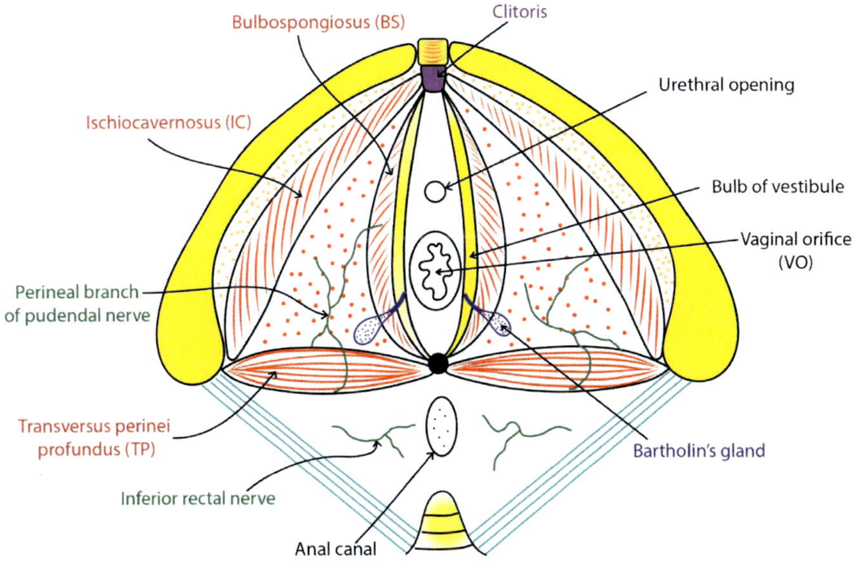

Figure 8.21. Vulva (external genitalia). It is bounded by the labia major and minor. Opening into it are the urethral opening and vagina (V). Greater vestibular gland (Bartholin's gland) opens at the side of the vaginal orifice (VO). There are three pairs of perineal muscles: ischiocavernosus (IC), bulbospongiosus (BS), and transversus perinei profundus (TP). Innervation is by the perineal branch of the pudendal nerve.

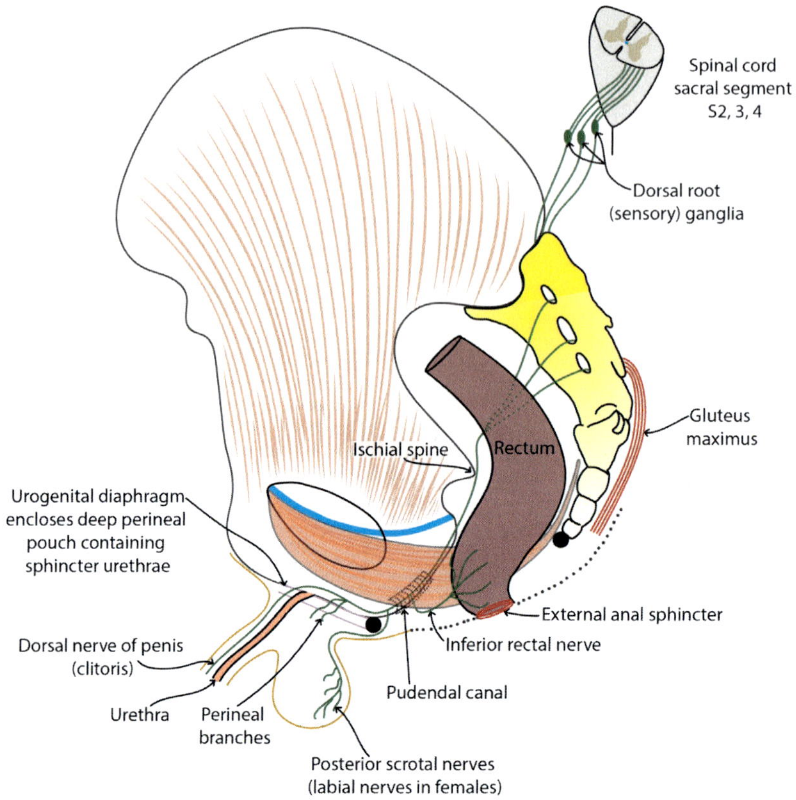

Figure 8.22. Pudendal nerve — its origin, course, and distribution. The nerve arises from the sacral nerve plexus with the root value (S2–4). It exits through the greater sciatic foramen below the piriformis. It then winds around the ischial spine and enters the pudendal canal medial to the ischial tuberosity. During its course, it gives off the inferior rectal nerve, dorsal nerve of the penis (clitoris), perineal nerves, posterior scrotal nerves (labial nerves in the female), etc. Note that the dorsal nerve of the penis pierces through the urogenital diaphragm, which encloses the deep perineal pouch.

PUDENDAL NERVE — ITS ORIGIN, COURSE, AND DISTRIBUTION (Fig. 8.22)

a. It arises from the sacral nerve plexus derived from the S2–S4 spinal cord segments.
b. It exits the pelvis through the greater sciatic foramen, inferior to the piriformis muscle. It then winds around the ischial spine and passes through the lesser sciatic foramen to enter the perineum. Subsequently, it travels along the lateral wall of the ischioanal fossa within the pudendal canal (Alcock's

canal), which lies medial to the ischial tuberosity. Within the canal, it is accompanied by the internal pudendal artery and vein.

c. Branches of the pudendal nerve innervate the anal canal and external genitalia. The branches consist of:
   - the inferior rectal nerve, innervating the anal canal and external anal sphincter,
   - perineal branches including posterior scrotal (or posterior labial) nerves and muscular branches innervating the muscles associated with the root of the penis (or clitoris), and
   - dorsal nerve of the penis (or clitoris), which provides sensory innervation to the external genitalia.

d. **Pudendal nerve block:** A pudendal nerve block may be performed via the lateral wall of the vagina during the second stage of labour. This procedure blocks the sensory supply to the lower vagina, perineum, and related structures, including the anal canal, thereby reducing pain during childbirth.

Pelvic Splanchnic Nerves

They arise from the sacral nerve plexus derived from the spinal cord segments S2–S4.

They contain parasympathetic nerve fibers that innervate the pelvic viscera, including the urinary bladder and the rectum. They also contribute to autonomic innervation of the erectile tissues of the penis (and clitoris), playing an important role in penile erection.

Chapter 9

MUSCULOSKELETAL SYSTEM

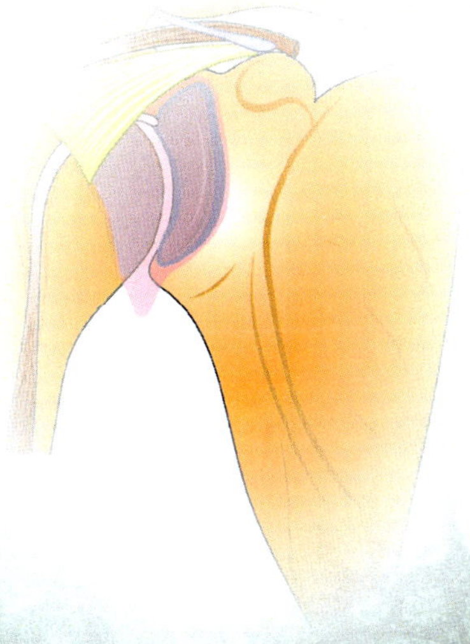

MUSCULOSKELETAL SYSTEM 1: UPPER LIMB AND BACK MUSCLES

The musculoskeletal system is primarily made up of bones, muscles, ligaments, tendons, and cartilage, providing a skeletal framework for the body and enabling movement.

GENERAL FEATURES

The upper limb is a highly specialized structure adapted for a wide range of motor activities, particularly precise and coordinated movements. This section summarizes the bones, muscles, innervation, arterial supply, venous drainage, and lymphatic drainage of the upper limb that contribute to movement.

A. **Movements of the Upper Limb:** The hand and forearm play a crucial role in prehensile functions involving various types of grip, including power grip, precision grip, pinch grip, and hook grip. These movements are essential for holding, grasping, and manipulating objects.

B. **Bones of the Upper Limb:** The upper limb consists of a skeletal framework made up of bones of varying shapes and sizes, enabling a wide range of movements. These bones articulate at multiple joints, which permit different degrees of mobility.

   The upper limb is connected to the axial skeleton via the pectoral (shoulder) girdle, which comprises the scapula (shoulder blade) and clavicle (collar bone). This arrangement provides structural support while allowing extensive mobility at the shoulder joint, including flexion, extension, abduction, adduction, medial and lateral rotation, circumduction, and elevation of the arm above the head.

C. **Muscles of the Upper Limb:** Movements of the bones of the upper limb and pectoral girdle are produced by coordinated actions of different muscle groups acting in synergy. For example, the flexor and extensor muscles of the forearm work in a coordinated manner to produce smooth movements such as flexion and extension at the wrist joint. Contraction of these muscles, which moves the upper limb, is under voluntary control.

D. Nerves of the Upper Limb: The muscles of the upper limb are innervated by nerves arising from the brachial plexus, which is derived from the anterior rami of spinal cord segments C5–C8 and T1. These nerves contain motor, sensory, and sympathetic fibers.

Injury to these nerves results in both motor and sensory deficits. Motor impairment may present as weakness (paresis) or complete loss of muscle function (paralysis), resulting in impaired joint movements. Sensory loss includes numbness over the skin and loss of proprioception. Furthermore, these nerves carry sympathetic nerve fibers, that supply the vascular smooth muscles and glands. Consequently, nerve injury can also affect blood vessel tone (causing vasodilation and warm skin), sweat gland activity (resulting in dry skin), and arrector pili muscle function.

E. Arteries of the Upper Limb: The main arterial supply to the upper limb originates from the subclavian artery. This continues as the axillary artery and then the brachial artery, which further divides into the radial and ulnar arteries to supply the distal parts of the upper limb (forearm and hand).

F. Venous Drainage of the Upper Limb: The venous drainage occurs through the superficial veins (cephalic vein and basilic vein) and the deep veins (brachial veins or venae comitantes of the accompanying artery). These veins drain into the subclavian vein, which returns blood to the right atrium of the heart via the superior vena cava.

G. Lymphatic Drainage of the Upper Limb: Lymph from the upper limb is carried by lymphatic vessels and passes through lymph nodes, particularly the axillary lymph nodes, where it is filtered before being returned to the venous circulation. Lymph nodes contain lymphocytes and macrophages (phagocytes), which play an essential role in immune defense.

BONES OF THE UPPER LIMB

These include the pectoral girdle (the clavicle and scapula) and the bones of the arm, forearm, wrist, and hand **(Fig. 9.1)**.

A. Clavicle (Fig. 9.1)

1. It is also called the collar bone. It is subcutaneous and can be palpated along its entire length.

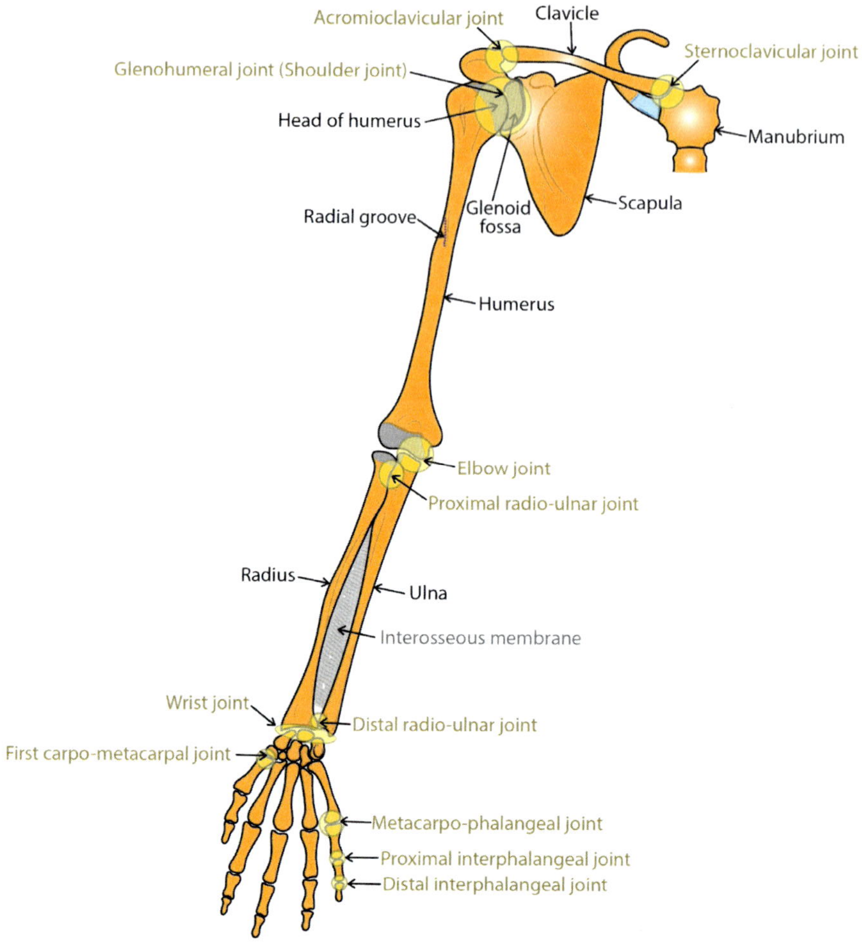

Figure 9.1. Bones and joints of the upper limb. The bones of the upper limb are attached to the trunk through the pectoral girdle comprising the clavicle and scapula. The medial end of the clavicle articulates with the manubrium via the sternoclavicular joint. Laterally, it articulates with the scapula at the acromioclavicular joint. The humerus articulates with the glenoid fossa (of the scapula), forming the shoulder (glenohumeral) joint. It articulates with the ulna and radius at the elbow joint. Note that the articulations between the proximal ends of the radius and ulna form the proximal radioulnar joint. Likewise, articulation also occurs between the distal ends of the radius and ulnar, forming the distal radioulnar joint. The distal ends of the ulna and the radius articulate with the proximal row of carpal bones at the wrist joint. Between the carpals and the metacarpals are the carpometacarpal joints. The metacarpals articulate with the proximal phalanx at the metacarpophalangeal joints. Between the phalanges are the interphalangeal joints.

2. It is S-shaped and its medial two-thirds is convex anteriorly, while the lateral one-third is concave anteriorly. The junction of the medial two-thirds and lateral one-third is the common site of fracture **(Fig. 9.2)**. Fractures at this site may potentially damage the underlying neurovascular bundles.
3. The medial end of the clavicle articulates with the manubrium of the sternum at the sternoclavicular joint; hence, it is called the sternal end of the bone.

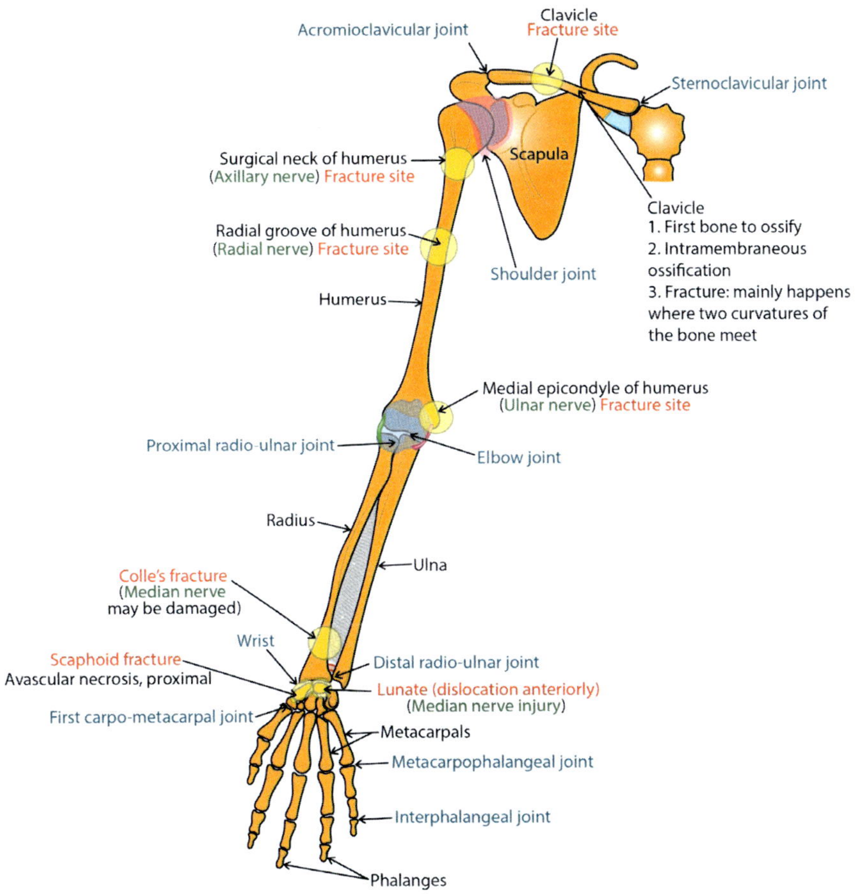

Figure 9.2. Common sites of bone fracture and joint dislocation in the upper limb. 1. Clavicle. Fracture at the junction between the lateral one-third and medial two-thirds. 2. Humerus. Fracture at the surgical neck, mid-shaft, and medial epicondyle. 3. Humerus. Dislocation (anterior) of the head of the humerus. 4. Medial epicondyle. 5. Radius. Fracture at its distal end, Colles' fracture. 6. Radius. Dislocation of the head involving the proximal radioulnar joint. 7 Scaphoid fracture. 8. Lunate dislocation. In most of the cases, the nerves closely related to the bones may be damaged.

4. The lateral end articulates with the acromion process of the scapula forming the acromioclavicular joint; hence, the lateral end is called the acromion end.
5. The clavicle is the first bone to begin ossification by intramembranous ossification. However, cartilage is found at both ends.
6. The clavicle acts as a strut, keeping the scapula and arm away from the trunk, thus allowing a greater range of movement.
7. The inferior surface of the medial part provides attachment for the subclavius muscle, which helps stabilize the clavicle.

B. Scapula (Fig. 9.1)

1. The scapula also called the shoulder blade, lies on the posterior aspect of the shoulder.
2. It is a triangular flat bone that provides attachment for many muscles.
3. Movements of the scapula greatly enhance the range of motion of the arm and contribute to overall upper limb mobility.
4. It has three borders: superior, lateral, and medial. The superior border has the suprascapular notch, which transmits the suprascapular nerve.
5. It has three angles: superior, inferior, and lateral. At the lateral angle is the glenoid fossa, which articulates with the head of the humerus forming the glenohumeral (shoulder) joint.
6. It has two surfaces: the ventral surface (subscapular fossa) and the dorsal surface. The dorsal surface is divided by the spine of the scapula into the supraspinous fossa and infraspinous fossa which provide attachment for the supraspinatus and infraspinatus muscles, respectively.

C. Humerus (Fig. 9.1; Fig. 9.2)

1. This is the only bone of the arm.
2. It is a long bone, consisting of the shaft (diaphysis) in the middle and two ends, the epiphyses. It develops through endochondral ossification.
3. The proximal end consists of the head which articulates with the glenoid fossa of the scapula to form the shoulder joint (glenohumeral joint). It also has the anatomical neck and the greater and lesser tuberosities (tubercles). The intertubercular (bicipital) groove, located between the tuberosities, accommodates the tendon of the long head of the biceps brachii.

4. The surgical neck lies between the head and the shaft and is a common site of fracture. The axillary nerve, which is closely related to this region, may be injured if surgical neck is fractured.
5. The shaft contains the radial groove along which the radial nerve winds around the humerus. This makes the nerve vulnerable in mid-shaft fractures of the humerus.
6. The distal end is expanded to form the lateral and medial epicondyles. The ulnar nerve passes posterior to the medial epicondyle.
7. The distal articular surface of the humerus includes the trochlea and capitulum. These articulate with the trochlear notch of the ulna medially and the head of the radius laterally, forming the humeroulnar and humeroradial joints, respectively. Together, they form the elbow joint.

D. Ulna (Fig. 9.1)

1. It is a long bone which develops through endochondral ossification.
2. Proximally, it has trochlea notch which is bounded anteriorly by the coronoid process and posteriorly by the olecranon process.
3. On lateral (radial) side of the ulna lies the radial notch which articulates with the head of the radius to form the proximal radioulnar joint.
4. The distal end of the ulna consists of the head and styloid process.
5. The head articulates with the ulnar notch on the radius distally, forming the distal radioulnar joint.
6. An intra-articular fibrocartilaginous disc (articular disc) is attached to the base of the styloid process and to the ulnar notch. This disc separates the synovial cavity of the distal radioulnar joint from that of the wrist joint.
7. The interosseous membrane (fibrous joint) spans between the shafts of the radius and ulna, connecting the two bones.

E. Radius (Fig. 9.1)

1. It is long bone that develops through endochondral ossification.
2. The head of the radius articulates superiorly with the capitulum of the humerus, forming the humeroradial joint.
3. The head of the radius articulates medially with the radial notch on the ulna, forming the proximal radioulnar joint.
4. Below the head is the neck and the radial tuberosity which provides attachment to the tendon of the biceps brachii muscle.

5. The distal end of the radius has a styloid process, which may be palpated on the lateral side of the wrist, just proximal to the anatomical snuff box.
6. Fracture of the distal radius (Colles' fracture) commonly occurs following a fall on an outstretched hand **(Fig. 9.2)**. The median nerve at the wrist may be affected in such injuries
7. Distally, the radius articulates with the proximal row of the carpal bones, scaphoid, and lunate, forming the wrist (radiocarpal) joint.

F. Carpal Bones (Fig. 9.1)

1. These bones form the wrist (carpus = wrist).
2. They enable the "cupping" of the hand, which is essential for various grips, such as holding a ball, tool, or pen.
3. The carpal bones are arranged in two rows: proximal and distal.
4. Proximal row carpal bones include the scaphoid, lunate, triquetrum and pisiform.
5. Distal row carpal bones include the trapezium, trapezoid, capitate and hamate.
6. A fall on an outstretched hand may cause a fracture of the scaphoid **(Fig. 9.2)**. Due to its distal-to-proximal blood supply, this can lead to avascular necrosis of the proximal fragment.
7. Such a fall may also result in anterior dislocation of lunate **(Fig. 9.2)**, which may compress the median nerve within the carpal tunnel (carpal tunnel syndrome).
8. The joints between the carpal bones are known as intercarpal joints.

G. Metacarpal bones (Fig. 9.1)

1. They are small, long bones. Each has a base (proximal), shaft, and head (distal). The heads form the visible knuckles.
2. They articulate distally with the proximal phalanges, forming the metacarpophalangeal (MCP) joints.

H. Phalanges (Fig. 9.1)

1. Each digit has three phalanges: proximal, middle, and distal.
2. The thumb is an exception as it has only two phalanges: proximal and distal.
3. The joints between phalanges are called interphalangeal (IP) joints.

CLASSIFICATION AND TYPES OF JOINTS

A joint is the articulation between two or more bones. Some joints produce varying degree of movements (e.g, shoulder) and some allow little or no movement (e.g., skull sutures).

Based on the bone articulations and movements, joints are classified into different types:

A. Cartilaginous Joint (Synchondrosis)

Bones are connected by cartilage.

1. **Primary cartilaginous joint:** It is found between the epiphysis and diaphysis of a long bone. Examples:
   - The epiphyseal plate in the humerus. The two bones are united by a hyaline cartilage plate and do not produce any movement.
   - The first costochondral joint (Thoracic cage) which does not produce movement.
2. **Secondary cartilaginous joint:** The articular cartilage is of the hyaline type, with an intervening fibrocartilage disc between the two articular surfaces. Examples:
   - pubic symphysis and
   - intervertebral joint.

   Limited movements are possible at these joints.

B. Fibrous Joints (Syndesmosis): The bones are joined by fibrous connective tissue. Examples:

- Sutures of the skull (frontal and parietal bones)
- Interosseous membrane between the radius and ulna

There is limited or no movement.

C. Synovial Joints (Diarthrosis): This allows a wide range of movement.

A typical synovial joint is characterized by synovial cavity between the articular bones containing the synovial fluid, which serves as a lubricant (rich in hyaluronic acid). These joints are classified based on shape, articulations and axis of movements. Examples:

1. **Ball and Socket type (Multiaxial joint)**
   - Example: Shoulder joint.
   - Movements: Flexion, extension, abduction, adduction, medial rotation, lateral rotation, and circumduction.

2. **Hinge type (uniaxial joint)**
    - Example: Elbow joint and interphalangeal joint
    - Movements: Flexion and extension.
3. **Condyloid (Ellipsoid) type (Biaxial joint)**
    - Example 1: Wrist joint. Movements: Flexion, extension, abduction (radial deviation), and adduction (ulnar deviation).
    - Example 2: Metacarpophalangeal joints. This joint is between the head of the metacarpal and the proximal phalanx. Movements: Flexion, extension, abduction, and adduction of the medial four fingers. Abduction is the movement of fingers away from an imaginary line along the middle of the middle finger, while adduction is a movement toward an imaginary line in the middle finger. This joint also allows limited rotation.
4. **Pivot type (Uniaxial joint)**
    - Example: Proximal and distal radioulnar joints.
    - Movements: Pronation and supination. The axis of movement extends from the head of the radius to the base of the styloid process of the ulna.
5. **Saddle type**
    - Example: First carpometacarpal joint (thumb). This is the joint of the thumb between the trapezium and first metacarpal.
    - Movements: Flexion and extension, adduction and abduction, and opposition.

JOINTS OF THE UPPER LIMB

A. Glenohumeral (Shoulder) Joint (Fig. 9.3)

1. **Type:** It is a synovial joint of the ball and socket type, allowing a wide range of movements.
2. **Articulations:** The head of the humerus (about one-third of a sphere) articulates with the glenoid cavity of the scapula, which is shallow and cup-shaped). Both articular surfaces are covered by a layer of hyaline cartilage (articular cartilage) which is devoid of perichondrium.
3. **Stability & Mobility:** The shallow glenoid cavity permits maximum mobility of the joint, making it the most mobile joint in the body. However,

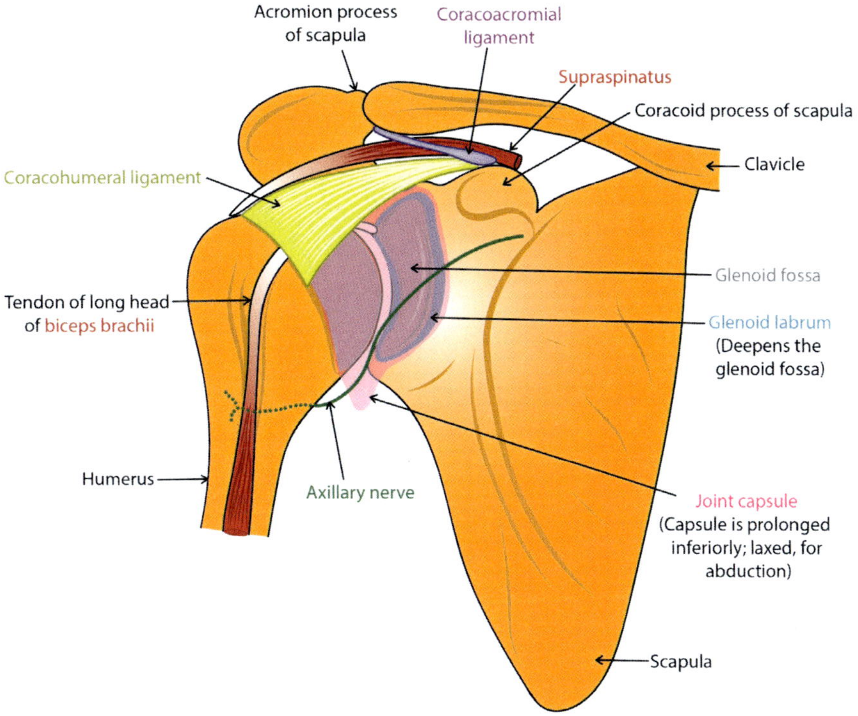

Figure 9.3. Shoulder joint (Glenohumeral joint). The bony articulation is between the glenoid fossa and the head of the humerus. The glenoid fossa is deepened by the glenoid labrum. The joint is surrounded by a layer of capsule, which is prolonged inferiorly. The joint is reinforced superiorly by the rotator cuff, coracohumeral and coracoacromial ligaments, and the long head of the biceps and anteriorly by the glenohumeral ligament (not shown).

the greater mobility reduces the stability. The glenoid cavity is deepened by the glenoid labrum, a fibrocartilaginous rim, making the joint more stable.

4. **Capsule:** The joint is covered by a layer of fibrous capsule (dense irregular connective tissue), which is attached to the articular margins of the glenoid fossa medially and to the anatomical neck laterally. Inferiorly, the capsule is laxed, allowing greater range for abduction.
5. **Ligaments:** The main ligaments stabilizing the joint are:
   - Glenohumeral ligaments (superior, middle, inferior): reinforce anterior aspect of the joint.
   - Coracohumeral ligament: strengthens superior aspect of the joint.

- Coracoacromial ligament: forms an arch preventing superior displacement of the joint.

Additionally, the long head of biceps tendon also contributes to stabilization of the joint.

6. **Rotator cuff:** The rotator cuff is formed by the fused tendons of supraspinatus, infraspinatus, teres minor, and subscapularis. It stabilizes the joint by holding the head of the humerus within the glenoid cavity.
7. **Innervation:** The shoulder joint is innervated by the axillary nerve, suprascapular nerve, and musculocutaneous nerve. These nerves provide motor innervation to the muscles, sensory innervation (pain, temperature, and touch) to the capsule, ligaments, and associated bursae and proprioception for detection of the joint position.

   Axillary nerve innervates the capsule covering the shoulder joint and winds around the surgical neck of the humerus and innervates the muscles that move the joint (e.g., deltoid, teres minor). It also innervates the joint itself (capsule, ligament) as well as the skin over the joint (upper lateral cutaneous nerve of arm).
8. **Movements (Fig. 9.5; Fig. 9.6):**
   - Flexion (arm moves forward): Coracobrachialis, pectoralis major (clavicular head), anterior fibers of the deltoid, and biceps brachii (weak action).
   - Extension (arm moves backward): Latissimus dorsi, teres major, long head of triceps, and posterior fibers of the deltoid.
   - Abduction (arm moves away from the body): Supraspinatus (initiates abduction first 15°) and deltoid (continues abduction from 15° to 90°).
   - Adduction (arm moves toward the body): Pectoralis major, latissimus dorsi and teres major
   - Medial rotation (internal rotation): Subscapularis, pectoralis major, and teres major.
   - Lateral rotation (external rotation): Infraspinatus and teres minor.
   - Circumduction (arm moves in a "cone-shaped" pattern): Combined movements produced by sequential action of flexors, extensors, abductors, and adductors.
9. **Applied anatomy:** Dislocation of the shoulder joint is most commonly anterior (anteroinferior dislocation). It typically occurs when the arm is

fully abducted and laterally rotated and may result in axillary nerve injury. In addition, the axillary nerve is vulnerable to injury if the surgical neck of the humerus is fractured (**Fig 9.2**).

B. Elbow Joint (Fig. 9.4)

1. It is a synovial joint of the hinge type, allowing uniaxial movement, flexion and extension.
2. In this joint, articulations occur between the trochlea of the humerus and trochlea notch of the ulna and between the capitulum of the humerus and the head of the radius.
3. Articular surfaces are lined by a layer of hyaline cartilage.
4. The synovial cavity of the elbow joint communicates with that of the proximal radioulnar joint.
5. The joint is covered by a joint capsule and strengthened by ulnar and radial collateral ligaments.
6. **Flexion:** Brachialis and biceps brachii (assisted by brachioradialis).
7. **Extension:** Triceps brachii (main muscle) and anconeus.
   Quiz: *Where is the axis of flexion and extension of the elbow joint?*

C. Radioulnar Joints (Proximal and Distal) (Fig. 9.4)

1. They are synovial joints of pivot type, responsible for the pronation and supination of the forearm. The axis of movement is a line extending from the head of the radius proximally to the base of the styloid process of the ulna distally.
2. **Proximal radioulnar joint:** Articulation occurs between the head of the radius and radial notch of the ulna. The synovial cavity of the proximal radioulnar joint communicates with the elbow joint. The joint is enclosed by a fibrous capsule. A strong annular ligament encircles the head of the radius and is attached to the anterior and posterior margins of the radial notch of the ulna. Annular ligament holds the radial head in position while allowing rotation during pronation and supination. Dislocation of the head of the radius (pulled elbow) is common in children.
   Quiz: *Why is it so?*
3. **Movements at proximal radioulnar joint:**
   - **Pronation:** Pronator teres and pronator quadratus
   - **Supination:** Biceps brachii (powerful when elbow is flexed) and supinator

4. **Distal radioulnar joint:** Articulation occurs between head of the ulna and ulnar notch on the radius. The synovial cavity of the distal radioulnar joint is separated from the wrist joint by an articular disc (fibrocartilage) which is attached to the base of ulnar styloid process and ulnar notch of the radius.

D. Wrist Joint (Fig. 9.4)

1. It is a synovial joint of ellipsoid (condyloid) type.
2. Articulations occurs between distal end of the radius and the articular disc with the proximal row of the carpal bones including scaphoid, lunate, and triquetrum.
3. **Movements:**
   - Flexion: Muscles that flex the wrist, e.g., flexor carpi radialis (lateral) and flexor carpi ulnaris (medial).
   - Extension: Muscles that extend the wrist, e.g., extensor carpi radialis longus and brevis and extensor carpi ulnaris.
   - Abduction (radial deviation): Flexor carpi radialis and extensor carpi radialis longus and brevis act together.
   - Adduction (ulnar deviation): Flexor carpi ulnaris and extensor carpi ulnaris act together.
   - Circumduction: Combined movements produced by sequential action of flexors, extensors, abductors, and adductors at the wrist joint.

E. First Carpometacarpal Joint (Fig. 9.4)

1. Articulation occurs between the trapezium and the first metacarpal bone.
2. It is a modified saddle type of synovial joint.
3. **Movements:**
   - Flexion: Flexor pollicis brevis and flexor pollicis longus (assist)
   - Extension: Extensor pollicis longus, extensor pollicis brevis and abductor pollicis longus
   - Abduction: Abductor pollicis longus and abductor pollicis brevis
   - Adduction: Adductor pollicis
   - Opposition: Opponens pollicis (assisted by flexor pollicis brevis and abductor pollicis brevis)
4. Muscles of the thenar eminence include flexor pollicis brevis, abductor pollicis brevis, and opponens pollicis.

Joints of the upper limb

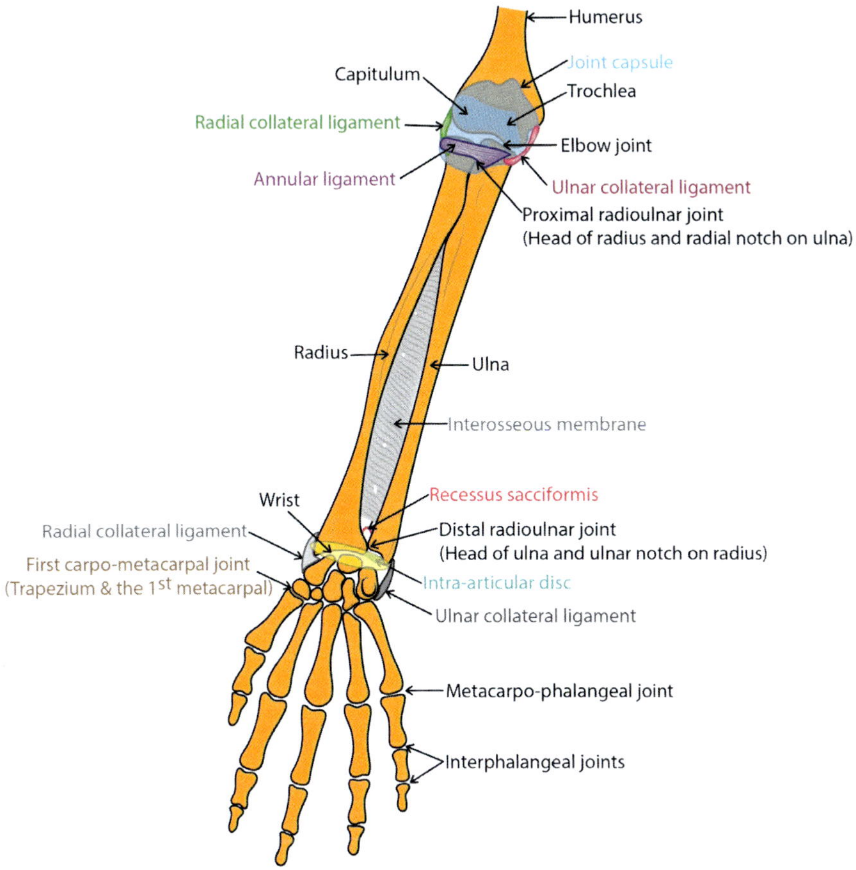

Figure 9.4. Elbow joint, radioulnar joint, and wrist joint. 1. The elbow joint is between the trochlea and capitulum of the humerus above and below with the trochlear notch (ulna) and the capitulum (radius). It is reinforced medially by the ulnar collateral ligament and laterally by the radial collateral ligament. 2. Proximal radioulnar joint is between the head of the radius and the radial notch. It is supported by the annular ligament. 3. Distal radioulnar joint is between the head of the ulna and the ulnar notch on the radius. Inferiorly, it is separated from the wrist joint by an intra-articular disc. 4. Wrist joint. The articulation is between the distal end of the radius and intra-articular disc with the proximal row of the carpal bones: scaphoid, lunate, and triquetral. **First carpometacarpal joint, metacarpophalangeal joint, and interphalangeal joint.**

1. The first carpometacarpal joint is between the trapezium and the first metacarpal.
2. Metacarpo-phalangeal joints are between the metacarpals and the proximal phalanges.
3. Interphalangeal joints are between the phalanges. The radius and ulna are held together by the interosseous membrane.

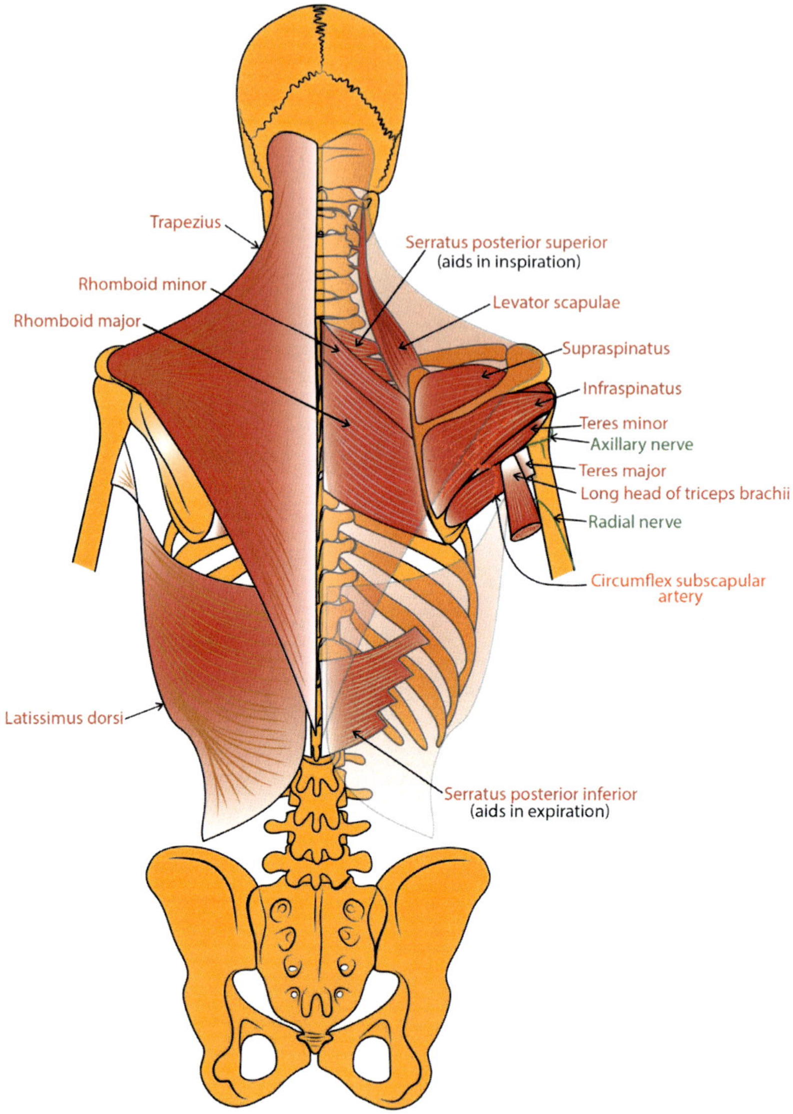

Figure 9.5. Muscles of the scapular region. These include the muscles that elevate/raise the scapula: trapezius, levator scapulae, serratus posterior superior, and rhomboids. On the dorsal surface of the scapula are the supraspinatus, infraspinatus, teres minor, and teres major. Also showing is the latissimus muscle, which arises from the lumbar fascia and lumbar vertebrae and is inserted to the bicipital groove of the humerus.

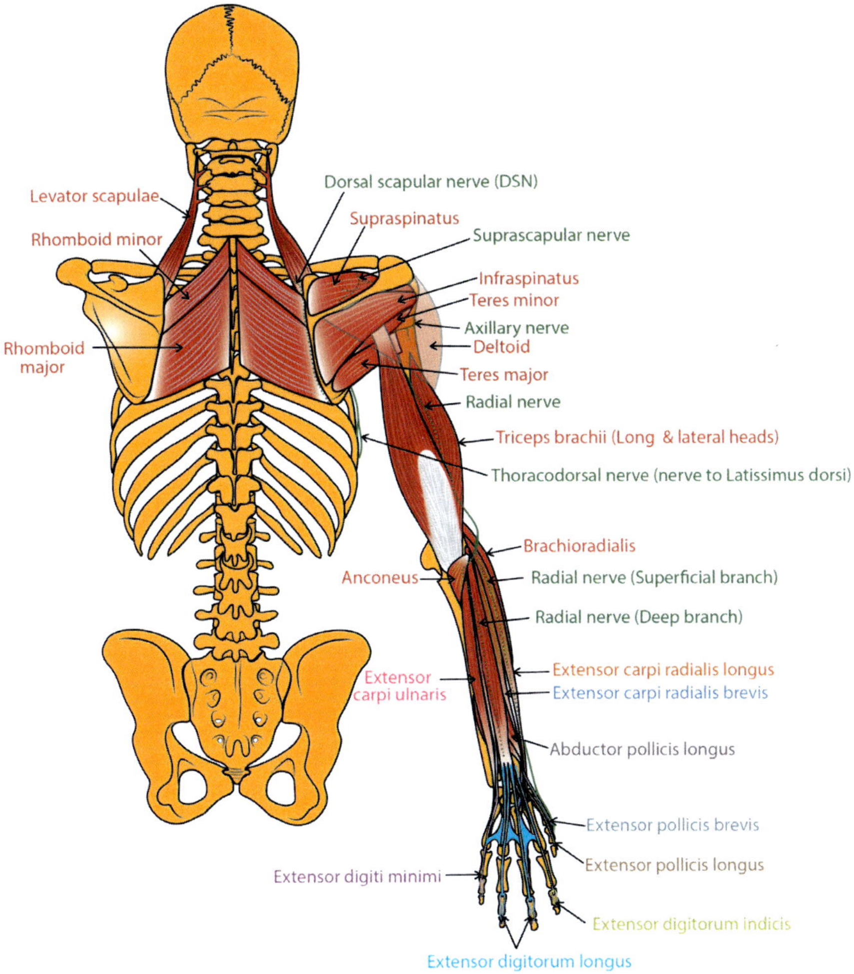

Figure 9.6. Muscles that move the scapula and shoulder joint and extend the arm, forearm, and hand and their innervation.

1. Muscles that arise from the midline and attach to the medial border of the scapula comprise the levator scapulae (dorsal scapular nerve, DSN) and rhomboids (dorsal scapular nerve, DSN). The muscles move the scapula.
2. Muscles crossing over and acting on the shoulder joint include the deltoid (axillary nerve), supraspinatus (suprascapular nerve), infraspinatus (suprascapular nerve), teres minor (axillary nerve), and teres major (subscapular nerve).
3. Muscles at the back of the arm are the long/lateral/medial heads of the triceps (radial nerve). They are extensors of the elbow joint.
4. Muscles at the back of the forearm include the extensors of the wrist joint and digits: the extensor carpi ulnaris (deep radial nerve), extensor digitorum and extensor carpi radialis longus (radial nerve), and brevis (deep radial nerve). They arise from the lateral epicondyle of the humerus (common extensor origin). In addition to these are the brachioradialis and supinator, which are also supplied by the radial nerve.

F. Metacarpophalangeal Joint (Fig. 9.4)

1. This joint is commonly known as knuckles. Articulation occurs between the head of the metacarpal bone and base of the proximal phalanx.
2. It is a synovial joint of condyloid type.
3. **Movements:**
   - Flexion: Lumbricals and interossei (assisted by long flexors including flexor digitorum superficialis and flexor digitorum profundus)
   - Extension: Extensor digitorum
   - Abduction: Dorsal interossei
   - Adduction: Palmar interossei
   - Circumduction: present but limited

G. Interphalangeal Joint (Fig. 9.4)

1. It is a synovial joint of hinge type.
2. **Movements:**
   - Flexion: Flexor digitorum superficialis (proximal interphalangeal joint) and flexor digitorum profundus (distal interphalangeal joint)
   - Extension: Extensor digitorum via extensor expansion (assisted by lumbricals and interossei)
3. The interossei also help in extension because they are inserted into the dorsal digital expansion (extensor hood), allowing them to extend the IP joints while primarily acting at MCP joints.

MUSCLES OF THE UPPER LIMB AND BACK

The muscles of the upper limb are described based on regions including pectoral, scapula, shoulder, arm, forearm, and hand.

A. Pectoral Region

This is the chest region. The muscles of this region move the arm (humerus), scapula, and clavicle.

1. **Pectoralis major:** Medial rotates and adducts the arm. Its clavicular head assists in flexion of arm.
2. **Pectoralis minor:** It draws the scapula forward and downward (protraction).
3. **Subclavius:** It stabilizes the medial end of the clavicle and protects sternoclavicular joint.

B. Scapular Region (Fig. 9.5; Fig. 9.6)

This is the back region over the scapula. Muscles arising from the axial skeleton (vertebrae and ribs) are attached to the medial border, spine, and inferior angle of the scapula. Movements of the scapula by these muscles enhance the range of movement (ROM) of the arm.

1. **Elevation of the scapula:** Trapezius (superior fibers), levator scapulae, and rhomboids (major and minor).
2. **Depression of the scapula:** Trapezius (inferior fibers). It is also assisted by pectoralis minor.
3. **Protraction of the scapula:** Serratus anterior and pectoralis minor.
4. **Retraction of the scapula:** Rhomboids (major and minor) and trapezius (middle fibers)

The serratus anterior has eight muscular slips that originate from the upper eight ribs and are inserted along the anterior surface of the medial border and inferior angle of the scapula **(Fig. 9.7)**. It rotates the scapula pivoting at the acromioclavicular joint (between the lateral end of the clavicle and acromion process). The serratus anterior muscle **(Fig. 9.7)** helps to hold the scapula firmly against the chest wall and also assists in deep inspiration. It is innervated by the long thoracic nerve (C5, 6, 7). Injury to the long thoracic nerve causes weakness of serratus anterior muscle, resulting in a "winged scapula".

Quiz: *Why is the long thoracic nerve prone to injury?*

C. Shoulder Region (Fig. 9.5; Fig. 9.6)

The shoulder muscles originate from the scapula and are inserted to the humerus. The main action of these muscles is to move the arm at the shoulder joint. These muscles and their action are described in the section of joints of the upper limb.

D. Arm (Fig. 9.6; Fig. 9.8)

The muscles of the arm are divided into anterior (flexor) and posterior (extensor) compartments, separated by the medial and lateral intermuscular septa. Proximally, these muscles attach to the scapula or humerus and distally insert into the ulna or radius. Muscles that cross the elbow joint produce flexion or extension, with some also acting on the shoulder and radioulnar joints. The anterior

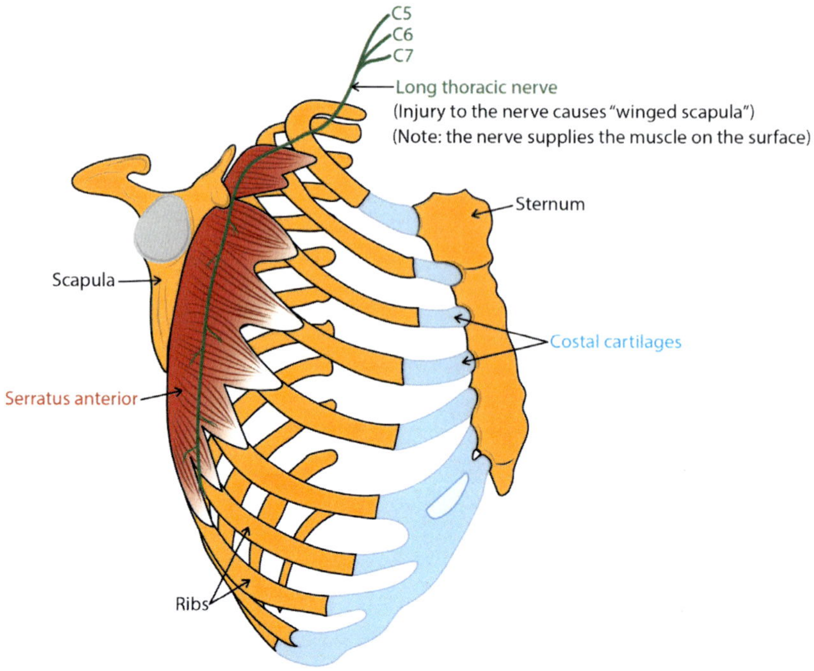

Figure 9.7. Serratus anterior and long thoracic nerve. The muscle arises from the medial border of the scapula. It has eight muscle slips, with most of the slips attached to its inferior angle. Anteriorly, the muscle slips are attached to the upper eight ribs. As such, the serratus anterior muscle keeps the scapula to the chest wall. It also helps with the upward rotation of the scapula in tandem with the upper fibers of the trapezius. It is supplied by the long thoracic nerve that arises from the ventral rami of the C5, 6, 7 spinal cord segments. It descends over the superficial surface of the serratus anterior muscle and supplies it. Injury to the nerve causes a "winged scapula."

compartment consists of the biceps brachii, brachialis, and coracobrachialis while the posterior compartment contains triceps brachii.

1. **Biceps brachii:** It has two heads, long head and short head. The tendon of the long head originates from supraglenoid tubercle of the scapula, passes through capsule of the shoulder joint (intracapsular, but extrasynovial) and intertubercle groove of the humerus. The short head originates from the coracoid process of the scapula. Both long and short heads join together to form a fusiform belly and is attached laterally on the radial tuberosity. The bicipital aponeurosis extending from the distal tendon of biceps brachii blends with the antebrachial fascia medially.

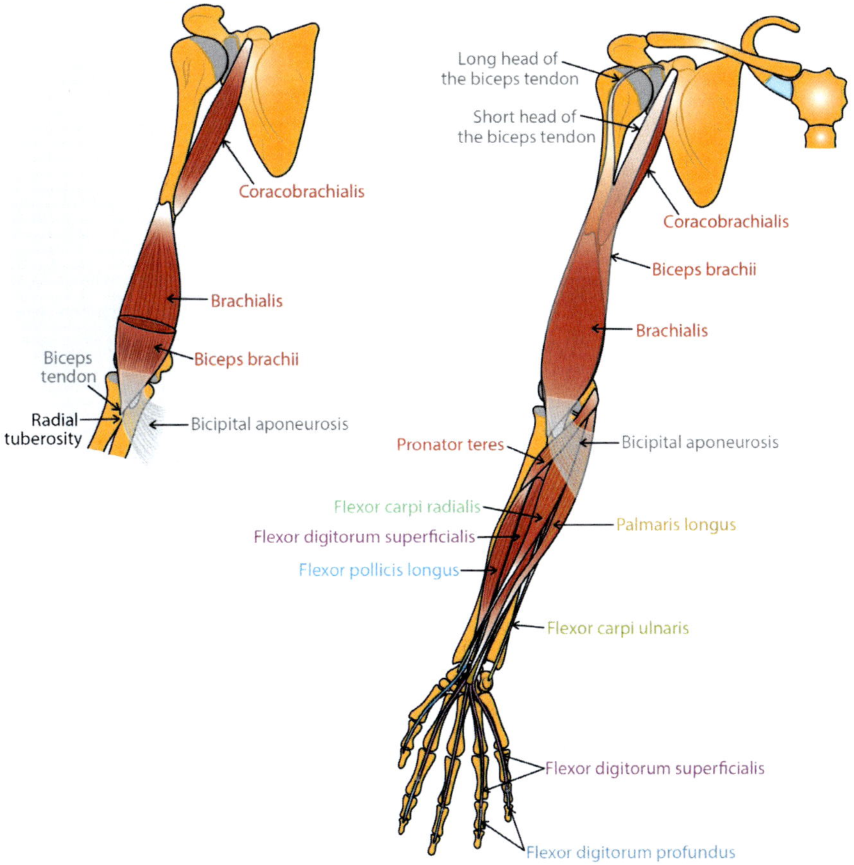

Figure 9.8. Muscles (flexors) of the arm and forearm and their innervation. In the arm are the coracobrachialis (musculocutaneous nerve), biceps brachii (long and short heads), and brachialis. In the forearm, the superficial layer muscles include the pronator quadratus (median nerve), flexor carpi radialis (median nerve), palmaris longus (median nerve), and flexor carpli ulnaris (ulnar nerve). The flexor muscle deep to them is the flexor digitorum superficialis (median nerve). In the deepest layer of the forearm are the flexor pollicis longus (median nerve) and flexor digitorum longus (median/ulnar nerves). Between the radius and ulna at the lower part is the pronator quadratus (median nerve).

Actions: Flexion at the elbow joint and supination of the forearm (powerful when elbow is flexed). It also helps in the flexion at the shoulder joint (weak action).

2. **Coracobrachialis:** It originates from the coracoid process of the scapula and inserts into the medial surface of the humerus.
   Action: Flexion and adduction (weak action) of the arm.

3. **Brachialis:** It originates from the distal half of the anterior surface of the humerus and is inserted into the coronoid process and ulnar tuberosity of the ulna.
   Action: Flexion at the elbow joint.
4. **Triceps brachii:** It has three heads: long, lateral, and medial heads. The long head arises from the infraglenoid tubercle of the scapula, while the lateral and medial heads arise from the posterior surface of the humerus above and below the radial groove, respectively. All three heads converge into a common tendon that inserts onto the olecranon process of the ulna.
   Action: It is the main extensor of the elbow joint. Its long head also assists in extension and adduction of the arm at the shoulder joint (weak action). The lateral head is the common site for an intramuscular injection.

   ***Quiz* 1:** *What is the histology of the tendon? Does it have a nerve supply?*
   ***Quiz* 2:** *What is the biceps tendon reflex? Describe its neural pathway.*
   ***Quiz* 3:** *What is the segmental innervation of the muscles that flex and extend the elbow joint?*

E. Forearm

The muscles are divided into anterior (flexor and pronator) and posterior (extensor and supinator) compartments. The flexor muscles arise mainly from the common flexor origin (medial epicondyle of the humerus), while the extensor muscles arise mainly from the common extensor origin (lateral epicondyle of the humerus).

Basis of nomenclature for the muscles of forearm:

The nomenclature of forearm muscles is based on their location, function, and depth. Muscles are named according to their position relative to the forearm bone; for example:

- *Flexor carpi ulnaris lies on the ulnar side, while flexor carpi radialis lies on the radial side.*
- *The term "flexor digitorum" refers to muscles that flex the medial four digits (digits 2–5), whereas "flexor pollicis longus" specifically denotes the muscle that flexes the thumb (pollex).*
- *Additionally, the terms "superficialis" and "profundus" describe the relative depth of the muscles, with superficialis indicating a more superficial position and profundus indicating a deeper location within the forearm.*

1. Anterior compartment of the forearm (Flexors and pronators) (Fig. 9.8; Fig. 9.9)

The flexor muscles are inserted into the carpals, metacarpals, and phalanges and produce flexion of the wrist joint, metacarpophalangeal (MCP), and interphalangeal (IP) joints. They also contribute to pronation of the forearm. The muscles are arranged in three layers: superficial, intermediate, and deep.

a. Superficial layer (Fig. 9.8; Fig. 9.9)

i. **Flexor carpi radialis:** It crosses both elbow and wrist joints and is inserted into the base of 2nd metacarpal. It mainly flexes the wrist joint and abducts the wrist (radial deviation).

ii. **Flexor carpi ulnaris:** It originates from the medial epicondyle (humeral head) and olecranon of the ulna (posterior side) and crosses both elbow and wrist joints. It is inserted into the carpal bones (pisiform and hamate) and base of the 5th metacarpal bone. It mainly flexes the wrist joint and adducts the wrist (ulnar deviation).

iii. **Pronator teres (Fig. 9.8):** It has two heads originating from the medial epicondyle of the humerus and coronoid process of ulna and is inserted into the lateral surface of the midshaft of the radius. It pronates the forearm and assists in elbow flexion (weak action).

iv. **Palmaris longus:** It is inserted into the palmar aponeurosis. It flexes at the wrist joint (weak action) and tense the palmar aponeurosis.
Quiz: *What is the histology of "aponeurosis"?*

b. Intermediate layer (Fig. 9.8; Fig. 9.9)

i. **Flexors digitorum superficialis:** It originates from the medial epicondyle (humerus), coronoid process (ulna) and proximal radius and is inserted into the sides of middle phalanges of medial four digits (2–5). It flexes the medial four digits at the proximal interphalangeal joints. It also assists in flexion at metacarpophalangeal joints and wrist joint (weak action).

c. Deep layer (Fig. 9.8; Fig. 9.9)

i. **Flexor digitorum profundus:** It arises from the proximal ulna and interosseous membrane and is inserted into the base of distal phalanges of medial four digits. It flexes the distal interphalangeal joints and is important in power (hook) grip.

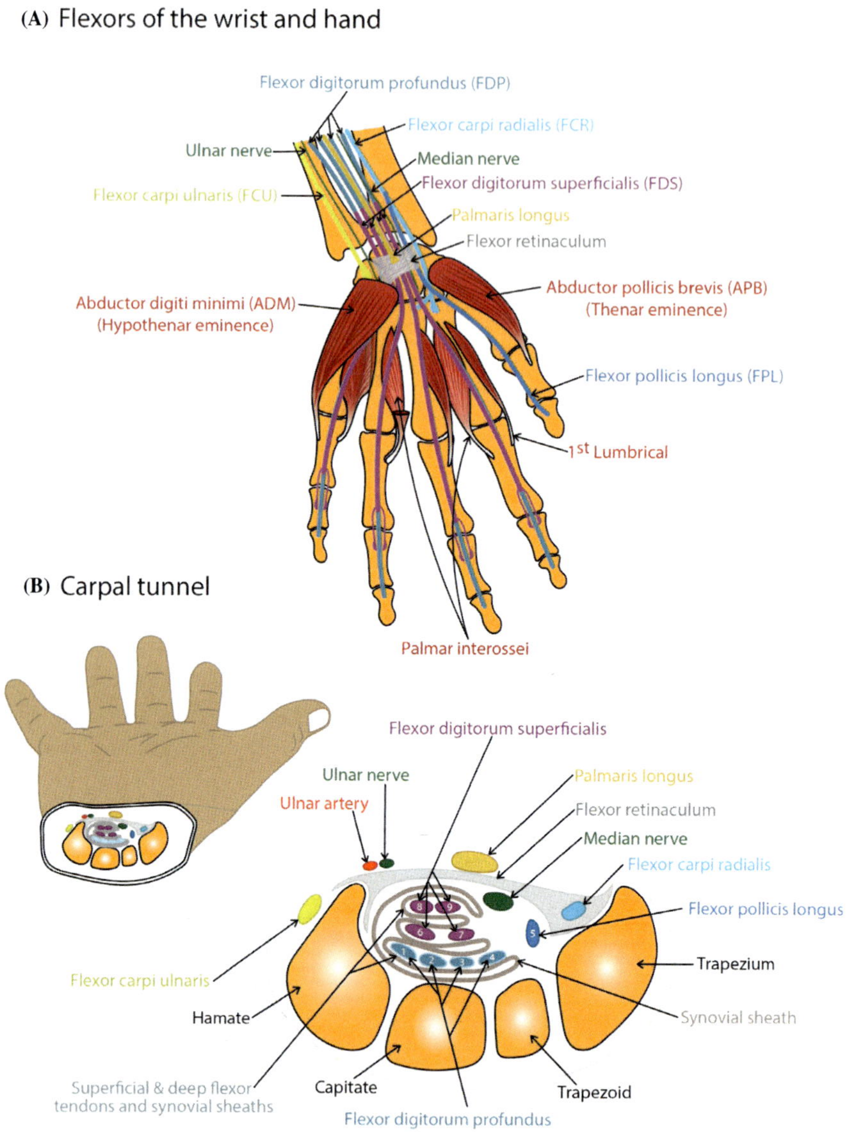

Figure 9.9. A. flexors of the forearm.
They are mainly to flex the wrist (carpus) and the five digits:

1. Flexor carpi radialis (FCR). It is inserted to the base of the second and third metacarpals.
2. Flexor carpi ulnaris (FCU). It is inserted to the pisiform bone.
3. Palmaris longus. It is inserted in the palm as the palmar aponeurosis.
4. Flexor digitorum superficialis (FDS). It is inserted to the intermediate phalanx.
5. Flexor digitorum profundus (FDP). It is inserted to the distal phalanx.
6. Flexor pollicis longus (FPL). It is inserted to the distal phalanx of the thumb.

ii. **Flexor pollicis longus:** It arises from anterior surface of the radius and interosseous membrane and is inserted into the base of distal phalanx of the thumb. It flexes the interphalangeal joint of the thumb.

iii. **Pronator quadratus:** It is a deep muscle extending from the distal ulna to distal radius. It is the primary pronator of the forearm, especially during slow movements.

2. Posterior compartment of the forearm (Extensors and Supinator) (Fig. 9.6; Fig. 9.10)

The extensor muscles of the forearm produce extension at the wrist, metacarpophalangeal (MCP), and interphalangeal (IP) joints. They arise mainly from the common extensor origin (lateral epicondyle of the humerus), along with contributions from the posterior surfaces of the radius and ulna. Their tendons are inserted into the carpals, metacarpals, and the respective distal phalanges through the dorsal digital expansion (extensor hood). This extensor hood also receives insertions from short muscles, lumbricals and interossei. The muscles in the posterior compartment are arranged in superficial and deep layers.

a. Superficial layer

i. Brachioradialis (Fig. 9.6): It arises from the lateral supracondylar ridge of the humerus and is inserted into distal end of the radius. It is a strong flexor of the elbow joint in the mid-prone position. It does not act on the wrist joint.

ii. Extensor carpi radialis longus: It arises from the lateral supracondylar ridge of the humerus and is inserted into the base of 2nd metacarpal. It extends and abducts the wrist.

iii. Extensor carpi radialis brevis: It arises from the lateral epicondyle of the humerus and is inserted into the base of 3rd metacarpal. It extends and abducts the wrist.

Figure 9.9. *(Continued on facing page)* In the hand are muscles of the thenar eminence, which includes the abductor pollicis brevis (APB), opponens pollicis, etc. In the hypothenar eminence are the abductor digiti mimini (ADM), etc. In the middle are the lumbricals and palmar interossei (between the metacarpals).
B. Carpal tunnel — a section through the carpal bones. Note that all flexors pass through the carpal tunnel except for the palmar aponeurosis and FCU. Also passing through the tunnel is the median nerve, excluding the ulnar nerve and ulnar artery. **C**: capitate; **H**: hamate; **T**: trapezoid; **TP**: trapezium.

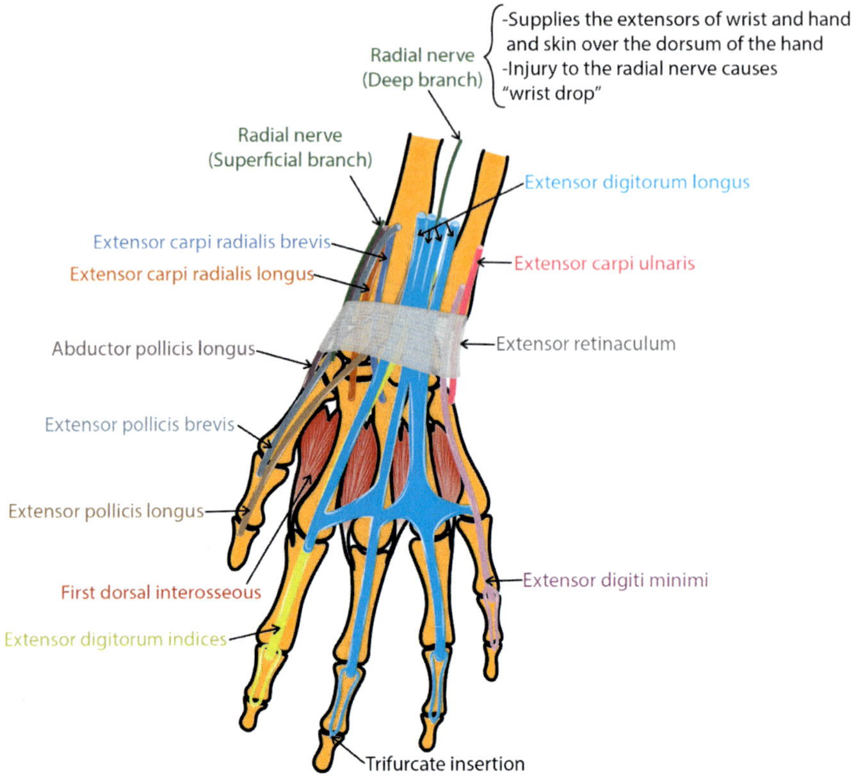

Figure 9.10. Extensors of the forearm — insertion. The tendons of the extensors are grouped into six compartments: 1. Abductor pollicis longus and brevis are inserted to the radial side of the proximal phalanx of the first digit. 2. Extensor carpi radialis longus and brevis are inserted to the base of the second and third metacarpals. 3. Extensor pollicis longus is inserted to the distal phalanx of the first digit. 4. Extensor digitorum longus is inserted to the intermediate phalanx of the medial four digits as dorsal digital expansion. 5. Extensor digiti minimi is inserted to the fifth digit. 6. Extensor carpi ulnaris is inserted to the base of the fifth metacarpal. All the tendons are held to the underlying bones by the extensor retinaculum. The extensors are supplied by the radial nerve via the posterior interosseus nerve (deep radial nerve).

iv. **Extensor digitorum:** It arises from lateral epicondyle and is inserted into extensor expansions of medial four digits (2-5). It extends digits from 2nd to 5th at the MCP joints and assists in interphalangeal extension.

v. **Extensor digiti minimi:** It arises from the lateral epicondyle of the humerus and is inserted into extensor expansion of the 5th digit. It extends the 5th digit (little finger) and assists in interphalangeal extension.

vi. **Extensor carpi ulnaris:** It arises from the lateral epicondyle of the humerus and posterior ulna and is inserted into the base of the 5th metacarpal. It extends and adducts the wrist.

b. Deep layer

i. **Supinator:** It arises from the lateral epicondyle of the humerus, radial collateral ligament, annular ligament, and supinator crest of ulna, and is inserted into the proximal radius (**Fig. 9.8**). It supinates the forearm, acting with the biceps brachii.

ii. **Abductor pollicis longus:** It arises from the posterior surfaces of the ulna, radius and interosseous membrane and is inserted into the base of the 1st metacarpal. It abducts and extends the thumb at the carpometacarpal joint.

iii. **Extensor pollicis longus:** It arises from the posterior surface of the midshaft of ulna and interosseous membrane and is inserted into the base of the distal phalanx of the thumb. It mainly extends the IP joint of the thumb and assists in extension at the metacarpophalangeal and carpometacarpal joints.

iv. **Extensor pollicis brevis:** It arises from the posterior surface of distal radius and interosseous membrane and is inserted into the base of the proximal phalanx of the thumb. It extends the metacarpophalangeal joint and assists in extension at the carpometacarpal joint.

v. **Extensor indicis:** It arises from the posterior surface of the distal ulna and interosseous membrane and is inserted into the extensor expansion of the 2nd digit. It extends the 2nd digit (index finger) independently and assists in wrist extension.

***Quiz* 1:** *What is meant by the "mid-prone" position of the forearm?*

***Quiz* 2:** *Where is the axis of pronation and supination?*

F. Hand

Thenar Muscles (Fig. 9.9A)

These are small intrinsic muscles that originate from the carpal bones and flexor retinaculum. They mainly produce movements at the carpometacarpal joint (between the trapezium and first metacarpal), which is a synovial joint of saddle type (biaxial and rotation), the metacarpophalangeal joint, and the interphalangeal joint of the thumb (1st digit) **(Fig. 9.11)**. The thenar muscles include:

1. **Flexor pollicis brevis**: It arises from the tubercle of trapezium and flexor retinaculum and is inserted into the base of proximal phalanx of the thumb. It produces flexion at the metacarpophalangeal joint of the thumb.
2. **Abductor pollicis brevis:** It arises from the tubercles of scaphoid, trapezium and flexor retinaculum and is inserted into the base of proximal phalanx of the thumb. It produces abduction at the carpometacarpal joint of the thumb.
3. **Opponens pollicis:** It arises from the tubercle of trapezium and flexor retinaculum and is inserted into 1st metacarpal of the thumb. It produces opposition of the thumb towards the other fingers at the carpometacarpophalangeal joint.
4. **Adductor pollicis:** It has 2 heads, the oblique and transverse heads which arise from capitate and 2nd and 3rd metacarpals and insert into the proximal phalanx of the thumb. It produces adduction of the thumb.

Thenar muscles including flexor pollicis brevis, abductor pollicis brevis and opponens pollicis form thenar eminence which are mainly responsible for opposition of the thumb.

Muscles of the hypothenar (Fig. 9.9A)

The hypothenar muscles move the little finger **(Fig. 9.11)**.

1. **Flexor digiti minimi brevis:** It arises from hook of hamate and flexor retinaculum and is inserted into the proximal phalanx of the little finger (5th digit). It produces flexion of little finger at metacarpophalangeal joint.
2. **Abductor digiti minimi:** It arises from the pisiform and tendon of flexor carpi ulnaris and is inserted into the proximal phalanx of the little finger (5th digit). It produces abduction of the little finger at metacarpophalangeal joint.
3. **Opponens digiti minimi:** It arises from hook of hamate and flexor retinaculum and is inserted into the 5th metacarpal. It produces opposition at 5th carpometacapal joint (little finger).

Short intrinsic muscles of the hand (Fig. 9.9; Fig. 9.10)

1. **Lumbricals:** They arise from the tendons of flexor digitorum profundus and insert into the dorsal digital expansion on the radial side (extensor

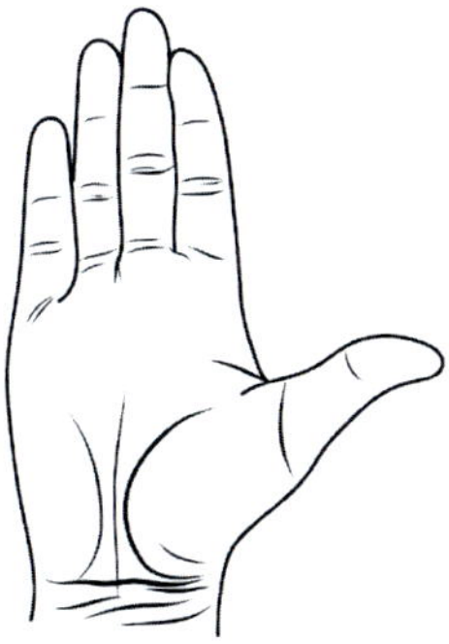

Extension - Away from the plain of palm
Extensor pollicis longus (Radial nerve)
Extensor pollicis brevis (Radial nerve)

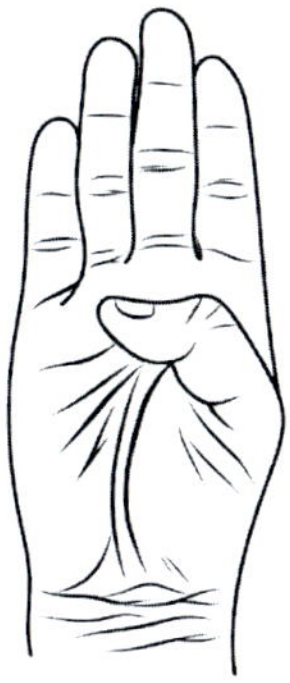

Flexion - Across the plain of palm
Flexor pollicis brevis (Median nerve)

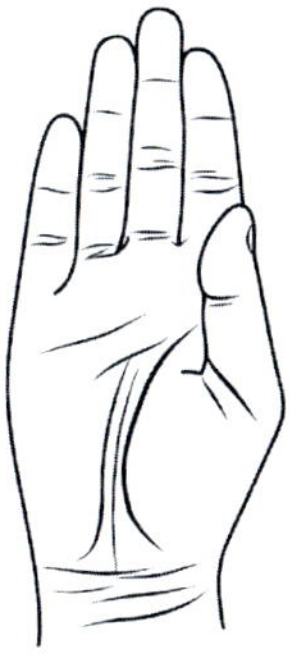

Adduction
Adductor pollicis (Ulnar nerve)

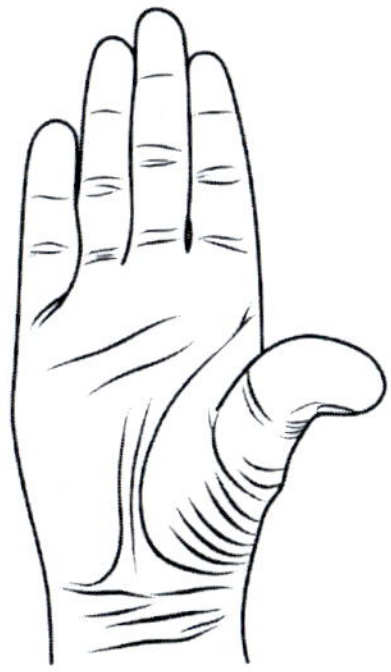

Abduction - Right angle to the plain of palm
Abductor pollicis longus (Radial nerve)
Abductor pollicis brevis (Median nerve)

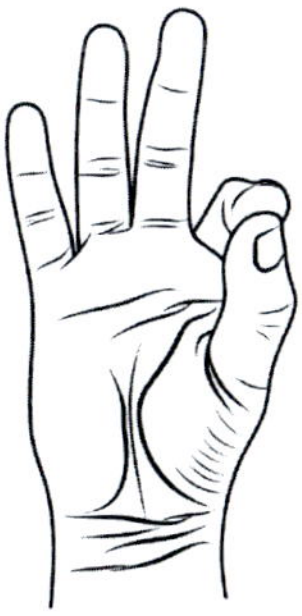

Opposition - Precision grip
Opponens pollicis (Median nerve)

Figure 9.11. Movements of the thumb. Showing the muscles involved in different movements of the thumb and their nerve supply.

expansion). They flex the fingers at the metacarpophalangeal joints and extend them at the interphalangeal joints.

2. **Palmar interossei:** They arise from the contiguous sides of the 2nd, 4th & 5th metacarpals and insert into base of proximal phalanges and extensor expansions. They adduct the index, ring, and little fingers toward an imaginary line along the long axis of the middle finger.
3. **Dorsal interossei:** They are bipennate muscles, arising from the adjacent sides of two metacarpals. They insert into base of proximal phalanges and extensor expansions. They abduct the index, middle, and ring fingers away from an imaginary line along the long axis of the middle finger.

G. Flexors at the Wrist

Flexor retinaculum and carpal tunnel (Fig. 9.9)

The flexors acting on the fingers and thumb pass through the carpal tunnel before reaching their insertion. The flexor retinaculum (a strong fibrous tissue) forms the roof of the carpal tunnel spanning the anterior aspect of the wrist. It is attached to the carpal bones as follows:

- Laterally: Trapezium and scaphoid
- Medially: Hamate and pisiform.

The concavity formed by the carpal bones together with the flexor retinaculum (roof) convert the osseofibrous passage into the "carpal tunnel". The following tendons with their synovial sheaths and the median nerve pass through the tunnel:

1. Four tendons of flexors digitorum superficialis
2. Four tendons of flexors digitorum profundus
3. One tendon of flexor pollicis longus and
4. Median nerve

Clinical anatomy

Inflammation of the synovial sheaths of the flexor tendons within the carpal tunnel (e.g., due to tenosynovitis or synovitis) increases the pressure inside this confined space. Because the carpal tunnel is rigidly bounded by carpal bones and the flexor retinaculum, any swelling reduces available space and compresses the median nerve. Compression of the median nerve leads to the clinical condition known as Carpal Tunnel Syndrome.

Arteries of the Upper Limb (Fig. 9.12)

Origin and course of the subclavian and brachial arteries (Fig. 9.12A)

1. The subclavian artery is the main artery supplying the upper limb. The right subclavian artery is a branch of the brachiocephalic trunk, while the left subclavian arises directly from the arch of the aorta.

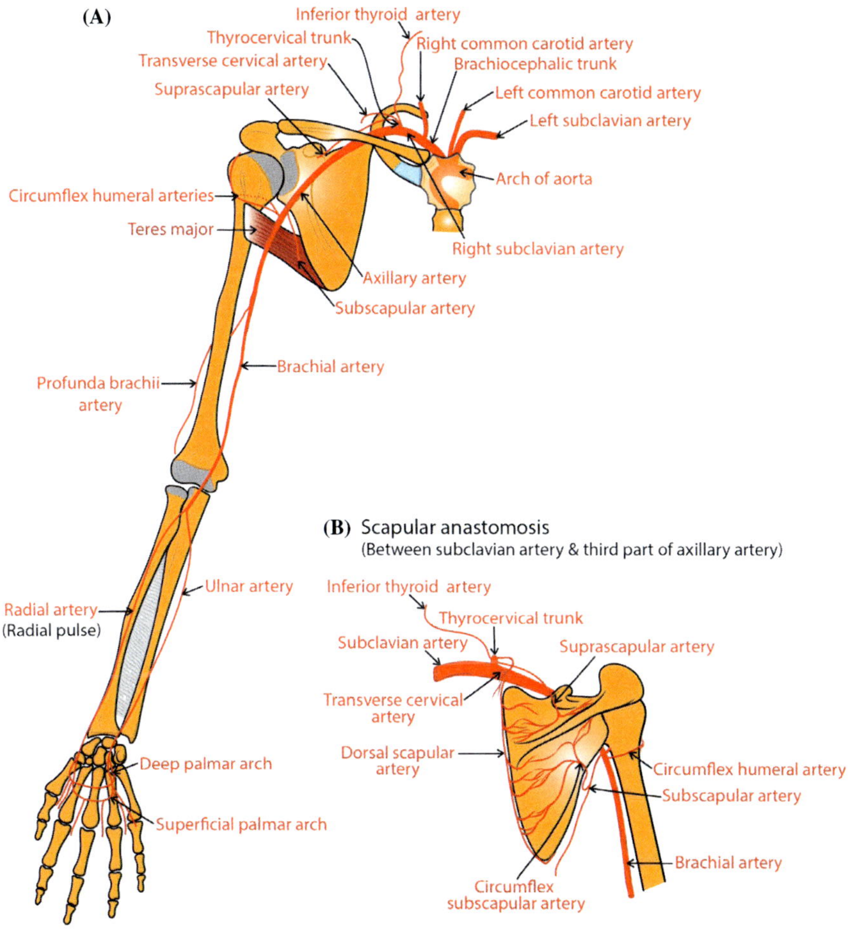

Figure 9.12. Arteries of the upper limb. **(A)** The main source of arterial supply is the subclavian artery. It crosses over the first rib and continues as the axillary artery till the lower border of the teres major. After this, it continues as the brachial artery, which divides into the ulnar and radial arteries in the forearm. The ulnar artery gives rise to the superficial palmar arch; the radial artery gives rise to the deep palmar arch. From the palmar arches are the digital arteries. **(B)** The scapular anastomosis is formed by the suprascapular artery, dorsal scapular artery (both from the thyrocervical trunk), and the subscapular artery (from the axillary artery).

2. The subclavian artery crosses over the first rib and continues as the axillary artery at the lateral border of the first rib.
3. At the inferior border of the teres major muscle, the axillary artery becomes the brachial artery.
4. The brachial artery descends along the medial aspect of the arm and gives off the profunda brachii artery (deep artery of the arm).
5. In the upper arm, the brachial artery lies medial to the humerus, while distally it lies anterior to the humerus within the cubital region.
6. In the cubital fossa, the brachial artery bifurcates into the radial and ulnar arteries, which descend along the lateral (radial) and medial (ulnar) aspects of the forearm, respectively.
7. The ulnar artery enters the hand anterior to the flexor retinaculum (palm) and forms the superficial palmar arch, which gives rise to the common palmar digital arteries, further dividing into digital arteries.
8. The radial artery passes through the anatomical snuff box, then enters the palmar surface between the first dorsal interosseous muscle to form the deep palmar arch, giving rise to palmar metacarpal arteries.

Distribution

1. The subclavian artery, through its branches (i.e., thyrocervical trunk) supplies the scapular and shoulder regions.
2. The axillary artery and its branches, including the humeral circumflex arteries, supply the pectoral region, axilla and scapular/shoulder regions.
3. The brachial artery and its main branch, profunda brachii artery (deep artery of the arm), supply the arm.
4. The radial and ulnar arteries supply the elbow region, forearm and hand, contributing to arterial anastomoses around the elbow and forming the palmar arches in hand.

Applied Anatomy

1. Subclavian artery may be compressed against the first rib to control severe bleeding in the upper limb.
2. Brachial artery is commonly used for measuring blood pressure using a sphygmomanometer.

3. *Scapular anastomosis* **(Fig. 9.12B):** This links branches of the subclavian artery (e.g., suprascapular artery) with branches of the third part of the axillary artery (e.g., subscapular artery). It provides collateral circulation between the subclavian artery and brachial artery, if the axillary artery is compressed, occluded, or ligated, maintaining blood flow to the upper limb.
4. The radial pulse may be palpated at the distal forearm, on the anterior aspect of the radius, lateral to the tendon of flexor carpi radialis.
5. The radial artery is commonly cannulated for arterial access (e.g., angiography or angioplasty).

   Quiz: *Describe the passage for the cannula to reach the coronary arteries in this invasive procedure.*
6. Superficial palmar arch can be surface marked as a curved line across the palm at the level of the distal border of the fully extended thumb.

Veins of the Upper Limb (Fig. 9.13)

1. The upper limb is drained by both superficial and deep veins.
2. The deep veins accompany the arteries as venae comitantes (e.g., radial, ulnar, and brachial veins).
3. Superficial veins include the cephalic vein and basilic vein.
4. The cephalic vein arises from lateral part of the dorsal venous network of the hand (near the anatomical snuff box). It ascends along the lateral side of the forearm and arm, passes through the deltopectoral groove, and drains into the axillary vein.
5. The basilic vein originates from the medial part of the dorsal venous network, ascends on the medial side of the forearm and arm, pierces the deep fascia in the mid-arm, and joins the brachial veins to form the axillary vein at the lower border of the teres major muscle.
6. In the cubital fossa, the median cubital vein connects the cephalic and basilic veins, forming an important superficial venous communication.
7. The veins contain valves, which facilitate unidirectional blood flow toward the heart and assist venous return, especially against gravity.

Applied anatomy

The median cubital vein is the most commonly used site for venepuncture.

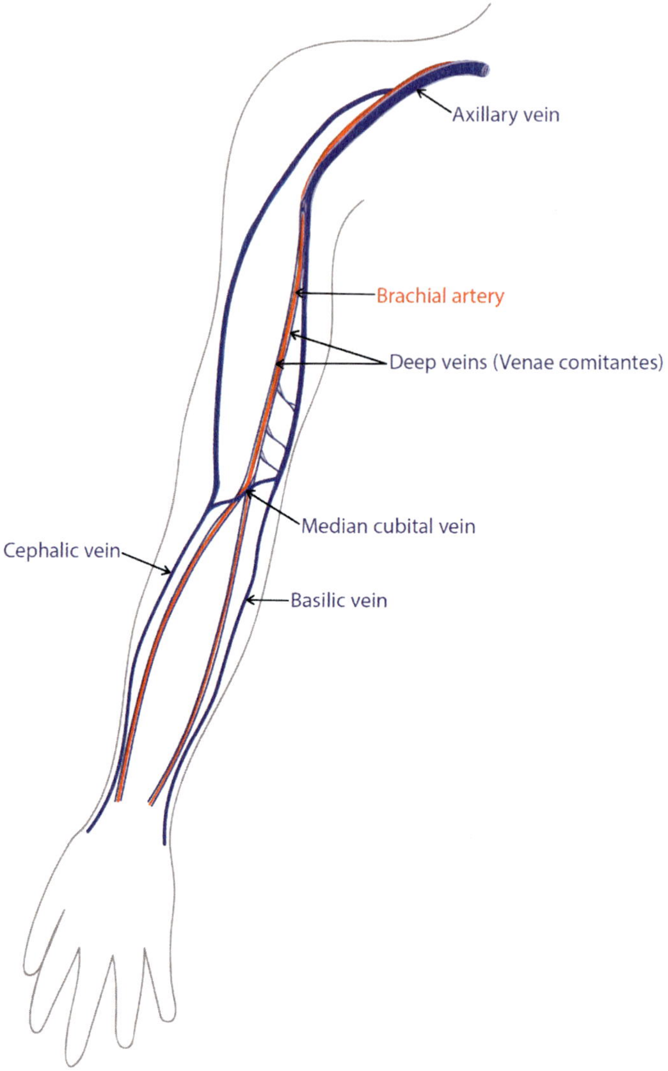

Figure 9.13. Venous drainage of the upper limb. The drainage is by both superficial and deep veins. The main superficial veins are the cephalic vein (which begins at the anatomical "snuff box") and the basilic vein, which begins from the medial side of the forearm. The cephalic vein drains into the axillary vein after passing through the deltopectoral groove. The basilic vein drains into the venae comitantes (brachial veins) of the brachial artery and ultimately drains into the axillary vein. The median cubital vein connects the cephalic and basic veins across the cubital fossa. The deep venous drainage of the hand and forearm follows the arteries.

Brachial nerve plexus (Fig. 9.14)

1. The brachial nerve plexus provides both motor and sensory innervation to the upper limb as well as contributions to the pectoral, shoulder, and scapular regions.
2. The brachial nerve plexus is a bundle of nerves that originate from the anterior (ventral) rami of spinal nerves C5-C8, T1.
3. The plexus begins in the root of the neck, passes between the anterior and middle scalene muscles, and continues into the axilla. During its course, it is organized into roots (C5-T1), trunks (upper, middle, lower), divisions (anterior and posterior), cords (lateral, medial, posterior) and terminal branches (nerves).
4. The brachial nerve plexus gives rise to several nerves to supply muscles, joints, and skin, for example:
   a. Long thoracic nerve originates from the spinal root (C5–C7)
   b. Suprascapular nerve originates from the upper trunk.
   c. Musculocutaneous nerve originates from the lateral cord.
   d. Ulnar nerve originates from the medial cord.
   e. Medial nerve originates from the lateral & medial cords.
   f. Axillary and radial nerves originate from the posterior cord.

Nerves of the Upper Limb

1. **Long thoracic nerve (Fig. 9.15):** It arises from the anterior (ventral) rami of C5–C7 and innervates the serratus anterior muscle which holds the scapula against the thoracic wall. Injury to the nerve results in a "winged scapula" where the inferior angle of the scapula protrudes posteriorly, especially when pushing against resistance.
2. **Suprascapular nerve (Fig. 9.15):** It arises from the upper trunk (C5, 6) and innervates the supraspinatus which initiates abduction of the shoulder joint and infraspinatus which acts as a lateral rotator of the shoulder joint.
3. **Axillary nerve (Fig. 9.15; Fig. 9.16):** It arises from the posterior cord (C5, C6) of the brachial plexus and passes posteriorly beneath the shoulder joint capsule. It then winds around the posterior aspect of the surgical neck of the humerus through the quadrangular space. It supplies motor fibers to

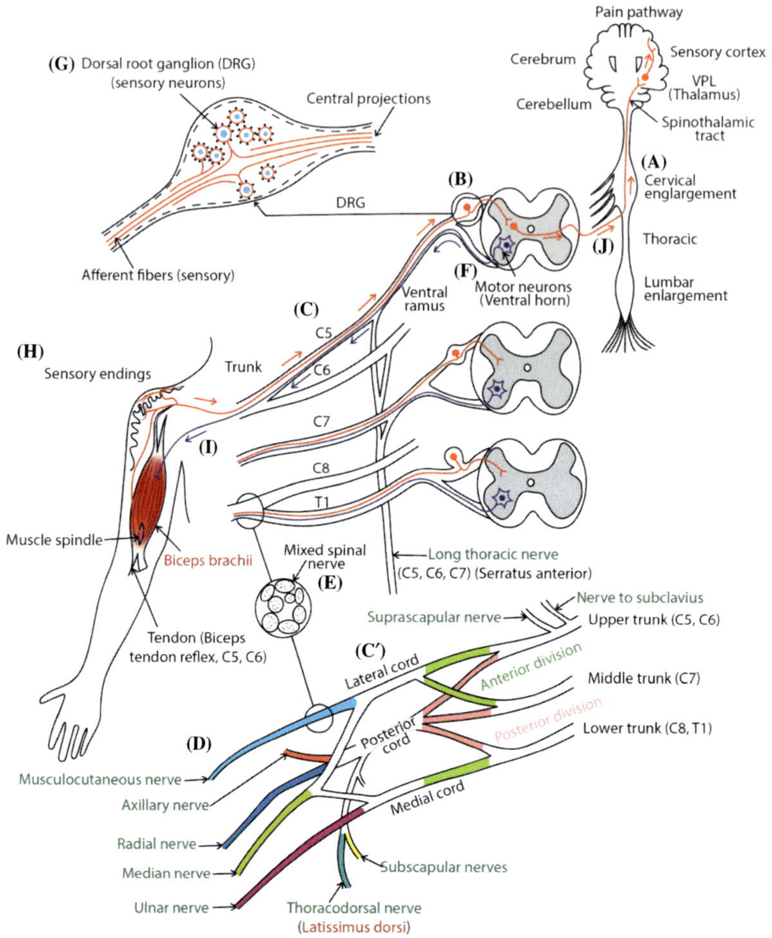

Figure 9.14. Brachial nerve plexus — its origin, organization, and distribution. The plexus is formed by the spinal nerves of the cervical and thoracic segments (C5, 6, 7, 8, T1) of the spinal cord. Note the cervical cord enlargement at this level **(A)**. Each spinal nerve is attached to the side of the cord by the dorsal and ventral roots (rootlets), conveying the sensory and motor fibers, respectively **(B)**. The ventral rami of C5–8/T1 unite and reorganize among themselves, forming the different parts of the brachial plexus — rami, trunks, cords, divisions, and nerves **(C, C′)**. The nerves **(D)** originate from different parts of the brachial nerve plexus (musculocutaneous, radial, median, ulnar, and long thoracic nerves) and, therefore, are composed of a mixture of sensory and motor fibers **(E)**. The sensory fibers (representing the peripheral process of the sensory neurons) supply the skin, muscle spindle **(H)**, joint capsule, etc., while the motor fibers (axons) supply the muscles **(I)** of the upper limb for various motor activities (contraction) (follow the direction of blue arrows). Note that the cell body of the sensory fibers (afferent fibers) is housed in the dorsal root ganglion (DRG) **(B)**, while the cell body of the motor fiber (axons) is localized in the ventral horn of the spinal cord of the above-named spinal cord segments **(F)**. Note that the sensory signal (e.g., pain) is conducted to the brain via the DRG — spinothalamic tract (crossed tract) — thalamus (VPL) — sensory cortex (follow the red arrows) **(J)**.

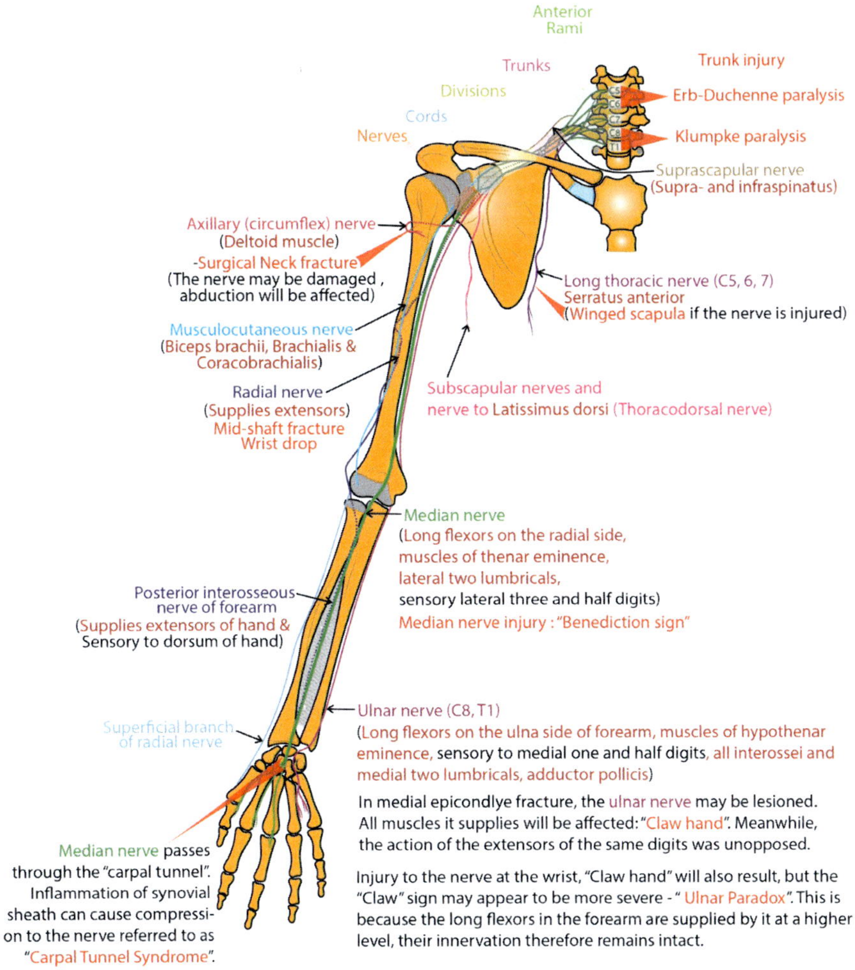

Figure 9.15. Nerves of the upper limb. 1. Long thoracic nerve (from C5, 6, 7 rami). 2. Suprascapular nerve (from the upper trunk). 3. Axillary nerve (from the posterior cord). 4. Radial nerve (from the posterior cord). 5. Musculocutaneous nerve (from the lateral cord). 6. Median nerve (from the lateral and medial cords). 7. Ulnar nerve (from the medial cord). 8. Subscapular nerves (from the posterior cord). (*Refer to the text for a more detailed description of the nerves.*)

deltoid and teres minor muscles and sensory innervation to the shoulder joint capsule and the skin over the lateral aspect of the shoulder joint.

In accordance with Hilton's law, the nerve supplying a joint also supplies the muscles moving the joint and the skin overlying it. Injury to the axillary nerve due to fracture of the surgical neck of the humerus results in weakness

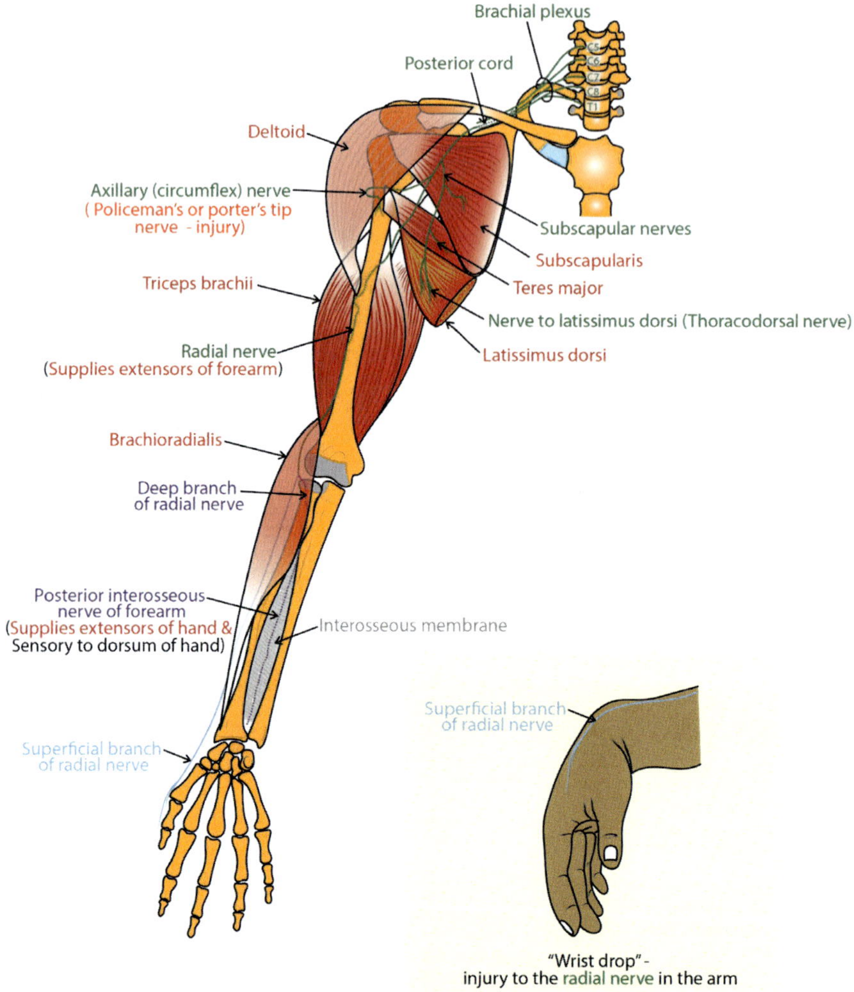

Figure 9.16. Nerves of the upper limb. 1. Long thoracic nerve (from C5, 6, 7 rami). 2. Suprascapular nerve (from the upper trunk). 3. Axillary nerve (from the posterior cord). 4. Radial nerve (from the posterior cord). 5. Musculocutaneous nerve (from the lateral cord). 6. Median nerve (from the lateral and medial cords). 7. Ulnar nerve (from the medial cord). 8. Subscapular nerves (from the posterior cord). (*Refer to the text for a more detailed description of the nerves.*)

of shoulder abduction (especially beyond 15°) and loss of sensation over the "regimental badge" area.

4. **Radial nerve (Fig. 9.15; Fig. 9.16)** It arises from the posterior cord (C5–C8, T1) of the brachial plexus in the axilla and descends into the arm,

where it lies in the radial (spiral) groove of the humerus. It supplies all three heads of the triceps brachii in the posterior compartment of the arm. The nerve then enters the lateral aspect of the cubital fossa where it divides into superficial and deep branches. Before its division, the radial nerve innervates the brachioradialis and extensor carpi radialis longus.

The deep branch pierces and innervates the supinator muscle and continues as the posterior interosseous nerve, which innervates all the extensor muscles of the forearm.

The superficial branch continues as a sensory (cutaneous) nerve, innervating the skin over the dorsum of the lateral hand.

A fracture of the mid-shaft of the humerus may injure the radial nerve, leading to paralysis of the extensor muscles and resulting in wrist drop.

5. **Musculocutaneous nerve (Fig. 9.15; Fig. 9.17)** It arises from the lateral cord (C5 – C7) of the brachial plexus. In the arm, it pierces the coracobrachialis muscle and runs between the biceps brachii and brachialis. It innervates the flexor muscles of the arm including coracobrachialis, biceps brachii, and brachialis. It terminates as the lateral cutaneous nerve of the forearm and innervates the skin over the lateral aspect of the forearm. Injury to the musculocutaneous nerve results in weak elbow flexion and loss of sensation over the lateral forearm.
6. **Median nerve (Fig. 9.15; Fig. 9.17):** It is formed by the contributions from both the medial and lateral cords of the brachial plexus (C5–C8, T1). In the arm, the nerve descends into the anterior compartment and crosses anterior to the brachial artery from lateral to medial. In the cubital fossa, it lies medial to the tendon of biceps brachii and enters the flexor compartment of forearm by passing between the two heads of the pronator teres. At the wrist, it lies between the tendons of the flexor carpi radialis and palmaris longus and passes through the carpal tunnel along with the long flexor tendons.

   The median nerve does not innervate any muscles in the arm. In the forearm, it innervates all the flexor muscles except the flexor carpi ulnaris and the medial (ulnar side) half of flexor digitorum profundus. It also innervates the pronator teres and pronator quadratus. In the hand, it innervates the muscles of the thenar eminence and lateral two lumbricals. Its sensory nerve fibers innervate skin of the lateral three and a half digits (palmar side) and their nail beds (dorsal side). Compression of the median nerve in the carpal tunnel leads to carpal tunnel syndrome.

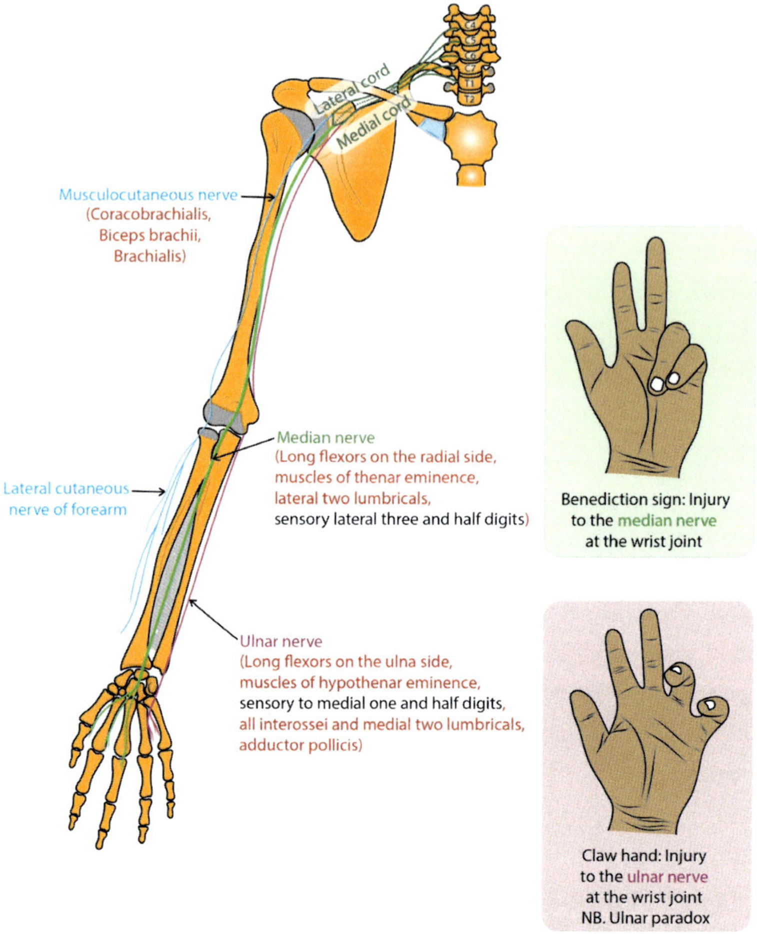

Figure 9.17. Nerves of the upper limb. 1. Musculocutaneous nerve. It arises from the lateral cord of the brachial nerve plexus. It pierces the coracobrachialis and supplies it. In addition, it supplies the biceps brachii and brachialis. It courses lateral to the cubital fossa and continues into the forearm as the lateral cutaneous nerve of the forearm. 2. Median nerve. It arises from both the medial and lateral cords. It descends into the arm first on the medial side and below it crosses anterior to the brachial artery. It passes through the cubital fossa medial to the biceps tendon. It enters the forearm after passing through the pronator teres. It supplies the long flexors on the radial side. At the wrist, it passes through the "carpal tunnel," enters the palm, and supplies the muscles of the thenar eminence, lateral two lumbricals, and sensory to the lateral three and a half digits. 3. Ulnar nerve. It arises from the medial cord of the brachial plexus. It descends on the medial side of the arm, lying posterior to the medial epicondyle. It passes through the flexor carpi ulnaris, which it supplies. In addition, it supplies the medial part of the flexor digitorum profundus. It lies superficial to the flexor retinaculum (outside of the carpal tunnel). In the hand, it supplies the muscles of the hypothenar eminence and all interossei and medial two lumbricals. It sends sensory branches to the medial one and a half digits, including the nail beds. Injury to the median nerve and ulnar nerve results in "Benediction sign" and "Claw hand," respectively. (*For details, see the description in the text.*)

7. **Ulnar nerve (Fig. 9.15; Fig. 9.17):** It arises from the medial cord (C8, T1, with a minor contribution from C7) of the brachial plexus and descends along the medial side of the arm. At the elbow, it passes posterior to the medial epicondyle of the humerus. It then pierces and runs between the heads of the flexor carpi ulnaris muscle. In the forearm, it innervates the flexor carpi ulnaris and the medial (ulnar side) half of the flexor digitorum profundus. At the wrist, it crosses superficial to the flexor retinaculum (through Guyon's canal) to enter the hand.

   In the hand, it innervates muscles of the hypothenar eminence, medial two lumbricals, all palmar and dorsal interossei muscles, and adductor pollicis. It provides sensory innervation to the skin of the medial one and a half digits on both the palmar and dorsal sides of the hand.
8. **Subscapular nerve and nerve to the latissimus dorsi (Fig. 9.15; Fig. 9.16)** The subscapular nerve arises from the posterior cord of the brachial plexus and innervates the subscapularis and teres major. The nerve to the latissimus dorsi (thoracodorsal nerve) arises from the posterior cord of the brachial plexus and innervates the latissimus dorsi muscle.

Applied anatomy (Fig. 9.15)

1. ***Upper trunk injury (Erb Duchenne palsy/paralysis)*** **(Fig. 9.15):** This may result from traction injuries such as birth trauma, falls, or traffic accidents affecting the superior trunk (C5, C6) of the brachial plexus. In this injury suprascapular, axillary, and musculocutaneous nerves are affected, resulting in paralysis of deltoid, biceps brachii, brachialis and brachioradialis. As a result, the patient will have weakened shoulder abduction and lateral rotation as well as weakened elbow flexion and forearm supination. The arm becomes adducted and medially rotated and forearm becomes extended and pronated. This characteristic posture is called the "waiter's tip" deformity.
2. ***Lower trunk injury (Klumpke's palsy)*****(Fig. 9.15):** This may occur due to excessive upward traction of the upper limb (as in breech delivery) or trauma (motor accident) causing injury to the inferior trunk (C8, T1) of the brachial plexus. The ulnar nerve is commonly involved. Usually, short intrinsic muscles of the hand (lumbricals and interossei) are paralyzed and the medial side of the flexor digitorum profundus is weakened. This produces a characteristic "claw hand" deformity. There is also sensory loss over the medial one and a half digits.

3. ***Axillary nerve injury*** **(Fig. 9.16):** This occurs following dislocation of the shoulder joint or fracture of the surgical neck of the humerus, resulting in the weakening or paralysis of deltoid and teres minor muscles leading to impaired shoulder joint stability. Abduction of the arm is also weakened, and there is sensory loss over the lateral shoulder.
4. ***Radial nerve injury*** **(Fig. 9.15; Fig. 9.16):** The radial nerve is injured following a mid-shaft fracture of the humerus. This results in paralysis of the extensor muscles of the forearm thereby, producing "wrist drop" (inability to extend the wrist and fingers).

   Quiz: *Why is supination of the forearm not totally lost when the radial nerve is injured in the arm?*
5. ***Median nerve injury — carpal tunnel syndrome*** **(Fig. 9.9; Fig. 9.15; Fig. 9.17):** Inflammation of the flexor tendons (tendonitis) or their synovial sheaths (tenosynovitis) within the carpal tunnel may compress the median nerve, leading to carpal tunnel syndrome. This results in pain and paresthesia over the lateral three and a half digits of the hand and weakness of thenar muscles of the thumb contributing to impaired flexion and opposition of the thumb. In median nerve injury at the elbow or wrist, the lateral two lumbricals (1st & 2nd) are paralyzed, impairing flexion of the lateral two fingers (index and middle finger) at MCP joints. When the affected individual attempts to make a fist, the lateral two fingers remain extended, producing the characteristic "hand of benediction" sign.
6. ***Ulnar nerve injury*** **(Fig. 9.15; Fig. 9.17):** The ulnar nerve may be injured in fracture of the medial epicondyle of the humerus or by lacerations at the wrist, where it passes superficial to the flexor retinaculum through Guyon's canal, lateral to the pisiform bone. The ulnar nerve lesion results in significant motor and sensory deficits in the hand.

   Injury at the proximal region (elbow): An injury at the level of medial epicondyle of the humerus results in paralysis of all muscles in both the forearm (flexor carpi ulnaris, medial half of the flexor digitorum profundus) and hand (most intrinsic hand muscles) that are associated with ring and little fingers and are innervated by the ulnar nerve. This leads to hyperextension at the MCP joints of the medial two fingers (4th and 5th digits). However, the flexion of the medial two fingers at the IP joints is less pronounced due to paralysis of medial half of flexor digitorum profundus.

Injury at the distal region (wrist): In contrast, lesion of ulnar nerve distally at the wrist causes paralysis of only the intrinsic hand muscles supplied by the ulnar nerve, while the flexor carpi ulnaris and medial half of flexor digitorum profundus remain functional as they receive their innervation proximally. This results in sensory loss over the medial one and a half fingers and produces a characteristic "claw hand" deformity due to hyperextension at the MCP joints and flexion at the IP joints of the medial two fingers (4th and 5th digits).

Ulnar paradox: Ulnar paradox refers to the phenomenon in which the claw hand feature appears more pronounced in a distal ulnar nerve lesion at the wrist, despite fewer muscles (short intrinsic muscles) are paralyzed, compared with a proximal ulnar nerve lesion at the elbow, where more muscles (flexor carpi ulnaris, medial half of the flexor digitorum profundus and most intrinsic hand muscles) are paralyzed.

In short, paralysis of more muscles → less claw deformity while paralysis of fewer muscles → more pronounced claw deformity.

Distal lesion of ulnar nerve at the wrist causes paralysis of 4th and 5th lumbricals, leading to hyperextension at the MCP joints due to the unopposed action of extensor digitorum and flexion of the 4th and 5th digits at the IP joints as the medial half of the flexor digitorum profundus remains functional.

In contrast, a proximal lesion at the elbow also paralyzes the medial half of the flexor digitorum profundus. As a result, flexion at the IP joints of the 4th and 5th digits is diminshed, making the claw hand deformity less pronounced.

***Quiz**: Following a nerve lesion, e.g., median or ulnar nerve injuries at the wrist, apart from motor and sensory loss, will there be any other functional deficits? Explain.*

Cubital fossa (Fig. 9.18)

The cubital fossa is a triangular space located anterior to the elbow joint. It is bounded superiorly by an imaginary line connecting the medial and lateral epicondyles of the humerus, laterally by the brachioradialis, and medially by the pronator teres. The floor is formed by the brachialis and supinator muscles,

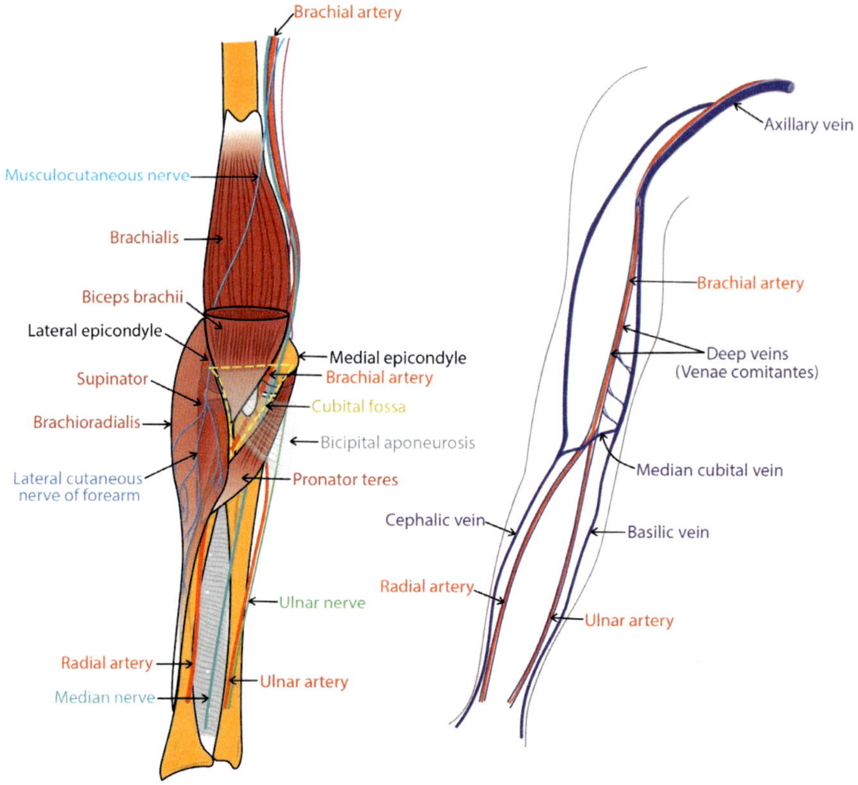

Figure 9.18. Cubital fossa. It lies anterior to the elbow joint. It is a triangular space bounded by an imaginary line joining the two epicondyles of the humerus, brachioradialis, and pronator teres. The floor is formed by the brachialis and supinator. The contents of the fossa include the biceps tendon, brachial artery, and median nerve. The musculocutaneous nerve and the radial nerve are at its lateral side. The fossa is "roofed" by the median cubital vein linking the cephalic vein and basilic vein **(Fig. 9.13)**. These superficial veins are common sites for withdrawing blood samples. In a venepuncture, the brachial artery may be damaged, causing Volkmann's ischemic contracture.

while its roof consists of skin, superficial fascia, deep fascia reinforced by the bicipital aponeurosis. The main contents of the cubital fossa, arranged from lateral to medial, are the biceps brachii tendon, brachial artery, and median nerve. The radial nerve courses through its lateral side, where it divides into superficial and deep branches.

The roof of the cubital fossa contains the median cubital vein connecting the cephalic and basilic veins superficially. These superficial veins, especially medial cubital vein are commonly used for venipuncture and blood sampling.

During venipuncture, accidental injury to the underlying brachial artery may occur. Severe vascular injury may result in ischemia of the forearm muscles and subsequently lead to Volkmann's ischemic contracture.

Back

Back muscles maintain the posture of the body, support the spine and trunk, and help in movement. The back muscles cover the neck and shoulder and run all the way down to your spine and lower back. There are three group of muscles: superficial (extrinsic), intermediate and deep (intrinsic). The superficial back muscles include trapezius, latissimus dorsi, rhomboids, levator scapulae and serratus anterior. The intermediate back muscles include serratus posterior superior and serratus posterior inferior. The deep muscles of the back are arranged in three layers: superficial layer (splenius capitis and splenius cervicis), intermediate layer, (spinalis, longissimus and iliocostalis) and deep layer (interspinales and intertransversarii, multifidus and rotatores). The intermediate layer of deep back muscles is collectively known as erector spinae muscles.

Back muscles over the suboccipital triangle **(Fig. 9.5; Fig. 9.19)**.

1. *Trapezius*: It is innervated by spinal accessory nerve (CN XI) and is involved in the elevation and upward rotation of the scapula.
2. *Splenius capitis*: It produces lateral flexion and rotation the head to the same side (ipsilaterally).
3. *Semispinalis capitis* **(Fig. 9.19)**: It extends the head (e.g., looking upward toward the ceiling) and help in lateral rotation of the head.
4. *Longissimus capitis*: It is located laterally and is mainly involved in extension and rotation of the head. (*See suboccipital region in the chapter on the Head and Neck.*)

Erector spinae (Sacrospinalis)

This group of muscles forms the intermediate layer of deep back muscles, located in the "gutter" on both sides of the spines of the vertebral column **(Fig. 9.19)**. These muscles are arranged into three longitudinal columns, extending from the iliac crest and sacrum to the suboccipital region.

They are antigravity muscles that maintain the body posture (straightening the back), stabilize the vertebral column, and assist in balance, coordination,

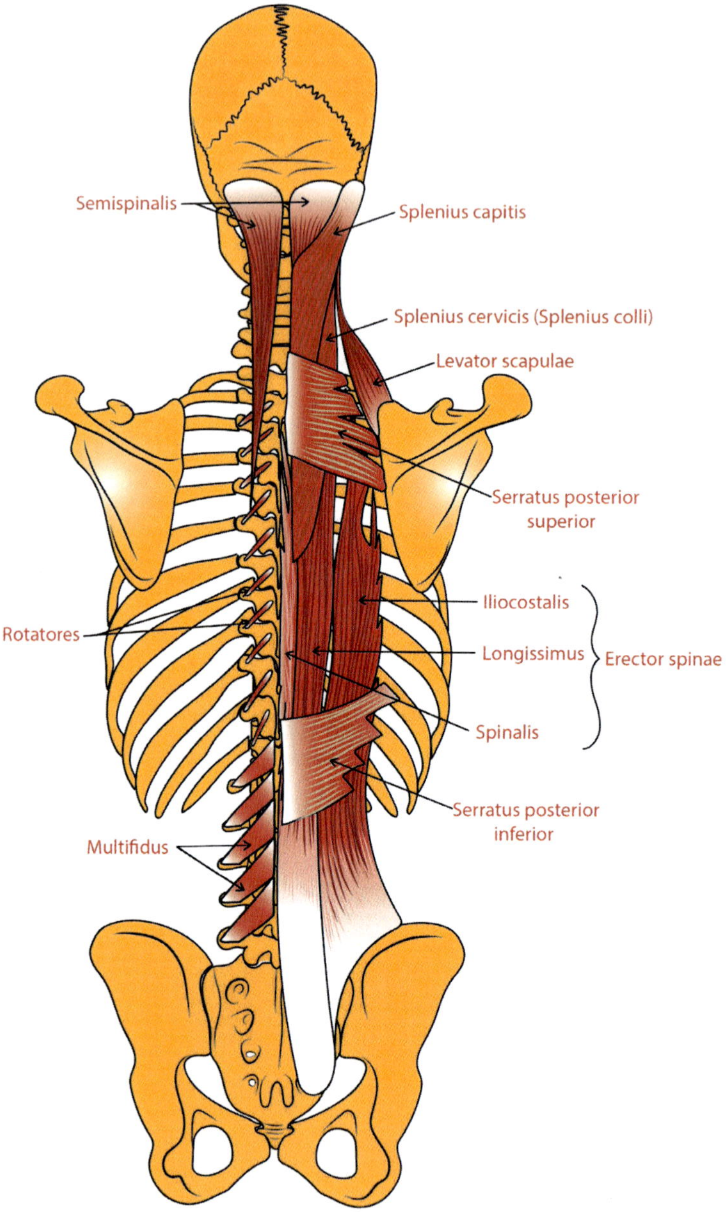

Figure 9.19. Muscles of the back. (*See the text for a detailed description.*)

and locomotion. They also help in extension, rotation, and lateral flexion of the trunk and head. Components of the erector spinae muscles include:

1. *Iliocostalis*: Iliocostalis lumborum, Iliocostalis thoracis, Iliocostalis cervicis.
2. *Longissimus*: This is the longest muscle of the erector spinae and include longissimus thoracis, longissimus cervicis, and longissimus capitis.
3. *Spinalis*: It comprises the spinalis thoracis, spinalis cervicis, spinalis capitis.

Deep to the erector spinae are smaller intrinsic muscles:

1. *Intertransversarii and interspinalis*: They extend between the transverse processes or spinous processes and help in stabilization of the vertebral column.
2. *Rotatores*: These are deepest intrinsic back muscles and form part of the transversospinalis group. They assist in rotation of the vertebral column.
3. *Multifidus*: It is also part of the transversospinalis group, extending from the mammillary process of the lumbar vertebrae to the spinous process of superior vertebrae. They also help in stabilization of the vertebral column, especially in the lumbar region.

Innervation

The muscles are mainly supplied by the posterior (dorsal) rami of the spinal nerves.

Spinal cord (Fig. 9.20)

The spinal cord begins at the level of the foramen magnum as a continuation of the medulla oblongata. As it descends within the vertebral (spinal) canal, it presents two enlargements: cervical enlargement and lumbar enlargement for innervation of the upper and lower limbs, respectively. The spinal cord terminates at the L1/L2 vertebral level in adults. Throughout its length, it is covered by three meninges: pia mater, arachnoid mater, and dura mater. The pia mater continues inferiorly as the filum terminale which anchors the spinal cord to the coccyx. Both the arachnoid mater and dura mater terminate at the S2 vertebral level. The spinal nerves (cervical/lumbar/sacral) pierce these meningeal layers before exiting through the intervertebral foramen. Below the termination of the spinal

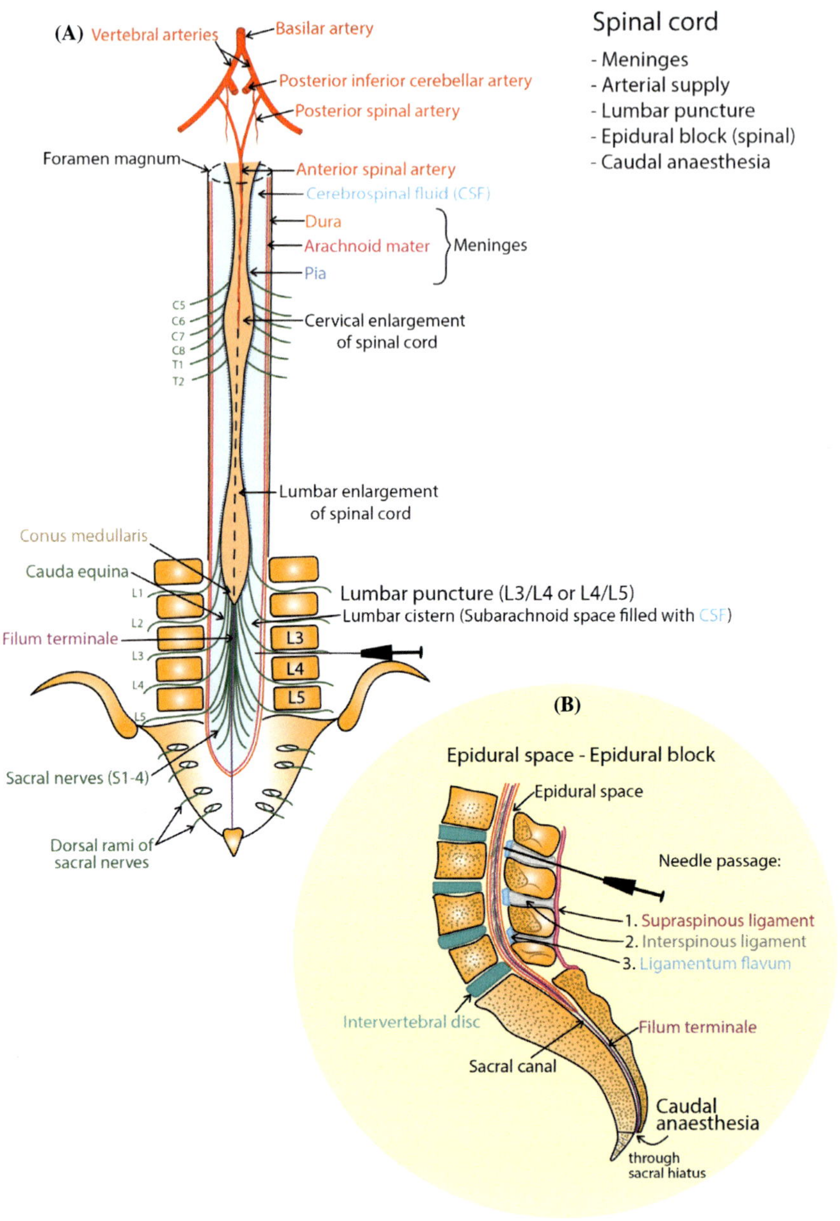

Figure 9.20. Spinal cord. **(A)** Its arterial supply and meninges — pia, arachnoid, and dura mater. **(B)** Showing the needle passage in an epidural block.

cord, the lumbar, sacral, and coccygeal nerve roots descend within the vertebral canal as a bundle known as the cauda equina (horse's tail). These nerves innervate the lower limbs, pelvic viscera, and perineum.

Blood supply: The spinal cord receives its arterial supply from the anterior and posterior spiral arteries, which arise from the vertebral and posterior inferior cerebellar arteries, respectively. In addition, the spinal cord receives segmental reinforcement from radicular and segmental medullary arteries arising mainly from the aorta.

Epidural block and caudal anesthesia **(Fig. 9.20)**: These are procedures used to anesthetize the caudal spinal nerves during specific surgical procedures such as cesarean section (C-section), pelvic surgeries, and procedures involving the perineum. In epidural anesthesia, anesthetic is injected into the epidural space surrounding the dura mater. In caudal anesthesia, the anesthetic is introduced through the sacral hiatus into the sacral epidural space.

Lumbar puncture: A lumbar puncture is usually performed below the L2 vertebral level (commonly between L3/L4 or L4/L5 vertebrae) to avoid injury to the spinal cord. The procedure is used for aspiration of cerebrospinal fluid (CSF) for diagnostic purposes or for administration of medications and anesthesia.

MUSCULOSKELETAL SYSTEM 2: LOWER LIMB

GENERAL FEATURES

The lower limb is a specialized structure of the human body adapted primarily for weight bearing, balance, posture, and locomotion. It supports the body during standing and walking cycle. It consists of the gluteal region, thigh, knee, leg, and foot, together with several major joints including the hip, knee, ankle, subtalar, and tarsal joints. The lower limb is mainly supplied by the femoral artery and the gluteal arteries, and its venous drainage is by the femoral vein and its tributaries, together with the superficial venous system. The skin, muscles, bones, and joints of the lower limb are innervated by branches of the lumbar and sacral plexuses. The lymphatic drainage of the lower limb occurs through both the superficial and deep lymphatic vessels. These drain into the popliteal and inguinal lymph nodes, and subsequently into the external and common iliac lymph nodes and the lumbar (para-aortic) lymph nodes. The lymph subsequently enters the thoracic duct, before returning to the venous circulation. This section summarizes the bones, joints, muscles, innervation, arterial supply, venous drainage, lymphatic drainage, and functions of the lower limb.

FUNCTIONS OF THE LOWER LIMB

Its major functions include:

1. Locomotion: enabling walking and running.
2. Weight-bearing: supporting and transmitting the body weight to the ground.
3. Maintenance of posture, balance, and coordination: helping maintain the erect posture and ensuring stability during standing and walking.

The alignment of the lower limbs helps maintain the body's line of gravity, ensuring efficient balance and weight distribution during standing and walking. In the normal erect posture **(Fig. 9.21)**, the line of gravity passes in relation to the major joints as follows:

a. At the neck: anterior to the atlanto-occipital joints
b. At the hip: posterior to the hip joints

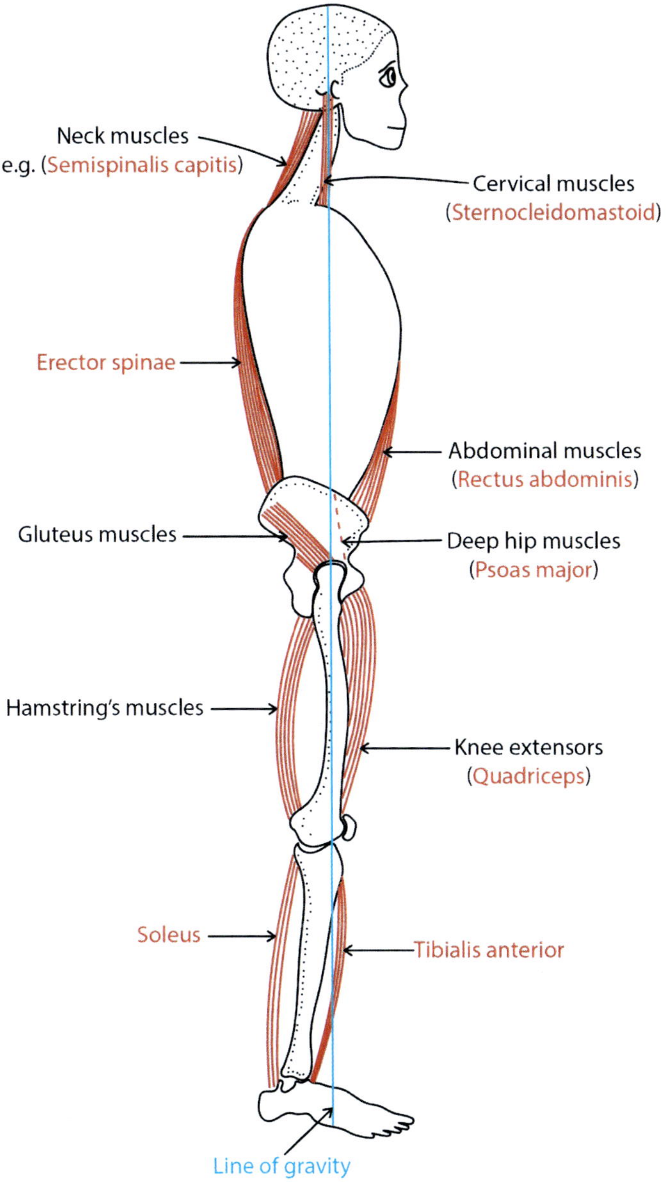

Figure 9.21. **Line of gravity.** At the neck, the line of gravity is anterior to the atlanto-occipital joint. At the hip, it is posterior to the hip joint. At the knee, it is anterior to the knee joint. At the ankle, it is anterior to the ankle joint. Note that the antigravity muscles are to counter the shift of the line of gravity.

c. At the knee: anterior to the knee joints
d. At the ankle: anterior to the ankle joints

Because the line of gravity does not pass directly through all joints, the body tends to sway under gravity. This tendency is resisted by the antigravity muscles, which contract continuously to maintain posture.

Quiz 1: *What are the cellular components of the lymph node, and what are their roles in lymph fluid filtration and immune response?*
Quiz 2: *Which muscles in the lower limb are considered "antigravity muscles"? Explain.*

BONES OF THE LOWER LIMB

The lower limb is made up of the following bones (**Fig. 9.22**):

1. The pelvic girdle: Hip bone (ilium, ischium, and pubis) and sacrum.
2. The femur: bone of the thigh.
3. The tibia and fibula: bones of the leg.
4. The tarsal bones: bones of the foot.
5. The metatarsals: bones of the foot
6. The phalanges: bones of the toes.

The body weight is transferred from the trunk (vertebral column) to the femur through the hip joints of the pelvic girdle.

1. **Pelvic Girdle** It is formed by the two hip bones, which articulate posteriorly with the sacrum at the sacroiliac joints, which are synovial joints with very limited mobility (**Fig. 9.22**). Anteriorly, the two hip bones are united at the pubic symphysis, a secondary cartilaginous joint (symphysis). Together with the sacrum and coccyx, the pelvic girdle forms the bony pelvis.
   a. **Sacrum:** It is a wedge-shaped and formed by the fusion of 5 sacral vertebrae. It has a sacral promontory which projects from the body of the first sacral vertebra (S1) and ala of sacrum, a wing like lateral expansion on either side of the sacral base.

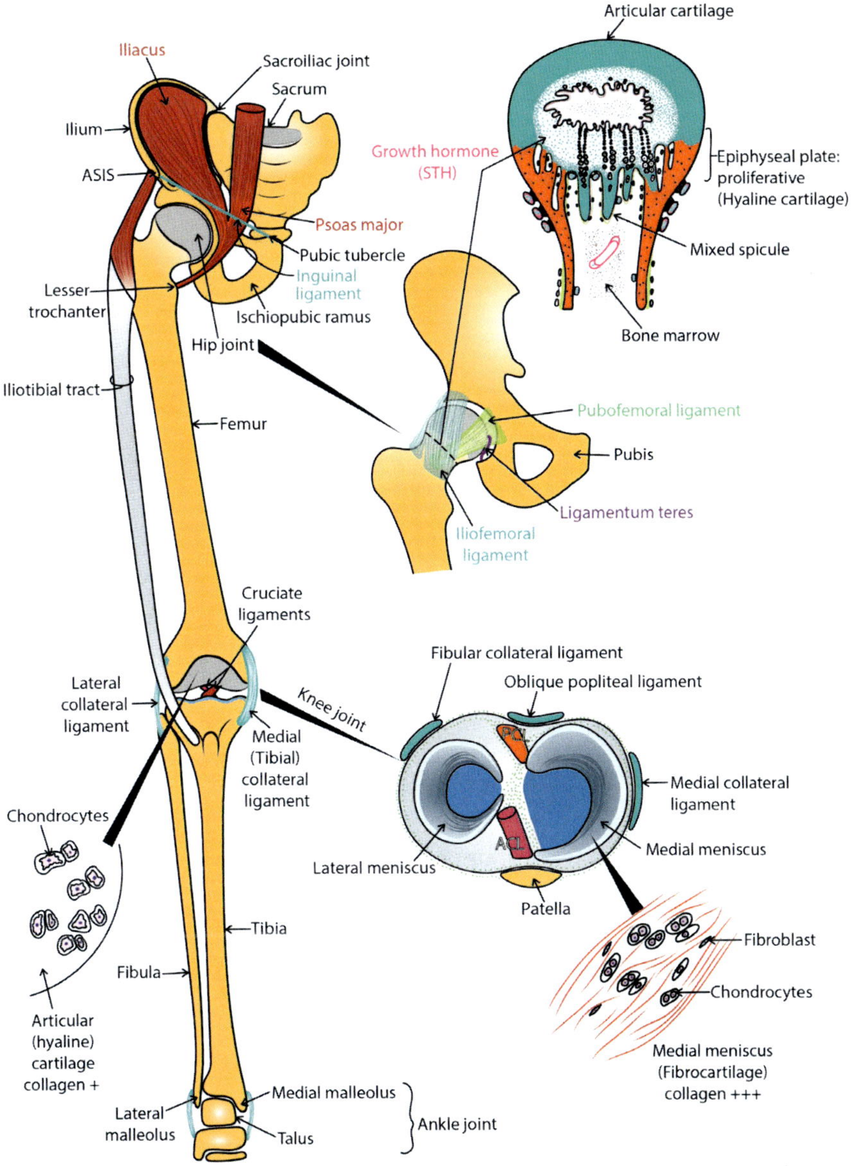

Figure 9.22. Bones and joints of the lower limb. The bones consist of the following: Hip bone (ilium, pubis, and ischium), femur, tibia and fibula, tarsal bones (talus, etc), metatarsals, and phalanges (not shown). The joints include the following main joints: hip joint, knee joint, and ankle joint (details will be described separately).

ASIS: Anterior superior iliac spine; **ACL**: Anterior cruciate ligament; **PCL**: Posterior cruciate ligament

b. **Ilium:** It is a part of the hip bone and has important landmarks including iliac crest, anterior superior iliac spine (ASIS), anterior inferior iliac spine (AIIS), iliac fossa and dorsum ilii (gluteal surface).

c. **Ischium:** It forms the posterior part of the hip bone and has body and ramus of the ischium, ischial tuberosity, ischial spine, and greater and lesser sciatic notch. The greater and lesser sciatic notches are converted into the greater and lesser sciatic foramina by the sacrospinous and sacrotuberous ligaments.

d. **Pubis:** It forms the anterior part of the hip bone and has the body of the pubis, pubic crest, public tubercle and ischiopubic ramus.

The ilium, ischium, and pubis fuse to form the acetabulum during development. Inferiorly, the acetabulum presents with the acetabular notch. The acetabulum articulates with the head of the femur to form the hip joint.

2. **Femur:** This is a bone of the thigh which is the longest and strongest bone in the body. It is formed by endochondral ossification. The proximal end of the femur consists of the head, neck, and the greater and lesser trochanters. The head of the femur is spherical and most of its surface is covered by hyaline (articular) cartilage **(Fig. 9.22)**, which lacks a perichondrium. There is a small depression on the head, the fovea capitis, providing attachment for the ligament of the head of the femur (ligamentum teres). The neck connects the head to the shaft of the femur. Below the head lie the greater trochanter which provides attachment for several gluteal muscles, while the lesser trochanter provides insertion for the iliopsoas muscle. Anteriorly, between the two trochanters is the intertrochanteric line; posteriorly, between them is the intertrochanteric crest. The shaft of the femur is slightly convex anteriorly. Posteriorly, it is reinforced mechanically by the linea aspera, a prominent longitudinal ridge, which serves as an important site for muscle attachment. The distal end of the femur consists of the medial and lateral femoral condyles, which articulate with the tibial condyles to form the knee joint. At the superior part of the medial epicondyle lies the adductor tubercle, a palpable bony prominence that marks the insertion of the adductor magnus muscle.

3. **Tibia and Fibula:** The tibia and fibula are the two long bones of the leg, both formed by endochondral ossification.

   a. **Tibia:** The tibia is the larger, weight-bearing bone located on the medial side of the leg. Proximally, it expands to form the medial and lateral tibial condyles which articulate with the corresponding femoral condyles to form the knee joint. The tibial tuberosity on its anterior surface is palpable and provides attachment for the ligamentum patella. Distally, the tibia articulates with the talus to form the ankle joint. Its medial projection, the medial malleolus, is palpable on the medial side of the ankle (**Fig. 9.22**).

b. **Fibula:** The fibula is a slender bone located on the lateral side of the leg and mainly provides attachment for muscles. Proximally, it consists of a head and neck. Distally, the fibula expands to form the lateral malleolus, which forms the lateral part of the ankle joint (**Fig. 9.22**).

4. **Tarsal Bones (Fig. 9.23; Fig. 9.24; Fig. 9.25):** Tarsal bones consist of 7 bones including the talus, calcaneum, navicular, cuboid and cuneiform (medial, intermediate, and lateral). The calcaneum is the largest tarsal bone and forms the heel. The talus articulates superiorly with the tibia and fibula to form the ankle joint.
5. **Metatarsal Bones (Fig. 9.23; Fig. 9.24; Fig. 9.25):** There are five metatarsal bones. Proximally, they articulate with the tarsal bones, and distally with the proximal phalanges at the metatarsophalangeal joints.
6. **Phalanges (Fig. 9.23; Fig. 9.24; Fig. 9.25):** The great toe (hallux) has proximal and distal phalanges, while the lateral four toes have proximal, intermediate, and distal phalanges.

JOINTS OF THE UPPER LIMB

1. Hip Joint (Fig. 9.22; Fig. 9.26)

a. **Type of joint and articulations:** It is a synovial joint of the ball and socket type. The head of the femur (approximately two-thirds of a sphere) articulates with the acetabulum of the hip bone.

b. **Articular surfaces:** The articular surfaces of both the head of the femur and the acetabulum are covered by hyaline cartilage (articular cartilage) which is devoid of the perichondrium. The hyaline cartilage provides smooth and low friction surface for movement. The acetabulum is deepened by a rim of fibrocartilage, the acetabular labrum, which increases the depth of the acetabulum and enhances stability of the joint. The acetabulum has a notch inferiorly which is bridged by transverse ligament. From the transverse ligament, ligamentum teres extends to the fovea capitis of the femoral head. ***Quiz:*** *Why is the perichondrium absent in the articular cartilage?*

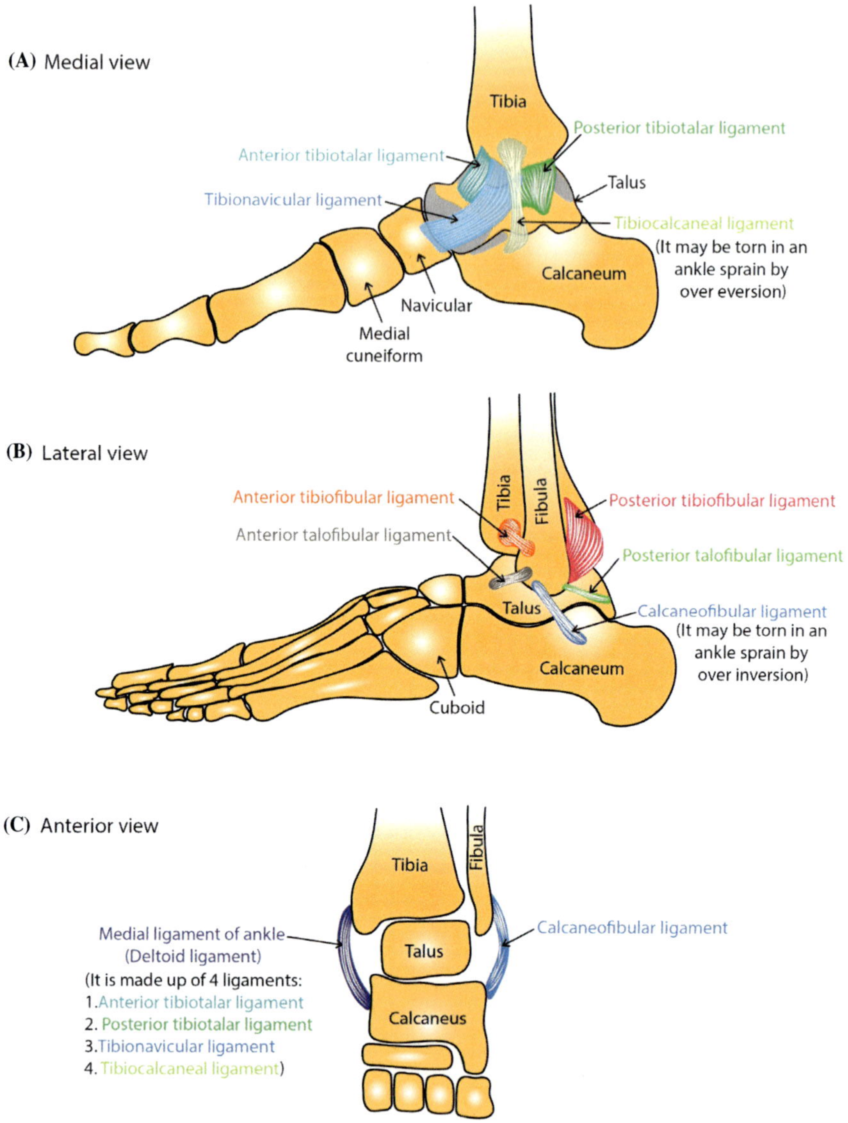

Figure 9.23. Ankle joint (right foot). **(A)** Medial aspect of the right ankle joint showing the medial ligament (deltoid ligament). **(B)** Lateral view of the right ankle joint showing the calcaneofibular ligament. **(C)** Posterior view of the joint showing the articulation of the right ankle joint between the lower ends of the tibia and fibula above and the talus below. Innervation of the joint is by the tibial nerve, deep peroneal nerve, and saphenous nerve.

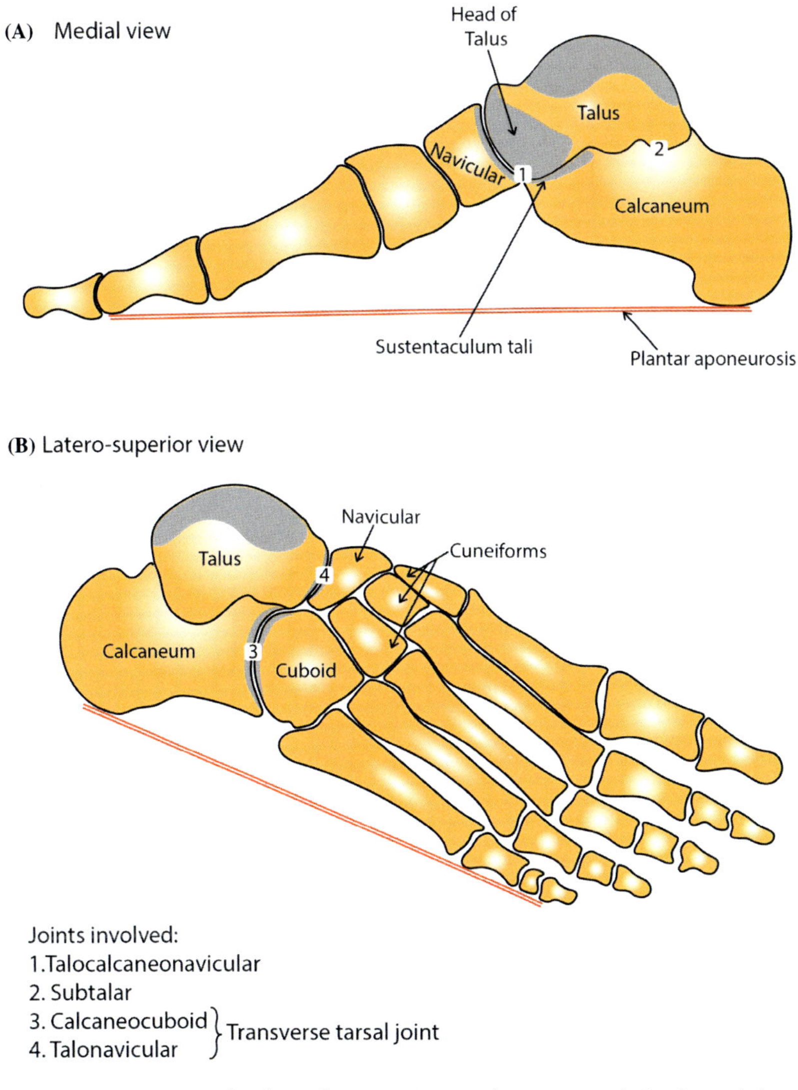

Figure 9.24. Joints involved in the inversion and eversion of the foot. **(A)** Medial side of the right foot. **(B)** Lateral view of the right foot. 1. Talocalcaneonavicular joint. 2. Subtalar joint. 3. Calcaneocuboid joint. 4. Talonavicular joint.

c. **Ligaments of the joint (Fig. 9.26):** The hip joint is reinforced primarily by three ligaments, namely, the iliofemoral ligament, pubofemoral, and ischiofemoral ligament. In addition, the ligamentum teres is attached to the fovea capitis and the transverse ligament, bridging the acetabular notch. All the ligaments provide support and stability to the joint.
Quiz: *What is the histology of ligaments associated with the joint?*

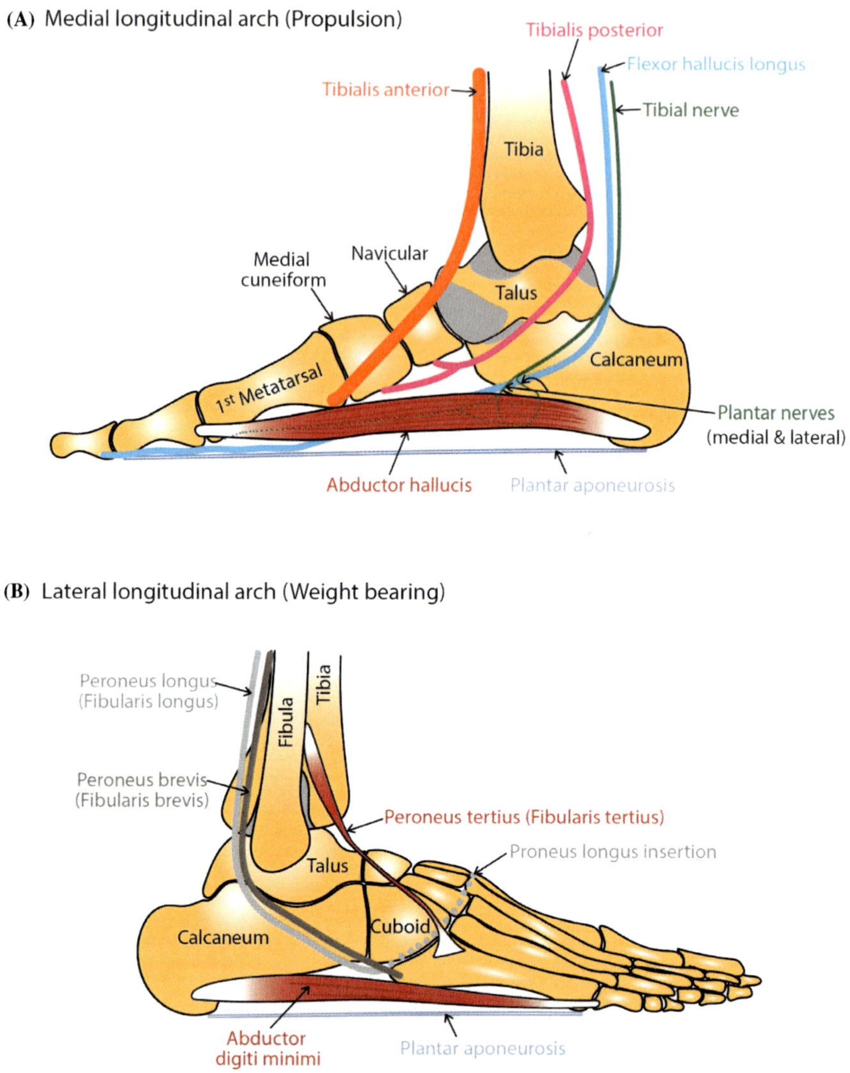

Figure 9.25. Arches of the foot. **(A)** Medial longitudinal arch. **(B)** Lateral longitudinal arch. For a detailed description regarding bones forming the arches and their support, refer to the text.

d. **Capsule of joint:** The hip joint is covered by a strong fibrous capsule, which is attached to the acetabular margin and transverse acetabular ligament proximally. Distally, it is attached to the intertrochanteric line anteriorly **(Fig. 9.26)**, and to the neck of the femur **(Fig. 9.26)** posteriorly (approximately halfway between the head and the intertrochanteric crest).

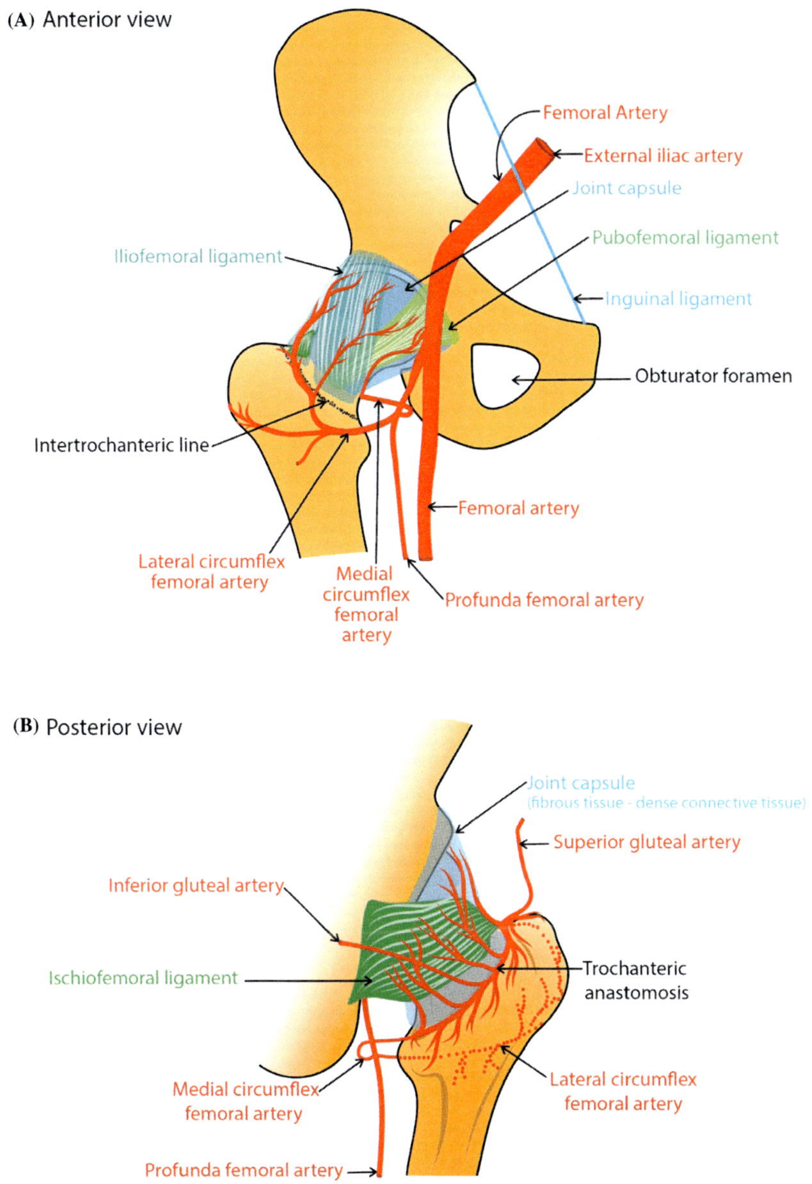

Figure 9.26. Hip joint. (A) Anterior view of the hip joint. The bony articulations are between the head of the femur and the acetabulum of the hip bone. **(B)** Note that the margin of the acetabulum is deepened by a rim of fibrocartilage, acetabular labrum. The joint has a capsule attached to the articular margin (anteriorly to the intertrochanteric line). **(A, B)** Three ligaments are associated with the joint: iliofemoral ligament, pubofemoral ligament, and ischiofemoral ligament. The head of the femur receives its arterial supply from the medial circumflex artery (from the profunda femoris) (trochanteric anastomosis) and obturator artery via the ligament teres attached to the fovea capitis and acetabular notch.

***Quiz* 1:** *What is the histology of the capsule?*

***Quiz* 2:** *Are there nerve endings in the capsule?*

***Quiz* 3:** *What are the roles of sensory nerve endings in the joint?*

***Quiz* 4:** *Where are the cell bodies of the sensory neurons located?*

e. **Arterial supply to the head of femur (Fig. 9.26):** It is mainly supplied by the medial circumflex femoral artery, a branch of the profunda femoris artery (from the femoral artery), giving rise to retinacular arteries (via the retinacula-reflected part of the capsule) that supply the head of the femur. Obturator artery (from the internal iliac artery) supplies the head of the femur via the ligamentum teres. Additional blood reaches the femur through nutrient arteries entering the shaft and passing through the marrow cavity.

f. **Innervation (Fig. 9.27; Fig. 9.28):** According to Hilton's law, the nerves supplying the muscles that move a joint also supply the joint and the skin overlying the muscle insertions. The hip joint is innervated by the femoral nerve, sciatic nerve, and obturator nerve.

***Quiz*:** *What structures in the joints (excluding the muscles) are supplied by the nerves? Do they supply the articular cartilage?*

g. **Movements (Fig. 9.27; Fig. 9.29)**

i. <u>Flexion</u> (brings the thigh anteriorly such as in stepping forward during walking or climbing stairs): Sartorius, rectus femoris, iliopsoas (which is the strongest flexor muscle) are involved.

ii. <u>Extension</u> (moves the thigh posteriorly, important in activities like rising from sitting, running, and climbing): Gluteus maximus (main extensor) and hamstrings (long head of the biceps femoris, semitendinosus, and semimembranosus).

iii. <u>Abduction</u> (moves the thigh laterally and helps clear the foot off the ground during walking): Gluteus medius and gluteus minimus are involved. The paralysis of gluteus medius and gluteus minimus causes the pelvis to drop on the opposite side during walking, which is known as Trendelenburg gait (dipping gait).

iv. <u>Adduction</u> (brings the thigh toward the midline e.g., activities like horseback riding or crossing the legs): Adductor longus, adductor brevis, adductor magnus, gracilis and pectineus muscles are involved.

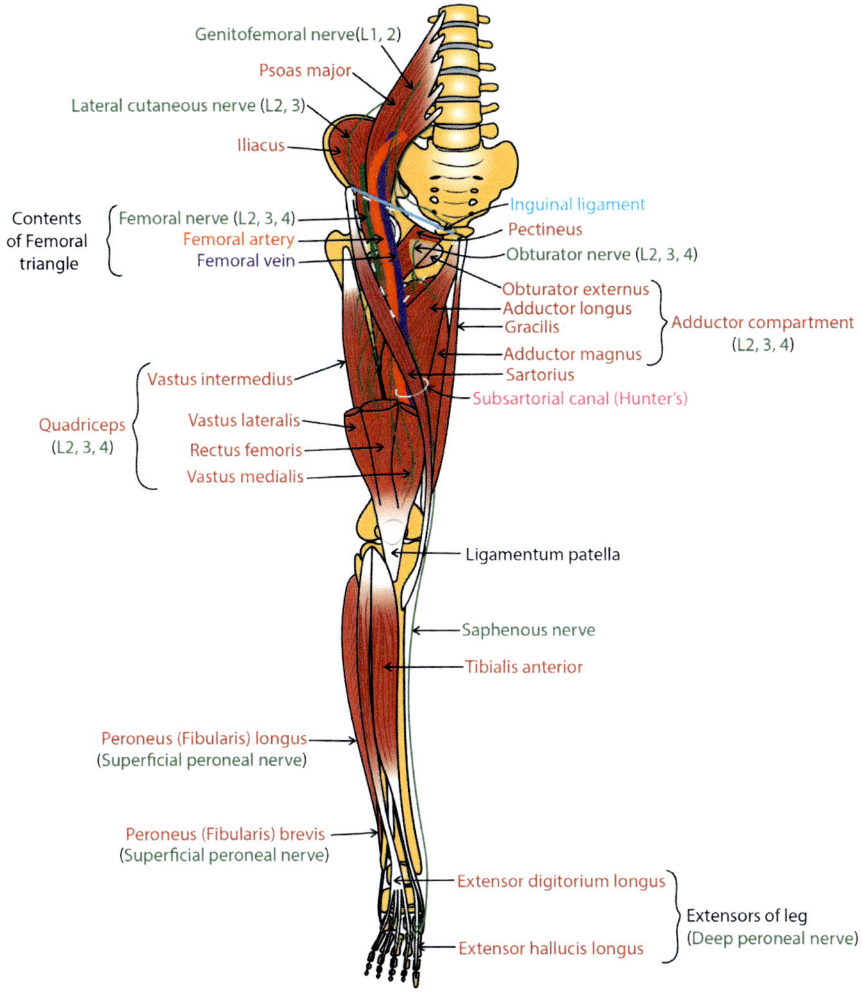

Figure 9.27. Hip joint and anterior and medial compartments of the thigh and leg. Anterior view of the hip joint showing the muscles that move the joint: sartorius (flexion), pectineus (flexion), rectus femoris (flexion), psoas major (flexion and medial rotation), adductor longus, magnus, and gracilis (adduction). The joint is innervated by the femoral nerve and obturator nerve from the lumbar nerve plexus (L2, 3, 4). In the lower part of the figure are the anterior and lateral compartment muscles of the leg. The anterior or extensor compartment consists of the tibialis anterior, extensor hallucis longus, and extensor digitorum longus. The lateral or peroneal compartment muscles include the peroneus (fibularis) longus and brevis. The extensor compartment muscles are supplied by the deep peroneal nerve, whereas the peroneal compartment muscles are supplied by the superficial peroneal nerve.

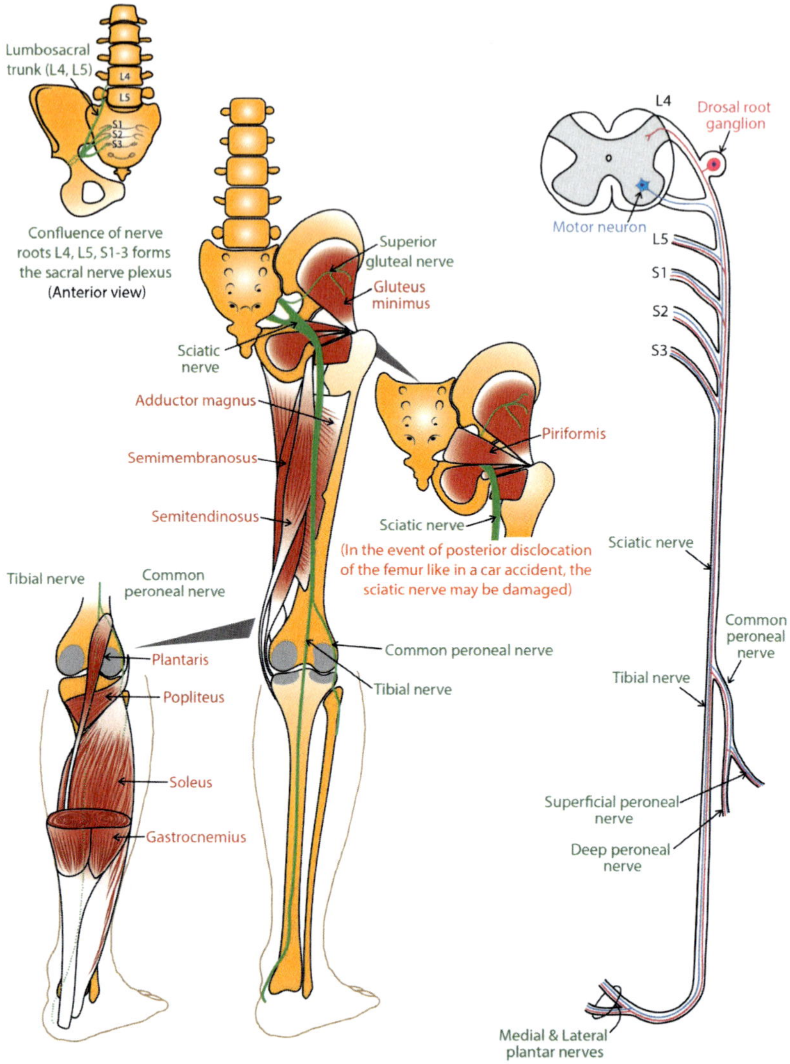

Figure 9.28. Origin, course, and distribution of the sciatic nerve. (A) The sciatic nerve arises from the sacral plexus L4–5, S1–4. It descends through the gluteal region and emerges below the piriformis muscle. It lies on the obturator internus tendon and the gamelli associated with it. In the thigh, it lies on the adductor magnus, and at the lower thigh, it divides into the common peroneal nerve and the tibial nerve. The common peroneal nerve divides into the superficial and deep peroneal nerve. The tibial nerve continues through the leg and supplies all the muscles in the back of the leg. In the foot, it divides into the medial and lateral plantar nerves. **(B)** The sciatic nerve is composed of both motor and sensory fibers. The motor nerve fibers (axons) originate from the ventral horn neurons from the lumbosacral spinal cord segments. The sensory nerve fibers originate from the dorsal root ganglion (DRG) cells.

Quiz: *What are the functional nerve fiber components present in the sciatic nerve, and what structures do they supply?*

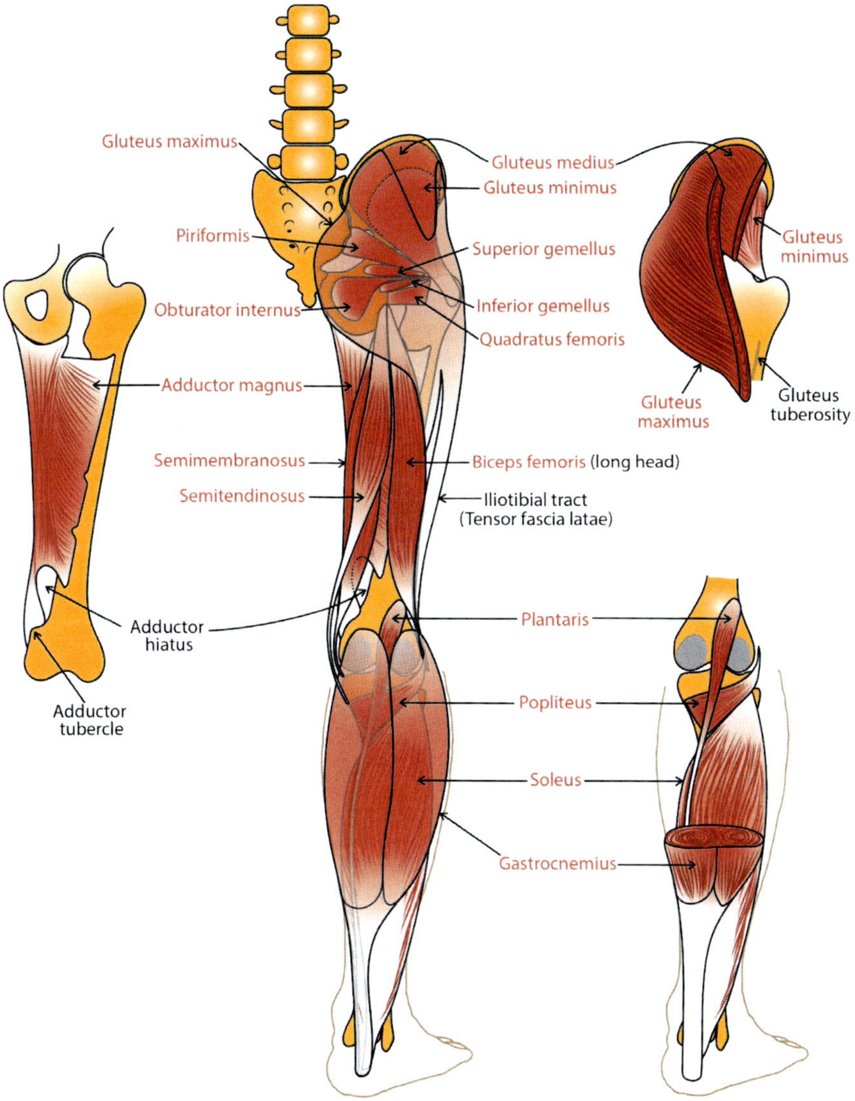

Figure 9.29. Hip joint, gluteal region, and back of thigh and leg. Posterior view of the hip joint and the gluteal region showing the muscles that move the joint: gluteus maximus (extension) and gluteus medius and minimus (abduction). Deep to the gluteal muscles are the piriformis, obturator internus, and quadratus femoris (lateral rotation). Note that the sciatic nerve is related to the joint posteriorly (see **Fig. 9.31**). Note also that the superior gluteal nerve supplies the gluteus medius and gluteus minimus, and the inferior gluteal nerve supplies the gluteus maximus. The back of the thigh consists of the hamstring (semimembranosus, semitendinosus, biceps femoris). The back of the leg (posterior compartment) consists of the gastrocnemius and soleus, with the common tendocalcaneum (Achille's tendon) inserted to the calcaneum.

v. Medial rotation (rotates the thigh inward, aligning the foot medially): Anterior fibers of gluteus medius and gluteus minimus are involved. It is also assisted by psoas major.

vi. Lateral rotation (rotates the thigh outward, important for stabilizing the hip during movement and standing): Small muscles such as piriformis, obturator internus, obturator externus, gemelli (superior and inferior), and quadratus femoris, and gluteus maximus are involved.

h. Factors contributing to the stability of the hip joint

i. Bony factor: The head of the femur fits snugly into the acetabulum, which is further deepened by the acetabular labrum, providing strong inherent stability.

ii. Ligamentous factor: Stability of the joint is reinforced by strong ligaments and a fibrous capsule. The ligaments restrict excessive movement and prevent dislocation.

iii. Muscular factor: All muscles associated with the hip joint, provide support and dynamic stability. In addition, muscle tone helps maintain joint congruency during standing and movement.

i. Applied anatomy

i. Fracture of the neck of femur is common in elders with osteoporotic bone after a fall causing the rupture of the retinacular arteries supplying the head of femur. This can lead to avascular necrosis of the head of femur, resulting in collapse of the bone and loss of joint function. In such cases, hip joint replacement (hip arthroplasty) is often required.

ii. Posterior dislocation of the head of femur occurs due to a high-energy impact on the flexed knee, such as in a motor vehicle accident (dashboard injury). The force drives the femoral head posteriorly out of the acetabulum resulting in injury of the sciatic nerve which lies posterior to the joint **(Fig. 9.28)**.

2. Knee Joint (Fig. 9.22; Fig. 9.30)

a. Type of joint: It is a synovial joint of the modified hinge type. It mainly allows flexion and extension, with a small degree of rotation when the knee is flexed. When you are standing with the foot on the ground, the knee is fully extended and said to be locked. This occurs because the femur rotates medially on the tibial condyles. In the locked position, all the cruciate and

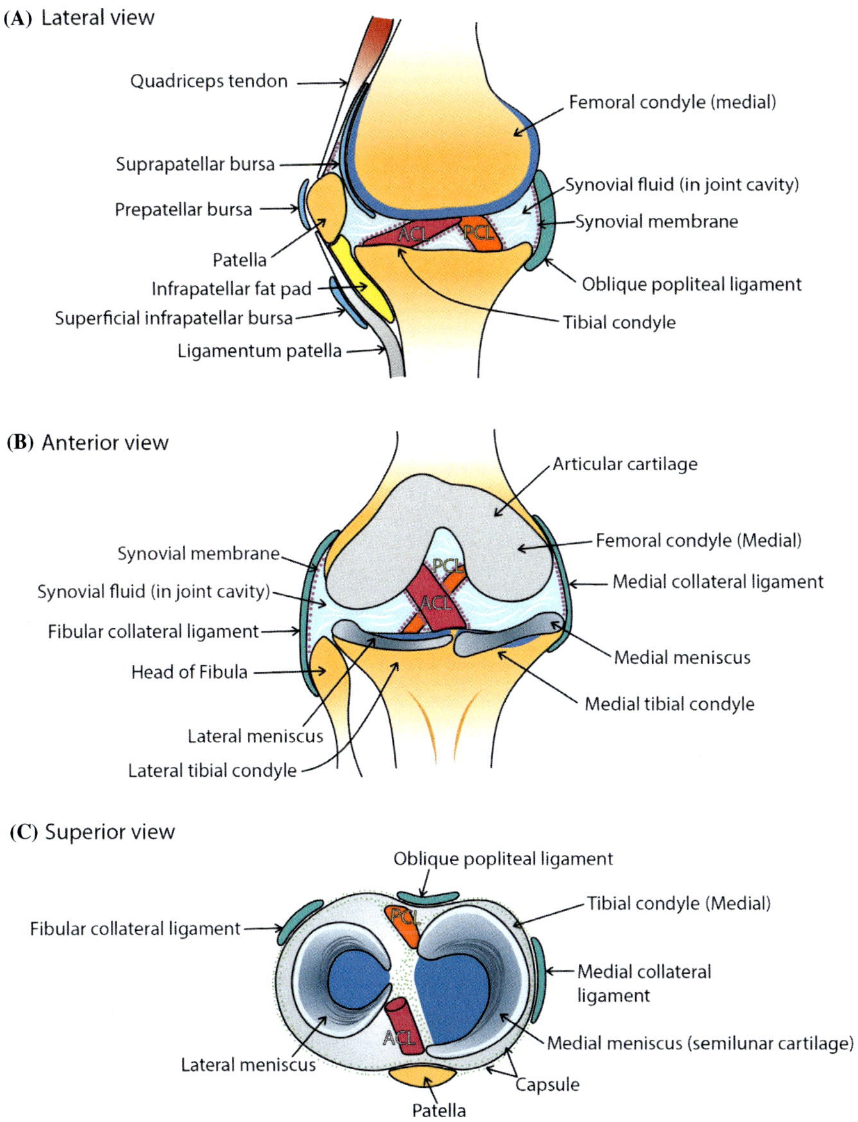

Figure 9.30. Knee joint (right). **(A)** Lateral view. **(B)** Anterior view. **(C)** Superior view of the tibial articular surface. The articulations are between the femoral condyles, tibial condyles, and patella. The femoral condyles are coated by a layer of articular cartilage **(B)**, whereas the superior surface of the tibial condyles is cushioned by the medial and lateral meniscus **(C)**. The joint is supported by the medial (tibial) collateral ligament, fibular collateral ligament (lateral) **(B)**, and posteriorly, by the oblique popliteal ligament **(A, C)**. Within the joint are the anterior cruciate ligament (ACL) and posterior cruciate ligament (PCL) **(A, B, C)**.

collateral ligaments associated with the joint are taut, making the joint highly stable and well adapted for weight bearing with minimal muscular effort. At the beginning of flexion (while you are walking or taking the foot off the ground), the popliteus muscle contracts to unlock the knee by rotating the femur laterally on the condyle of fixed tibia. Once unlocked, flexion can proceed normally. During walking, the knee undergoes repeated cycles of locking during terminal extension and unlocking at the onset of flexion, providing both stability during stance and mobility during the swing phase.

b. **Articulation:** The lateral and medial condyles of the femur articulate with the superior surface of the corresponding tibial condyles Anteriorly, the patellar surface of the femur articulates with the posterior articular surface of the patella. The articular surfaces of the femoral condyles, tibial condyles, and patella are covered by hyaline cartilage. The medial and lateral menisci (singular: meniscus), which are semilunar fibrocartilage, rest directly on the tibial plateaus.

c. **Capsule:** It is attached to the bony articular margins.

d. **Ligaments (Fig. 9.26; Fig. 9.30):** The knee joint is strengthened by the extracapsular and intracapsular ligaments. The extracapsular ligaments include:
   - Ligamentum patella (anterior): It is the extension of the tendon of quadriceps femoris and is attached on the tibial tuberosity.
   - Tibial (medial) collateral ligament (medial side): It extends from the medial epicondyle of the femur to the superior part of the medial surface of the tibia.
   - Fibular (lateral) collateral ligament (lateral side): It extends from the lateral epicondyle of the femur to the lateral surface of the head of the fibula.
   - Oblique popliteal ligament (posterior): This is a reflected part from the tendon of semimembranosus muscle, supporting the joint capsule posteriorly.

   The intracapsular ligaments include:
   - Anterior cruciate ligament (ACL): It runs from the anterior intercondylar region of tibia to the posteromedial surface of the lateral femoral condyle. It helps prevent hyperextension of the knee and resist posterior

displacement of the femur on a fixed tibia. It is weaker than the posterior cruciate ligament and is more commonly injured.

- Posterior cruciate ligament (PCL): It arises from the posterior intercondylar region of tibia and is attached the anterolateral surface of the medial femoral condyle. It helps prevent hyperflexion of the knee and resist anterior displacement of the femur on a fixed tibia.

  Both ligaments are prone to be ruptured in extreme movements, such as in a soccer game.

e. **Meniscus (semilunar cartilage) (Fig. 9.30):** The knee joint contains two crescent-shaped fibrocartilaginous menisci which are interposed between the femoral condyles and tibial plateaus. Both medial and lateral menisci deepen the articular surfaces, improve congruence between the bones, and help absorb shock during weight bearing.

   i. <u>Medial meniscus:</u> It is a C-shaped and less mobile. The medial collateral ligament firmly adheres to the medial meniscus. It is more commonly injured during a medial collateral ligament tear.

   ii. <u>Lateral meniscus:</u> It is more mobile and more circular in outline. The lateral collateral ligament is not directly attached to the lateral meniscus as the popliteal tendon runs between them. Consequently, it is less prone to injury.

f. **Posterior relations:** The posterior aspect of the knee joint is related to the contents of the popliteal fossa. These include the popliteal artery, popliteal vein, tibial nerve, common fibular nerve, and popliteal lymph nodes embedded in fat **(Fig. 9.29; Fig. 9.31)**.

g. **Movements**

   i. <u>Flexion (bending the knee):</u> This movement is primarily produced by the biceps femoris, semitendinosus, and semimembranosus muscles. The gastrocnemius, sartorius, gracilis and popliteus muscles also assist in the movement.

   ii. <u>Extension (straightening the knee):</u> This movement is mainly produced by quadriceps femoris muscle.

   iii. <u>Lateral rotation of the femur:</u> At the onset of flexion, the popliteus muscle contracts and rotates the femur laterally on the fixed tibia. This action unlocks the knee joint.

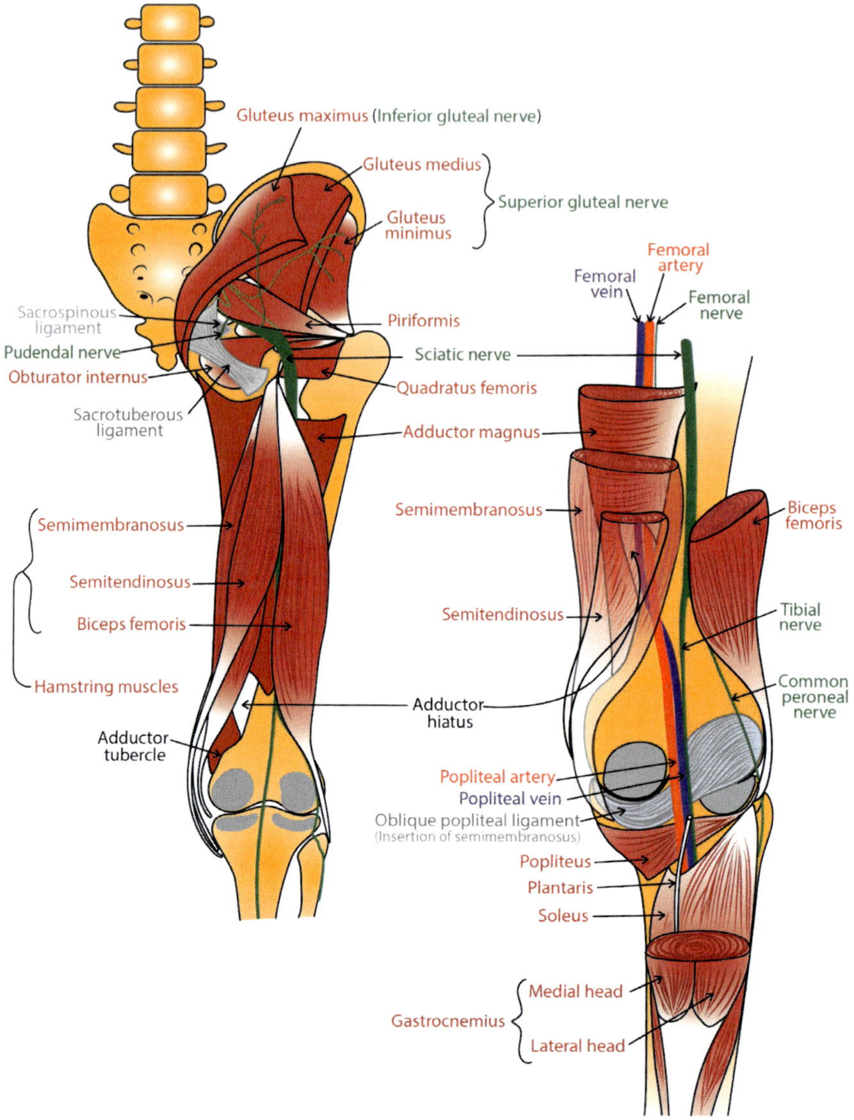

Figure 9.31. Gluteal region, back of the thigh, and popliteal fossa. The gluteal muscles include the gluteus maximus (supplied by the inferior gluteal nerve), gluteus medius and minimus (superior gluteal nerve), and tensor fascia latae (superior gluteal nerve). Deep to these are the small lateral rotators of the hip joint, which include the piriformis, obturator internus, etc. The back of the thigh is the hamstring muscles (semimembranosus, semitendinosus, and biceps femoris). The popliteal fossa is bounded above by the biceps femoris and semimembranosus and semitendinosus; inferiorly, it is bounded by the two heads of the gastrocnemius. The floor of the fossa is formed by the oblique popliteal ligament and popliteus muscle. The fossa contains the popliteal artery and vein and the tibial nerve. The popliteal artery is a continuation of the femoral artery after passing through the hiatus of the adductor magnus. It is most deeply placed in the popliteal fossa.

iv. Medial rotation (of the femur): During the end stage of extension, the femur rotates medially on the fixed tibia. This movement tightens the cruciate and collateral ligaments, placing the knee in a stable locked position.

h. **Nerve supply:** The knee joint receives articular branches from the femoral nerve, saphenous nerve (terminal branch of the femoral nerve), obturator nerve, tibial nerve, and common peroneal (fibular) nerve.

i. **Applied anatomy**

i. ACL injury: ACL rupture or tear can be assessed using the anterior drawer test, in which the knee is flexed, and the tibia is pulled anteriorly. Excessive forward movement of the tibia suggests ACL injury.

ii. PCL injury: PCL rupture or tear is evaluated by the posterior drawer test, where the knee is flexed, and the tibia is pushed posteriorly. Increased backward displacement of tibia indicates PCL damage.

iii. Degenerative knee disease: Thinning of the menisci and articular cartilage is characteristic of osteoarthritis of the knee joint, a common cause of pain and stiffness in the elderly. In advanced cases, total knee joint replacement may be required (**Fig. 9.30**).

3. Ankle Joint (Talocrural Joint) (Fig. 9.23)

a. **Type of joint:** It is a synovial joint of hinge type, allowing two main movements: dorsiflexion and plantarflexion.

b. **Articulation:** The distal ends of the tibia and fibula together form a mortise (socket) which articulates with the trochlea of the talus.

c. **Ligaments:** The ankle joint is strengthened by strong medial and lateral collateral ligaments.

i. Medial ligament: It is a triangular (deltoid) ligament which is composed of tibiocalcaneal ligament, anterior and posterior tibiotalar ligaments, and tibionavicular ligament.

ii. Lateral ligament: It consists of anterior and posterior talofibular ligaments and calcaneofibular ligament.

d. **Movements:**

i. **Dorsiflexion** (bending of the foot so that toes are pointing upward): Tibialis anterior, extensor hallucis longus, and extensor digitorum longus muscles are involved in dorsiflexion.

ii. **Plantarflexion** (bending of the foot so that toes are pointing downward): Soleus, gastrocnemius, and plantaris muscles are involved in plantarflexion.

e. **Innervation:** The ankle joint is innervated by tibial nerve, deep peroneal nerve, and saphenous nerve.

f. **Applied anatomy**

i. Ankle sprain: Excessive inversion commonly injures the lateral ligament, especially the anterior talofibular ligament.

ii. Deltoid ligament injury: Excessive eversion may tear the strong medial (deltoid) ligament, often associated with fractures of the medial malleolus.

iii. Ankle swelling after sprain: A sprained ankle often leads to swelling and pain due to tearing of ligaments and leakage of fluid and blood into surrounding tissues.

4. Joints Involved in Inversion and Eversion of the Foot (Fig. 9.24)

The movements of inversion and eversion occur mainly at the intertarsal joints of the foot, particularly:

a. Talocalcaneonavicular joint
b. Subtalar joint
c. Calcaneocuboid joint
d. Talonavicular joint
e. Transverse tarsal joint (midtarsal joint): This joint is formed by the combination of the calcaneocuboid joint and talonavicular joint.

Movements: The movements at the intertarsal joints of the foot allow the foot to adapt to uneven surfaces or slopes during walking.

- **Inversion of the foot** (The sole of the foot turns medially, so the plantar surface faces inward): Tibialis anterior, tibialis posterior, extensor hallucis longus, and extensor digitorum longus muscles are involved in inversion of the foot.
- **Eversion of the foot** (The sole of the foot turns laterally, so the plantar surface faces outward): Peroneus (fibularis) longus and peroneus (fibularis) brevis muscles are involved in eversion of the foot.

Axis of movement: It is an imaginary oblique line extending from the lateral calcaneum tubercle to the navicular bone through the sinus tarsi.

5. Arches of the Foot (Fig. 9.25)

The foot has three main arches that provides strength, resiliency, shock absorption and efficient transmission of body weight during standing and walking. These arches include:

a. Medial longitudinal arch
b. Lateral longitudinal arch
c. Transverse arch

a. Medial longitudinal arch (Fig. 9.25A)

This arch plays a major role in propulsion of the body during walking, running and splinting.

i. Bones that form the medial longitudinal arch include calcaneum, talus (head of the talus is the keystone), navicular, three cuneiforms, and medial three metatarsals.
ii. Ligamentous support: Plantar aponeurosis (which acts as the tie beam) and plantar calcaneonavicular ligament (spring ligament) support the head of the talus.
iii. Muscular support: The tendons of the tibialis anterior and tibialis posterior support the arch. In addition, small intrinsic muscles of the foot help maintain the integrity of the arch.

b. Lateral longitudinal arch (Fig. 9.25B) This arch provides weight-bearing capability and stability.

i. Bones that form the lateral longitudinal arch include calcaneum, cuboid, and lateral two metatarsals. The cuboid is the keystone.
ii. Ligamentous support: Plantar aponeurosis (which acts as the tie beam), long and short plantar ligaments support the arch.
iii. Muscular support: The tendons of the peroneus longus and brevis support the arch. In addition, small intrinsic muscles of the foot help maintain the arch integrity.

c. Transverse arch

Bones that form the transverse arch include cuboid, three cuneiforms, and metatarsals. The tendons of the peroneus longus and tibialis posterior crossing the foot, help maintain the arch. This arch provides weight bearing capability and helps distribute the body weight.

Applied anatomy

i. Pes Planus (Flat Foot): In flat foot, especially due to collapse of the medial longitudinal arch, the plantar ligaments and nerves may be overstretched, leading to pain and fatigue in the foot.
ii. Plantar Fasciitis: Inflammation of the plantar aponeurosis causes heel pain, particularly after prolonged standing or on first steps in the morning.

Muscles of the Lower Limb

1. Gluteal region (Fig. 9.28; Fig. 9.29; Fig. 9.31)

The gluteal region consists of the following muscles:

a. Gluteus maximus: The gluteus maximus is a large muscle and functions as the main extensor of the hip joint (during walking, climbing stairs, and standing up from a sitting position). It is innervated by the inferior gluteal nerve (L5, S1, S2).
b. Gluteus medius and gluteus minimus: They lie deep to the gluteus maximus and function as the abductors of the hip joint. They also help in medial rotation of the thigh and stabilization of the pelvis during walking. When standing on one leg, they prevent the pelvis from tilting on the unsupported side, allowing the opposite foot to clear the ground during walking. Both the gluteus medius and gluteus minimus are innervated by the superior gluteal nerve (L4, L5, S1).
c. Piriformis, obturator internus, superior and inferior gemelli, and quadratus femoris: These muscles act together to laterally rotate the thigh at the hip joint and stabilize the head of the femur within the acetabulum. The piriformis is innervated by the nerve to piriformis (S1, S2). The superior gemellus and obturator internus are innervated by the nerve to obturator internus (L5, S1). The inferior gemellus and quadratus femoris are supplied by the nerve to quadratus femoris (L5, S1).

2. Thigh Region

The muscles in the thigh are divided into three compartments, anterior, posterior, and medial (adductor) compartments by the intermuscular septa.

a. **Anterior compartment:** This compartment contains the quadriceps muscle group (rectus femoris, vastus anterior, vastus intermedius, vastus medialis) and the sartorius muscle **(Fig. 9.27; Fig. 9.32)**. Most of these muscles arise from the femur, except the sartorius and rectus femoris which originate from the hip bone and cross the hip and knee joints. The sartorius ("tailor's muscle") flexes, weakly abducts and laterally rotates the thigh at the hip joint. It also aids in flexion at the knee joint as in the traditional cross-legged sitting posture of tailors. The rectus femoris flexes the hip joint and extends the knee joint. The quadriceps is attached to the patella and continues inferiorly as the ligamentum patella which is inserted to the tibial tuberosity. The quadriceps femoris is the chief extensor of the knee joint and is involved in walking, running, jumping and climbing. Because of its powerful action in knee extension, it is often referred to as the "kicking muscle" (as soccer players do). Both the quadriceps and sartorius muscles are supplied by the femoral nerve (L2-4) of the lumbar nerve plexus.

Quiz: *Tapping the ligamentum patella elicits the knee-jerk (patellar) reflex. What is the neural pathway of this reflex arc?*

b. **Posterior compartment:** This compartment contains the hamstring muscles (semitendinosus, semimembranosus, and biceps femoris) **(Fig. 9.29; Fig. 9.31)**. These muscles arise mainly from the ischial tuberosity. They cross both the hip and knee joints, except for the short head of the biceps femoris which crosses only the knee joint. They extend the hip joint and flex the knee joint, and they are involved in climbing, walking, and running. Most hamstring muscles are supplied by the tibial division of the sciatic nerve. However, the short head of the biceps, is supplied by the common fibular (peroneal) division of the sciatic nerve.

c. **Adductor compartment:** This compartment contains the adductor longus, adductor brevis, adductor magnus, gracilis, and pectineus muscles (Fig. 9.27; Fig. 9.32).

   The adductor muscles primarily adduct the thigh at the hip joint, as occurs during horse riding. They arise mainly from the pubis and ischiopubic ramus and are inserted mainly into the linea aspera of the femur. The adductor muscles are supplied by the obturator nerve (L2-L4), which passes through the obturator foramen **(Fig. 9.27; Fig. 9.32)**. The pectineus is innervated by a branch from the femoral nerve (L2, L3).

d. **Tensor fascia latae (Fig. 9.29).** It is a small muscle, located in the lateral aspect of the thigh. It is enclosed within the iliotibial tract, a thickened band of fascia extending from the iliac crest to the lateral condyle of the tibia.

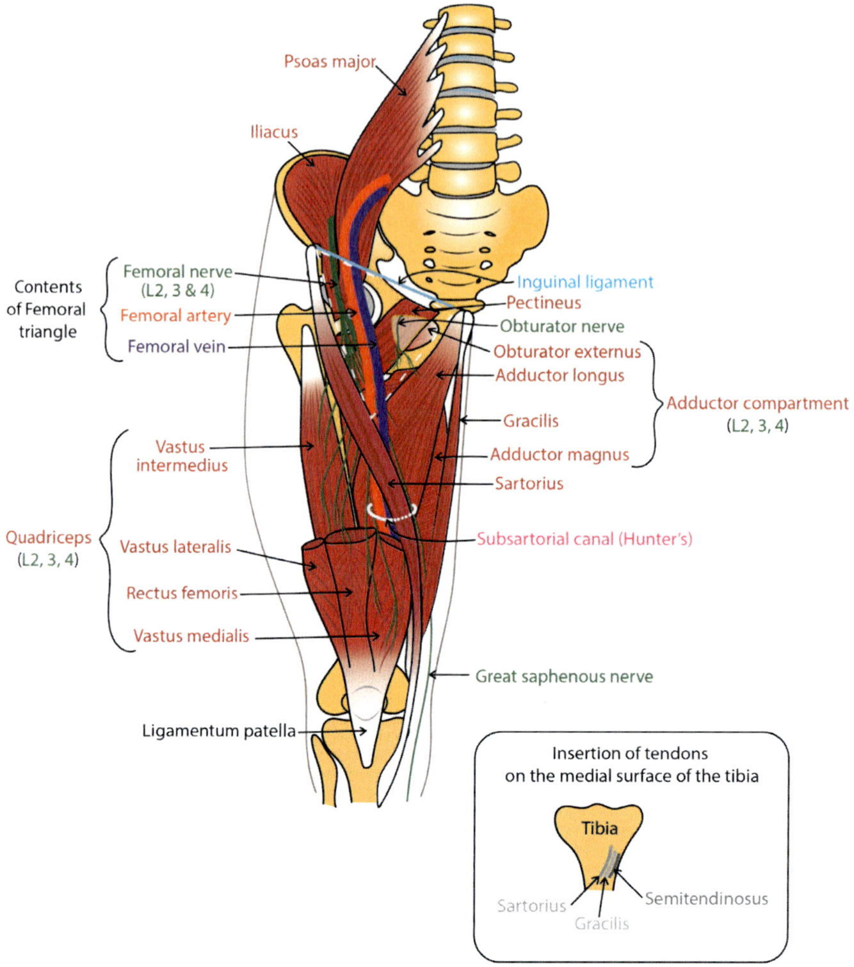

Figure 9.32. Muscle compartments of the thigh: anterior (extensor) and medial (adductor) compartments. The anterior muscle compartment consists of the sartorius and quadriceps (rectus femoris, vastus intermedius, vastus lateralis, and vastus medialis). All are supplied by the femoral nerve. The medial or adductor muscle compartment includes the adductors (obturator externus, adductor longus, adductor magnus, adductor brevis, and gracilis). All adductors of the thigh (hip joint) are supplied by the obturator nerve.

It contributes to stabilization and extension of the knee joint. It is innervated by the superior gluteal nerve.

e. Femoral triangle (Fig. 9.32; Fig. 9.33)

The femoral triangle is a triangular intermuscular space located in the upper anterior part of the thigh, just below the inguinal ligament. It is bounded

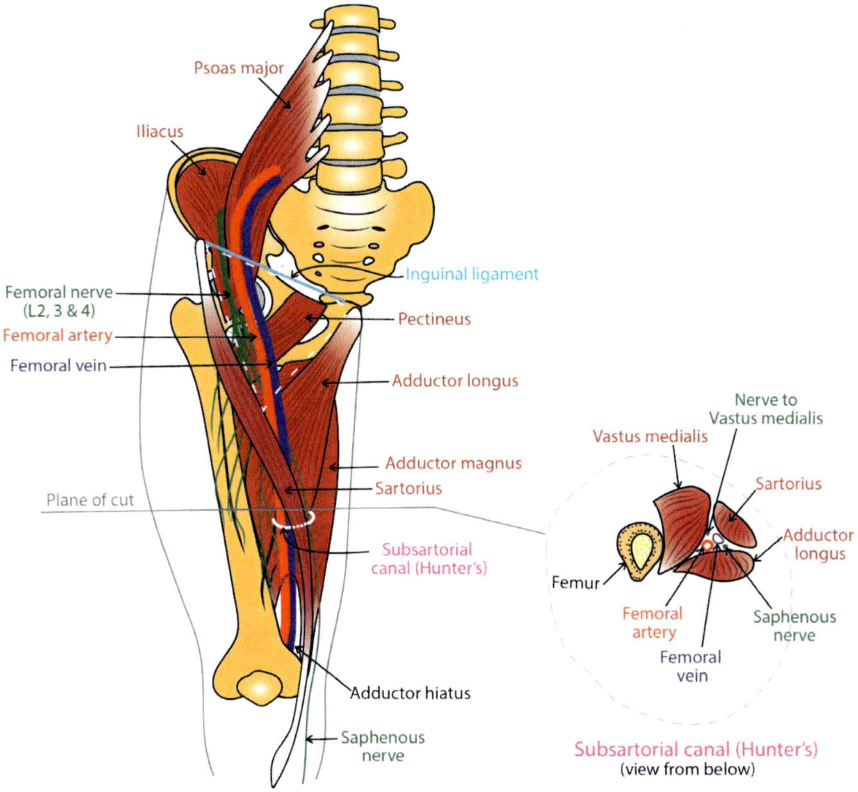

Figure 9.33. Femoral triangle and subsartorial canal. The femoral triangle is bounded by the inguinal ligament, sartorius and adductor longus. The floor is formed by the pectineus and iliopsoas tendon. It contains the femoral vein, femoral artery, and femoral nerve arranged medio-laterally. The neurovascular bundle leaves the triangle through its "apex" into the subsartorial canal (right of the figure), which is bounded by the sartorius, vastus medialis (femur), and adductor longus. The canal forms the passage for the femoral artery and vein, saphenous nerve, and nerve to the vastus medialis.

superiorly by the inguinal ligament extending from the anterior superior iliac spine to the public tubercle, laterally by the medial border of the sartorius muscle, and medially by the adductor longus muscle. The floor of the femoral triangle is formed by the iliopsoas muscle and pectineus muscle. The femoral triangle contains the femoral vein, femoral artery, and femoral nerve which are arranged from medial to lateral. Both the artery and vein are enclosed within the femoral sheath, whereas femoral nerve lies outside the sheath. The femoral canal containing the deep inguinal lymph nodes lies medial to the vein.

f. Applied anatomy

***Quiz* 1:** *The femoral artery in the femoral triangle can be catheterized when performing an angiogram/angioplasty procedure. Name the arteries in order by which the catheter passes through to reach the coronary arteries during an angiogram procedure.*

***Quiz* 2:** *How do you surface mark the femoral artery?*

***Quiz* 3:** *What are direct and indirect inguinal hernias?*

***Quiz* 4:** *What is "femoral hernia"?*

***Quiz* 5:** *How do you differentiate the femoral hernia from the inguinal hernia?*

3. Leg (Fig. 9.27; Fig. 9.29)

The muscles of the leg are organized into three compartments separated by the deep fascia and intermuscular septa: anterior, lateral, and posterior compartments.

a. Anterior compartment (Fig. 9.27)

i. This compartment contains the tibialis anterior, extensor hallucis longus (hallux = great toe), extensor digitorum longus, and peroneus (fibularis) tertius. They are involved in dorsiflexion of the foot at the ankle joint and extension of the toes. Tibialis anterior also is the main invertor of the foot. Extensor hallucis longus and extensor digitorum longus assist in inversion.

ii. Innervation: All muscles in the anterior compartment are innervated by the deep peroneal nerve, a branch of the common peroneal (fibular) nerve.

b. Lateral (peroneal compartment) (Fig. 9.27)

i. This compartment contains peroneus (fibularis) longus and peroneus (fibularis) brevis. They are evertors of the foot. They also assist in plantar flexion weakly.

ii. Innervation: Lateral compartment muscles are innervated by the superficial peroneal (fibular) nerve, a branch of the common peroneal (fibular) nerve.

c. Posterior compartment

i. This compartment consists of superficial and deep groups of muscles. Superficial group muscles include gastrocnemius (lateral and medial heads) **(Fig. 9.29)**, soleus, and plantaris. Gastrocnemius and soleus form the triceps surae (calf muscles). The deep group muscles include flexor digitorum longus, flexor hallucis longus, tibialis posterior and popliteus. Gastrocnemius arises from the medial and lateral condyles of femur. It is a powerful plantar flexor of the foot during running and sprinting. It also assists in flexion of the knee as it crosses both the knee and ankle joints.

ii. Soleus arises from the posterior surfaces of the tibia and fibula. It functions as an antigravity (postural) muscle during standing and acts as a peripheral heart pump because its contractions aid venous return from the lower limb. This function is facilitated by the extensive venous plexus embedded within the soleus muscle **(Fig. 9.34)**, which are compressed during its contraction and help propel blood toward the heart. The gastrocnemius and soleus unite to form the common tendon, "tendon calcaneum" (Achilles tendon), which inserts into the posterior surface of the calcaneum. Tibialis posterior, flexor hallucis longus, and flexor digitorum are plantar flexors of the foot at the ankle joint. The tibialis posterior and flexor hallucis longus muscles assist in the inversion of the foot. They also maintain the medial longitudinal arch of the foot **(Fig. 9.25A)**. Popliteus **(Fig. 9.29; Fig. 9.31)** lies on the posterior aspect of the tibia. Superiorly, its upper attachment is to the lateral femoral condyle and the lateral meniscus. It assists in the unlocking of the knee joint (lateral rotation of the femur) at the beginning of the knee flexion.

iii. Innervation: All muscles in the posterior compartment are innervated by the tibial nerve.

4. Foot

The muscles of the foot mainly consist of the intrinsic muscles located on the dorsum and the sole of the foot. They act on the toes producing movements at the metatarsophalangeal and interphalangeal joints.

Dorsum of the foot

a. Extensor digitorum brevis: It extends the second to fourth toes (except the small toe) and assists the extensor digitorum longus muscle.
b. Extensor hallucis brevis: It extends the great toe at the metatarsophalangeal joint and assists the extensor hallucis longus.

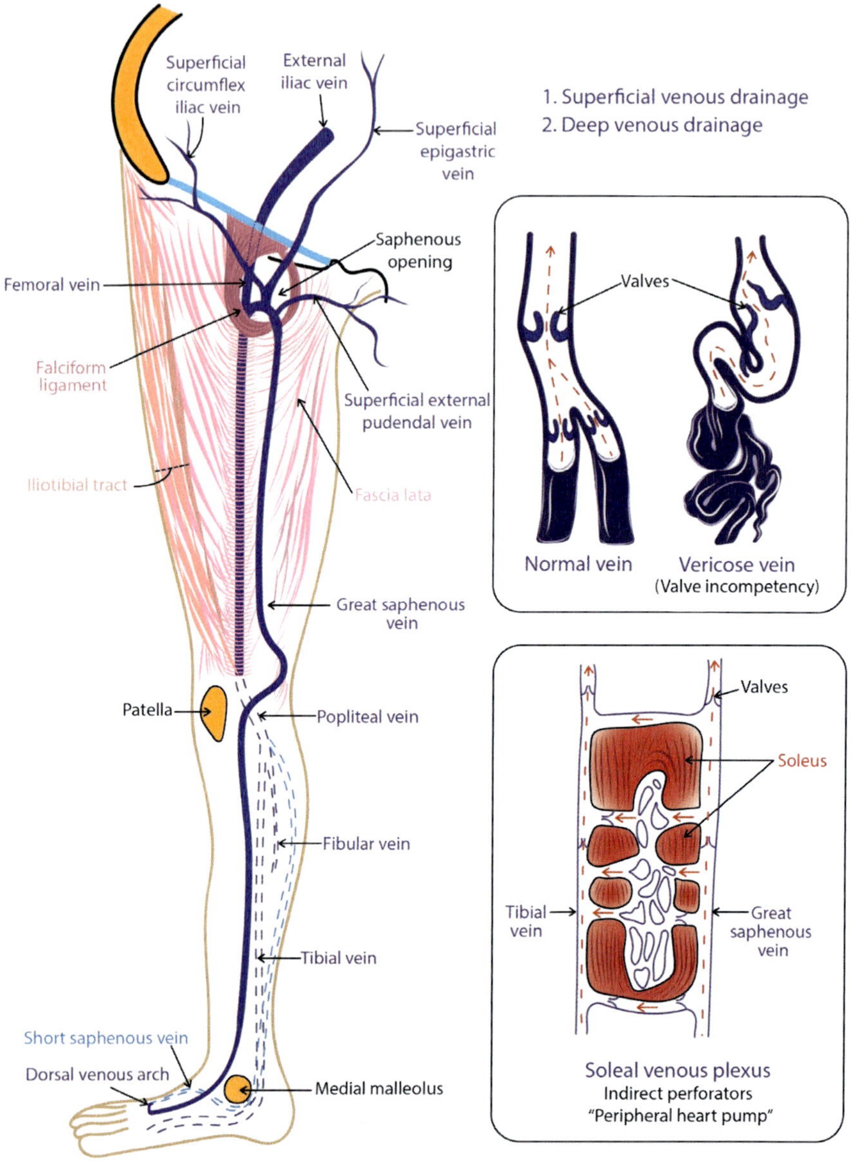

Figure 9.34. Venous drainage of the lower limb. It is facilitated by the superficial and deep venous drainage system. The superficial veins include the great saphenous vein and the short saphenous vein; both ultimately drain into the femoral vein. There are many tributaries, as indicated. Note that venous blood from the superficial vein may be drained into the deep veins, either directly or indirectly, through the perforators embedded in the muscle, such as the soleus. Varicose veins are due to the incompetency of valves.

Sole of the foot

Deep to the thick skin of the sole lies the plantar aponeurosis, a strong fibrous sheet that protects the underlying structures (**Fig. 9.25**). The intrinsic muscles of the sole are arranged in different layers. Their main function is to move the toes at the metatarsophalangeal and the interphalangeal joints. The following muscles of the foot are included for reference only.

a. Flexor digitorum brevis: It flexes the lateral four digits (second to fifth).
b. Flexor hallucis longus tendon: It flexes the great toe.
c. Flexor digitorum longus: It flexes the lateral four toes.
d. Plantar accessories (quadratus plantae): It assists the flexor digitorum longus in flexing the lateral four toes.
e. Four lumbricals: These muscles flex the metatarsophalangeal joints and extend the interphalangeal joints of the lateral four toes.
f. Muscles of the great toe (Abductor hallucis, flexor hallucis brevis, and adductor hallucis): These muscles are responsible for abduction, flexion and adduction of the great toe, respectively.
g. Plantar interossei (three muscles): They adduct the lateral three toes (third, fourth and fifth toes) toward an imaginary line along the axis of the second toe.
h. Dorsal interossei (four muscles): They assist abduction of the second, third, and fourth toes away from an imaginary line along the longitudinal axis of the second toe.
i. The interossei also stabilize the toes during walking and standing.

Nerves of the Lower Limb (Fig. 9.28; Fig. 9.35)

1. There are two major nerve plexuses supplying the lower limb: the lumbar nerve plexus (L1–L4), which gives rise to the femoral nerve and obturator nerve (**Fig. 9.35**) and the sacral nerve plexus (L4-S4) which gives rise to the sciatic nerve and its major branches.

   The femoral and obturator nerves supply mainly the muscles of the anterior and medial compartments of the thigh, respectively. The sciatic nerve (**Fig. 9.28**), the largest nerve in the body, arises from the sacral nerve plexus and provides motor and sensory innervation to the lower limb

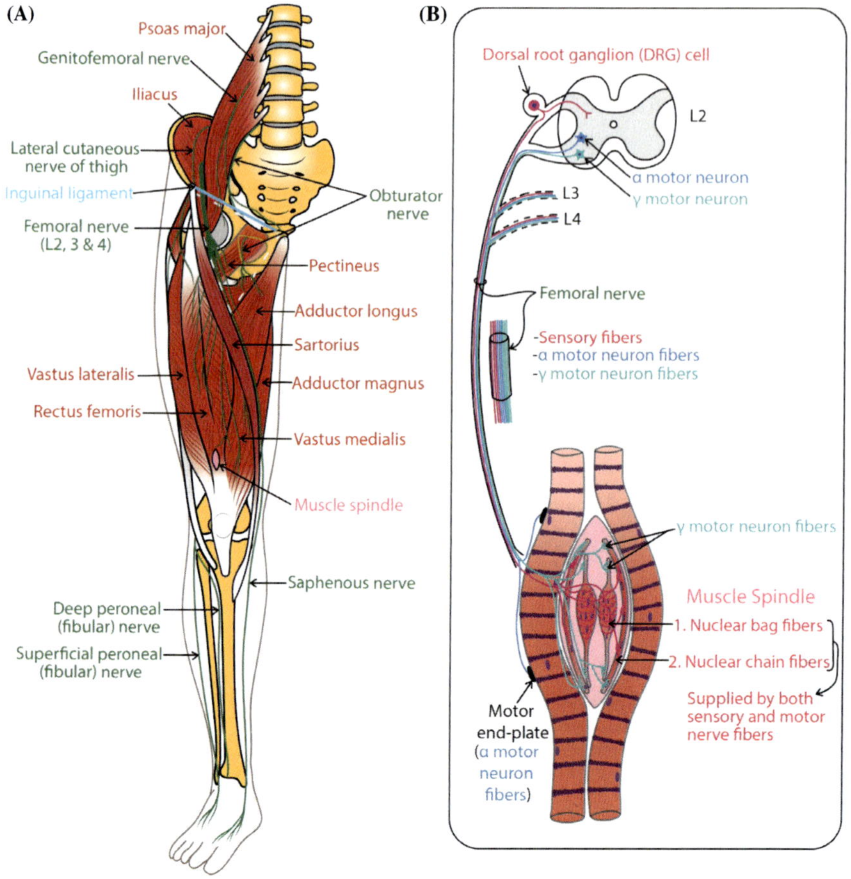

Figure 9.35. Origin, course, and distribution of the femoral nerve and obturator nerve. (A) The femoral nerve arises from the lumbar plexus (L2, 3, 4). It descends lateral to the iliopsoas major muscle. It enters the femoral triangle deep to the inguinal ligament. It then passes through the subsartorial canal and continues as the saphenous nerve, which runs along the medial side of the leg and terminates at the base of the big toe. The obturator nerve also arises from L2, 3, 4. It descends along the medial border of the iliopsoas major and passes through the obturator foramen, and supplies the adductors of the thigh. **(B)** The femoral nerve is composed of both motor and sensory nerve fibers originating from the motor neurons of the ventral horn at L2, 3, 4 and sensory fibers from the dorsal root ganglion cells at L2, 3, 4. The motor fibers (axons) supply the quadriceps and sartorius muscle fibers via their terminations — motor endplate. The sensory fibers supply the skin, capsule, and ligament, as well as the muscle spindles that elicit the knee-jerk reflex.

musculature, skin, and joints. The nerves contain not only the motor and sensory nerve fibers but also the postganglionic sympathetic nerve fibers supplying the smooth muscle of vascular walls (arteries, veins), sweat glands, and arrector pili muscle of the skin.

2. The cell bodies of the motor neurons are located in the ventral (anterior) horn of the lumbosacral segments of the spinal cord **(Fig. 9.28)**. Thus, the motor nerve fibers in the peripheral nerves represent the axons of these motor neurons.
3. The cell bodies of the sensory neurons are located in the dorsal root or sensory ganglia of the corresponding spinal nerves **(Fig. 9.28)**. These sensory neurons are classified as the pseudounipolar neurons. The sensory nerve fibers in the peripheral nerves represent the peripheral process (afferent fibers) of these neurons.
4. Accompanying the motor and sensory fibers are postganglionic sympathetic vasomotor nerve fibers. Their cell bodies are located in the paravertebral sympathetic ganglia (L1–L2). These nerve fibers regulate blood flow to the lower limb by controlling the calibre of blood vessels. Excessive vasoconstriction may contribute to Raynaud's disease, characterized by reduced blood flow to the lower extremities.

All peripheral nerves in the lower extremities are, therefore, mixed nerves containing motor, sensory and autonomic (sympathetic) fibers. Because many of these peripheral nerves travel long distance to supply their target structures, they are vulnerable to injury. For example, the common peroneal (fibular) nerve may be injured at the neck of the fibula. This may lead to paralysis of dorsiflexor muscles of the foot, resulting in a characteristic condition known as "foot drop."

Nerve Plexuses of the Lower Limb

1. **Lumbar nerve plexus (L1-L4):** The major nerves supplying the lower limb from the lumbar plexus are the femoral nerve and obturator nerve **(Fig. 9.35)**.
   a. **Femoral nerve:** It supplies the muscles of the anterior compartment of the thigh, including the sartorius and quadriceps femoris. It also provides sensory innervation to the anterior thigh. Its terminal branch is the saphenous nerve, which supplies the skin on the medial side of the leg and foot as far as the base of the great toe. It also supplies the knee joint and mediates the "knee-jerk" reflex (patellar reflex) (L2-L4) through the muscle spindle **(Fig. 9.35)**.
   b. **Obturator nerve:** It supplies the muscles of the adductor compartment of the thigh, including the adductor muscles and gracilis. It also supplies the hip and knee joints.

2. **Sacral nerve plexus (L4-S4) (Fig. 9.28)**

The sacral plexus gives rise to the sciatic nerve which divides into the tibial nerve and the common peroneal nerve, as well as superior and inferior gluteal nerves. There are several other nerves from this plexus supplying the lateral rotators of the hip joint in the gluteal region.

i. **Superior gluteal nerve (L4, 5, S1) (Fig. 9.28; Fig. 9.31):** It supplies the gluteus medius, gluteus minimus, and tensor fascia latae (enclosed in the iliotibial tract). These muscles are important for hip abduction and stabilization of the pelvis during walking. The tensor fasciae lata contributes to stabilization of the knee joint.

ii. **Inferior gluteal nerve (L5, S1, 2) (Fig. 9.28; Fig. 9.31):** It supplies the gluteus maximus.

iii. **Sciatic nerve (Fig. 9.28; Fig. 9.31):** It is the longest nerve in the body. It passes through the gluteal region and descends along the posterior compartment of the thigh. At the apex of the popliteal fossa, it divides into the tibial nerve and common peroneal (fibular) nerve. The tibial nerve continues through the popliteal fossa and posterior compartment of the leg. It passes deep to the flexor retinaculum (tarsal tunnel) and terminates as the medial and lateral planter nerves in the sole of the foot.

» *The tibial division in the thigh region* **(Fig. 9.28; Fig. 9.31)**
It supplies the semitendinosus, semimembranosus, long head of femoris and the hamstring part of adductor magnus. The short head of the biceps femoris is supplied by the common peroneal (fibular) division.

» *Common peroneal (fibular) nerve* **(Fig. 9.28; Fig. 9.31)**
It courses along the superolateral side of the popliteal fossa and winds around the neck of the fibula, where it divides into the superficial peroneal (fibular) nerve and deep peroneal (fibular) nerve. In the thigh, it supplies the short head of the biceps femoris.

» *Superficial peroneal (fibular) nerve* **(Fig. 9.35)**
It supplies the muscles of the lateral compartment of the leg including, the peroneus (fibularis) longus and peroneus (fibularis) brevis.

» *Deep peroneal (fibular) nerve* **(Fig. 9.35)**
It supplies the muscles of the anterior compartment of the leg, including tibialis anterior, extensor hallucis longus, extensor digitorum longus, and peroneus (fibularis) tertius. It continues into the dorsum of foot to innervate extensor digitorum brevis.

» *Medial plantar nerve* **(Fig. 9.28)**
It supplies the muscles of the foot on the medial side, including, flexor digitorum brevis, abductor hallucis, flexor hallucis brevis, first lumbrical. It provides sensory innervation to the medial three and a half toes and the adjacent plantar surface of the foot.

» *Lateral plantar nerve* **(Fig. 9.28)**
It supplies the muscles of the foot on the lateral side including the quadratus plantae, flexor digiti minimi, adductor hallucis, interossei and the lateral three lumbricals. It provides sensory innervation to the skin of the lateral third of the sole of the foot and the plantar surface of the lateral one and a half toes.

Applied anatomy

1. In poliomyelitis, the poliovirus selectively destroys the ventral horn motor neurons of the lumbosacral spinal cord segments, causing paralysis of the gluteal muscles. Weakness or paralysis of the gluteus medius and gluteus minimus prevents stabilization of the pelvis during walking. As a result. The pelvis drops on the unsupported side when the patient stands on the affected limb, producing a positive Trendelenburg sign and a characteristic a "dipping gait".
   Quiz: *Where is the safe site for intramuscular injection in the gluteal region? Why?*
2. The sciatic nerve arises from the sacral plexus (L4-S4). Herniation of the intervertebral disc (fibrocartilage) at the L4-L5 or L5-S1 levels may compress on the corresponding spinal nerve roots. This may produce sciatica, characterized by severe pain radiating from the lower back and gluteal region along the posterior aspect of the thigh and leg, extending into the foot.
3. The common peroneal (fibular) nerve is subcutaneous at the neck of the fibula, where it is vulnerable to injury from fractures or compression. Damage to this nerve results in paralysis of the extensor muscles of the anterior compartment of the leg, leading to loss of dorsiflexion of the foot (foot drop).
4. Plantar fasciitis: This is a common condition caused by inflammation of the plantar aponeurosis. It produces severe pain in the sole of the foot.
5. Segmental innervation of muscles/joints and Tendon Reflexes: Knowledge of segmental innervation is important in the clinical assessment of nerve root

function. Extension of the knee (L3-L4) is tested by eliciting the knee-jerk (patellar) reflex by tapping the ligamentum patella. Plantar flexion of the ankle (S1-S2) is tested by eliciting the ankle-jerk (Achilles) reflex by tapping the Achilles' tendon (calcaneal tendon).

Quiz* 1:** *What is a "stretch receptor" in a muscle? What are its functions? (See* **Fig. 9.35B)*

***Quiz* 2:** *Describe the neural pathway of the "knee-jerk reflex."*

Popliteal Fossa (Fig. 9.31)

The popliteal fossa is a diamond-shaped depression located posterior to the knee joint. It is bounded superomedially by the semitendinosus and semimembranosus muscles and superolaterally by the biceps femoris muscle. Inferiorly, it is bounded by the lateral and medial heads of the gastrocnemius muscle. The floor is formed by the posterior (popliteal) surface of the femur, oblique popliteal ligament (reflected part of the semimembranosus tendon), knee posterior capsule of the knee joint, and popliteus muscle. The popliteal fossa contains the tibial nerve, popliteal vein and popliteal artery, popliteal vein, and tibial nerve. It also contains popliteal lymph nodes, fat and connective tissue.

A fluid-filled cyst known as a Baker (popliteal) cyst may develop in the popliteal fossa.

Arteries of the Lower Limb

The lower limb receives its arterial supply mainly from two sources:

1. **Superior and inferior gluteal arteries:** Both are branches of the internal iliac artery and supply the gluteal region.
2. **Femoral artery (Fig. 9.26; Fig. 9.31; Fig. 9.32; Fig. 9.33):** It is the continuation of the external iliac artery. It enters the femoral triangle beneath the inguinal ligament and gives off its largest branch, the profunda (deep) femoris artery. The profunda femoris artery supply the deep muscles of the thigh and the hip joint (including the head and neck of the femur via the medial and lateral circumflex femoral arteries through the trochanteric anastomosis) **(Fig. 9.26)**. The femoral artery passes through the adductor hiatus and becomes the popliteal artery. At the lower part of the popliteal

fossa, the popliteal artery divides into the anterior tibial and posterior tibial arteries. The posterior tibial artery gives rise to the fibular (peroneal) artery. The anterior tibial artery supplies the anterior compartment of the leg and continues onto the dorsum of the foot as the dorsalis pedis artery. The posterior tibial artery descends in the posterior compartment of the leg alongside the tibial nerve and enters the sole of the foot, where it divides into the medial and lateral plantar arteries.

Applied anatomy

a. The arterial pulse may be palpated at the following sites in the lower limb:
   i. Femoral pulse: just inferior to the inguinal ligament within the femoral triangle;
   ii. Posterior tibial pulse: posterior to the medial malleolus;
   iii. Dorsalis pedis pulse: between the extensor hallucis longus and extensor digitorum longus tendons;
   iv. Popliteal pulse: deep within the popliteal fossa with the knee flexed.
b. Femoral artery catheterization: The femoral artery is commonly used for arterial catheterization and endovascular procedures such as minimally invasive angioplasty and angiography.
c. Popliteal Aneurysm: A localized dilatation of the popliteal artery may occur due to a weakening of the arterial wall. This may compromise distal blood flow.
   Quiz: *What is the clinical implication if the femoral pulse is diminished unilaterally or bilaterally?*

Venous Drainage of the Lower Limb (Fig. 9.34)

The venous drainage of the lower limb occurs by superficial and deep venous systems:

1. **Superficial venous drainage:** This venous drainage occurs via the great (long) saphenous vein and the small saphenous vein. The great saphenous vein originates from the medial end of the dorsal venous arch of the foot. It passes anterior to the medial malleolus, ascends along the medial aspect of the leg and thigh and then drains into the femoral vein through the saphenous opening. It is accompanied by the saphenous nerve.

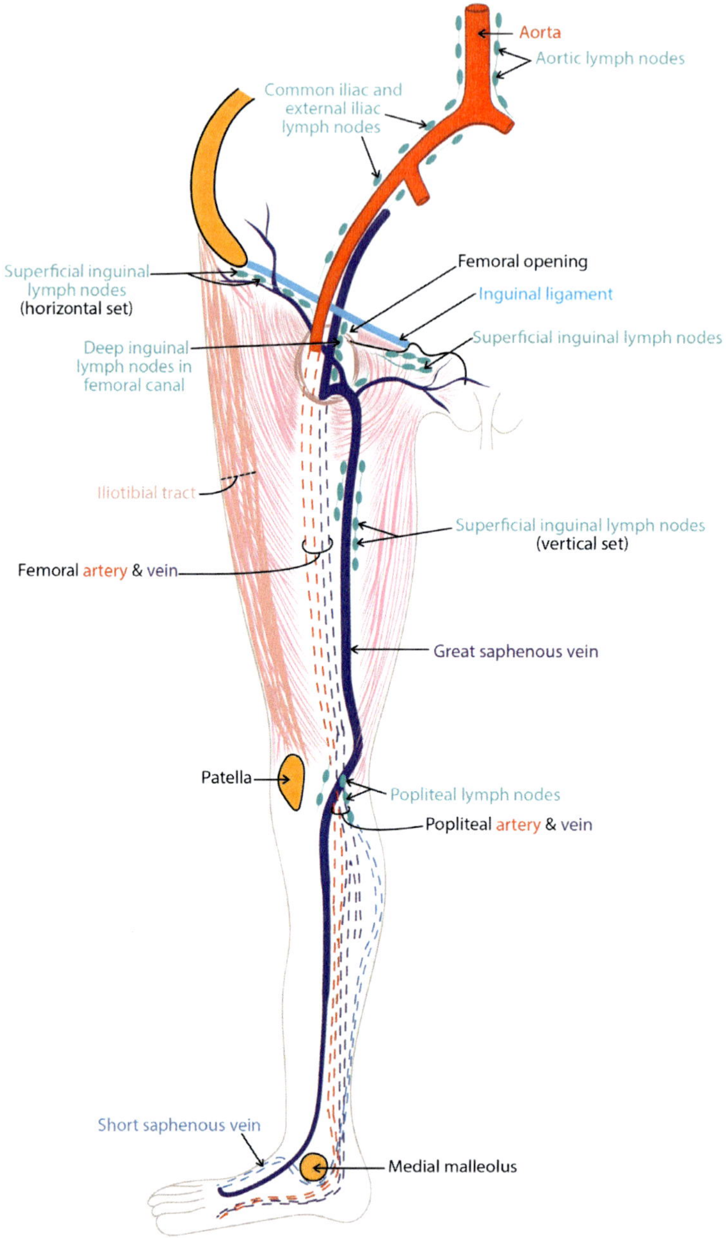

Figure 9.36. Lymphatic drainage of the lower limb. The superficial lymphatic drainage follows the superficial veins, while the deep lymphatic drainage follows the arteries. All drainage goes to the deep inguinal lymph nodes — external iliac nodes — common iliac nodes — aortic nodes — cisterna chyli — thoracic duct.

The small or short saphenous vein arises from the lateral end of the dorsal venous arch of the foot. It passes posterior to the lateral malleolus, ascends in the posterior aspect of the leg, penetrates the popliteal fossa, and drains into the popliteal vein. It is accompanied by the sural nerve.

2. **Deep venous drainage (Fig. 9.34):** The deep veins accompany the corresponding arteries and include the tibial veins, popliteal vein, femoral vein, and external iliac vein.

Perforating veins connect the superficial and deep veins are and normally direct blood flow from superficial to deep veins. Some perforating veins ramify within the soleus muscle as the soleal venous plexus.

Applied anatomy

a. The venous return of the lower limb is facilitated by a series of venous valves and contraction of the calf muscles, particularly the soleus muscle. Incompetency of the valves may lead to varicose veins **(Fig. 9.34)**.
b. Deep vein thrombosis (DVT): DVT (formation of blood clots in the deep venous plexus) may occur following prolonged immobilization, long-haul flight or an invasive surgery involving the knee or hip joint. Dislodgement of a thrombus may result in pulmonary embolism (deep vein thrombosis), which can be potentially fatal.

Lymphatic Drainage of the Lower Limb (Fig. 9.36)

1. Superficial lymphatic drainage follows the superficial veins, including great (long) saphenous and small (short) saphenous veins. Most vessels drain initially into the superficial inguinal lymph nodes.
2. Deep lymphatic vessels accompany the major arteries, including posterior tibial artery, popliteal artery and femoral artery and drain into popliteal, deep inguinal and external iliac lymph nodes.
3. Lymph from the lower limb passes through the deep inguinal lymph nodes in the femoral canal, external iliac nodes, common iliac nodes and aortic nodes.

The superficial inguinal lymph nodes are located near the termination of the great saphenous vein, inferior to the inguinal ligament.

Quiz: *What is the lymphatic drainage of the anal canal, scrotum, ovary, and testis?*

Chapter 10

HEAD AND NECK

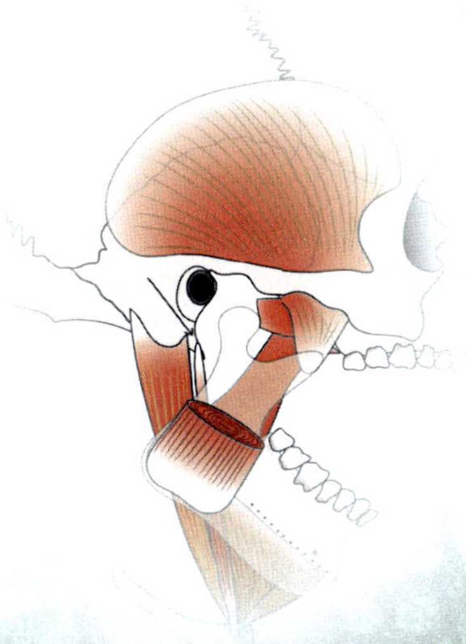

HEAD AND NECK

THE NECK

General Organization

The neck serves as a conduit for the passage of visceral structures such as the larynx, trachea, pharynx, esophagus, great vessels, and the spinal cord **(Fig. 10.1A)**.

The neck extends from the inferior border of the mandible, styloid process (temporal bone), mastoid process (temporal bone), superior nuchal line (occipital bone), and external occipital protuberance (inion) and is inferiorly bounded by the suprasternal notch (jugular notch), clavicle, and the spine of the scapula **(Fig. 10.1A)**. It supports and moves the head (through the cervical spine or vertebral column) and maintains posture and balance of the body. The outlying muscle layers protect the visceral structures and help the movement of the neck and head. In addition to the above are two major endocrine glands, namely, the thyroid and parathyroid glands, which are closely related with the larynx and trachea. In addition, there are deep cervical lymph nodes, which are closely associated with great vessels such as the internal jugular vein, carotid arteries, and four cranial nerves, namely, the glossopharyngeal (CN IX), vagus (CN X), accessory (CN XI), and hypoglossal (CN XII) nerves.

Cervical Spine (Vertebral Column)

The skeletal framework of the cervical spine comprises seven cervical vertebrae. The first cervical vertebra is the atlas, and the second, the axis. Superiorly, the atlas articulates with the two occipital condyles at the base of the skull, forming the atlantooccipital joint (this allows flexion and extension of the head). Inferiorly, the atlas articulates with the axis, forming the atlantoaxial joint (this allows rotation of the head).

The atlas (C1), axis (C2), and C7 cervical vertebrae are considered atypical, with the rest of the cervical vertebrae (C3–6) being typical. A typical cervical vertebra is identified by the presence of the following parts: the transverse process, foramen transversarium (for transmission of the vertebral artery and the vein), the body, and a bifid spine. The atlas is devoid of a spine and body; hence, it has

(A)

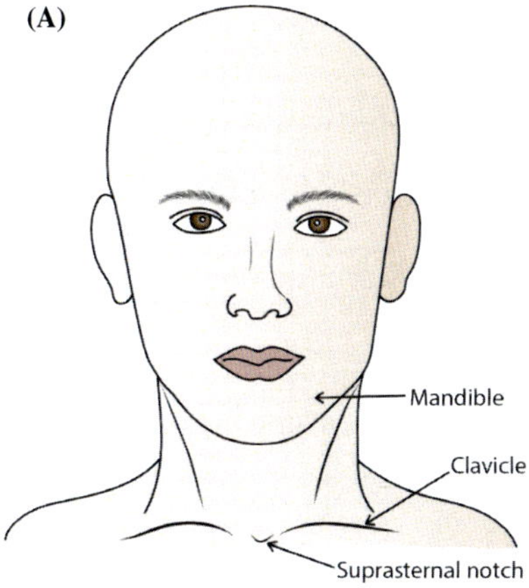

(B)

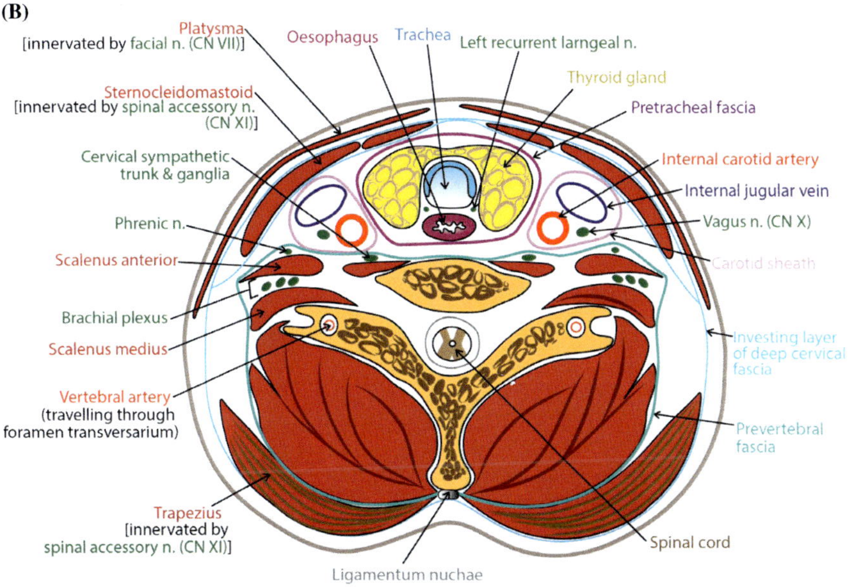

Figure 10.1. (A) Neck. The neck extends from the mandible superiorly to the clavicle and suprasternal notch inferiorly. The neck muscles help maintain the body posture and move the head. It serves as a conduit for the trachea, esophagus, and great vessels (carotids, internal jugular vein), the vagus nerve, and the spinal cord. **(B)** Transverse section of the neck showing the main muscles (sternocleidomastoid, trapezius, and strap muscles), great vessels (carotids and internal jugular vein), trachea, esophagus, and vagus nerve. Posteriorly are the cervical vertebrae and muscles associated with them (pre- and postvertebral muscles) and the cervical sympathetic trunk/ganglia.

"*no spine, no body*"! The axis is identified by an odontoid process (a tooth-like projection) that articulates with the anterior arch of the atlas. The C7 vertebra has a prominent, long spinous process. The vertebral (or spinal) canal transmits the spinal cord and its coverings (meninges).

Bony landmarks in the neck region that are palpable:

1. **Mandible**: Inferior border and angle of the mandible.
2. **Hyoid bone**: It lies at the level of the third cervical vertebra (C3).
3. **Thyroid cartilage**: It lies at the level of the fourth and fifth cervical vertebrae (C4/C5). The thyroid prominence, also called the Adam's apple, can be seen at the anterior surface of the thyroid cartilage.
4. **Cricoid cartilage**: It lies at the level of the sixth cervical vertebra (C6).
5. **Mastoid process**: It is a part of the temporal bone and lies behind the external ear.
6. **External occipital protuberance**: Also known as the "inion," and the superior nuchal line in the occipital bone forms the superior border of the neck posteriorly.

Muscles of the neck **(Fig. 10.1B)**

They are grouped into those associated with the cervical vertebrae (posterior), in the midline anteriorly, and those at the periphery, deep to the skin/deep cervical fascia:

1. *Pre- and postvertebral muscles*: They are involved in maintaining the body posture and movements of the head/neck, including flexion, extension, and rotation. Prevertebral muscles include the scalenus anterior and scalenus medius, and postvertebral muscles include the semispinalis capitis and longissimus capitis.
2. *Strap muscles*: They are midline muscles anterior to the trachea. They are named according to their attachments, namely, sternohyoid, sternothyroid, thyrohyoid, and omohyoid (*omo* refers to the shoulder). The "strap muscles" act to stabilize the hyoid bone so that the suprahyoid muscles, e.g., digastric muscles, can act on a firm base. The strap muscles are also called the "infrahyoid muscles." In addition to them is the cricothyroid muscle, which is a laryngeal muscle (*see the section on the Larynx*).

3. *Two superficial muscles*: The sternocleidomastoid and trapezius (*described previously in the Upper Limb region*) are involved in moving the head and the neck. Both the sternocleidomastoid and trapezius are enclosed by the investing layer of the deep cervical fascia.

<u>Deep cervical fascia</u>

The deep cervical fascia lies deep to the skin. It has three layers: (1) investing layer, (2) prevertebral fascia, and (3) pretracheal fascia and carotid sheath. The investing layer of deep cervical fascia surrounds the neck like a collar. Posteriorly, it attaches to the ligamentum nuchae and spinous processes of cervical vertebrae. Anteriorly, it splits to enclose the sternocleidomastoid and trapezius muscles. The prevertebral layer encloses the prevertebral muscles. The pretracheal layer attaches superiorly to the thyroid cartilage and hyoid bone and encloses the thyroid gland, trachea, and esophagus. Laterally, all three layers contribute to the formation of the carotid sheath, which encloses the carotid artery, internal jugular vein, and vagus nerve.

<u>Anterior and posterior triangles of the neck</u>

In a lateral view **(Fig. 10.2)**, the neck is divided into anterior and posterior triangles by the sternocleidomastoid muscle. The anterior triangle is bounded anteriorly by the midline of the neck, the inferior border of the mandible, and the anterior border of the sternocleidomastoid muscle. The posterior triangle is bounded by the posterior border of the sternocleidomastoid muscle, the anterior border of the trapezius muscle, and the clavicle.

Sternocleidomastoid muscle ***(Fig. 10.2; Fig. 10.3A)***

The sternocleidomastoid is a key muscle involved in the flexion and rotation of the neck and head.

1. <u>*Attachments*</u>: Superiorly, it is attached to the mastoid process (temporal bone) and superior nuchal line (occipital bone). Inferiorly, it is attached to the clavicle (fleshy) and manubrium (tendinous).
2. <u>*Superficial relations*</u> **(Fig. 10.2)**: Crossing superficial to the muscle are the external jugular vein, great auricular nerve (sensory), transverse cervical nerve (sensory), and platysma muscle ("skin muscle" attached to the inferior border of the mandible and skin).

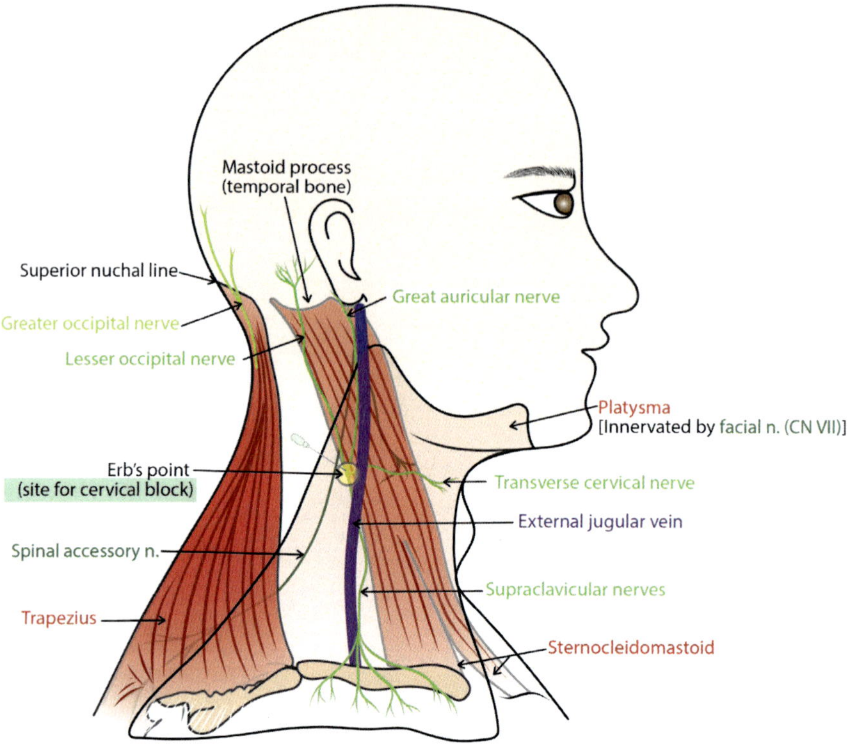

Figure 10.2. Neck. The neck is divided anatomically into the anterior and posterior triangles. The anterior triangle is bounded by the anterior midline, the anterior border of the sternocleidomastoid muscle, and the mandible. The posterior triangle is bounded by the sternocleidomastoid, trapezius, and clavicle. Note that the cervical nerve plexus (C2–4) and its branches (transverse cervical, great auricular, lesser occipital, and supraclavicular nerves) emerge at the midpoint of the posterior border of the sternocleidomastoid muscle.

3. *Deep relations*: Deep (posteromedial) to the muscle are the great vessels (carotid arteries, internal jugular vein, and vagus (X) nerve), trachea/esophagus, and thyroid gland.
4. *Action*: It turns the head to the opposite side, with the chin approximating the shoulder tip. When both muscles act in concert, they protract the head, like lifting one's head during a yoga push-up.
5. *Innervation*: Spinal accessory nerve (XI), a nerve that is purely motor. The motor neurons are localized in the ventral horn of the upper cervical spinal cord segments (C1–3).

6. The muscle may be damaged or ruptured, e.g., in a breech delivery. The affected muscle may become fibrotic and shortened. As a result, the head may be tilted toward the affected side, causing "congenital torticollis" or wryneck.
7. The cervical nerve plexus and its branches (C2–4) (sensory) emerge at the midpoint on the posterior border of the sternocleidomastoid muscle. This is the site where anesthetics may be injected to numb the skin during a surgical procedure of the neck.

Posterior triangle of the neck **(Fig. 10.2)**

It is bounded by the posterior border of the sternocleidomastoid muscle, anterior border of the trapezius muscle, and clavicle. The two muscles are enclosed by the investing layer of the deep cervical fascia. The external jugular vein pierces the fascia at the lower part and drains into the subclavian vein. The spinal accessory nerve and C2 and C3 nerves (proprioceptive) from the cervical plexus cross the triangle to innervate the trapezius. The floor of the triangle is formed by the scalenus anterior, scalenus medius, levator scapulae, and splenius capitis. At the lower part, the brachial nerve plexus passes between the two scalene muscles.

Quiz 1: *If the spinal accessory nerve is damaged or injured in the posterior triangle of the neck, which movement of the upper limb would be affected? Explain.*

Quiz 2: *Besides the motor innervation, the skeletal muscles, such as the trapezius, also receive a sensory nerve supply. Where do the sensory nerve fibers terminate in the muscle, and what are their functions?*

Anterior triangle of the neck **(Fig. 10.3A)**

1. At the midline, the hyoid (C3 level), thyroid cartilage (C4/5 level) and its notch, cricoid cartilage (C6 level), and trachea are palpable.
2. Above the hyoid are the suprahyoid muscles: the digastric muscles and the mylohyoid.
3. Infrahyoid muscles or "strap muscles," including the thyrohyoid, sternothyroid, sternohyoid, and omohyoid, lie anterior to the trachea and extend from the hyoid to the thyroid cartilage and to the manubrium. Ansa cervicalis innervates the "strap muscles" **(Fig. 10.4)**.

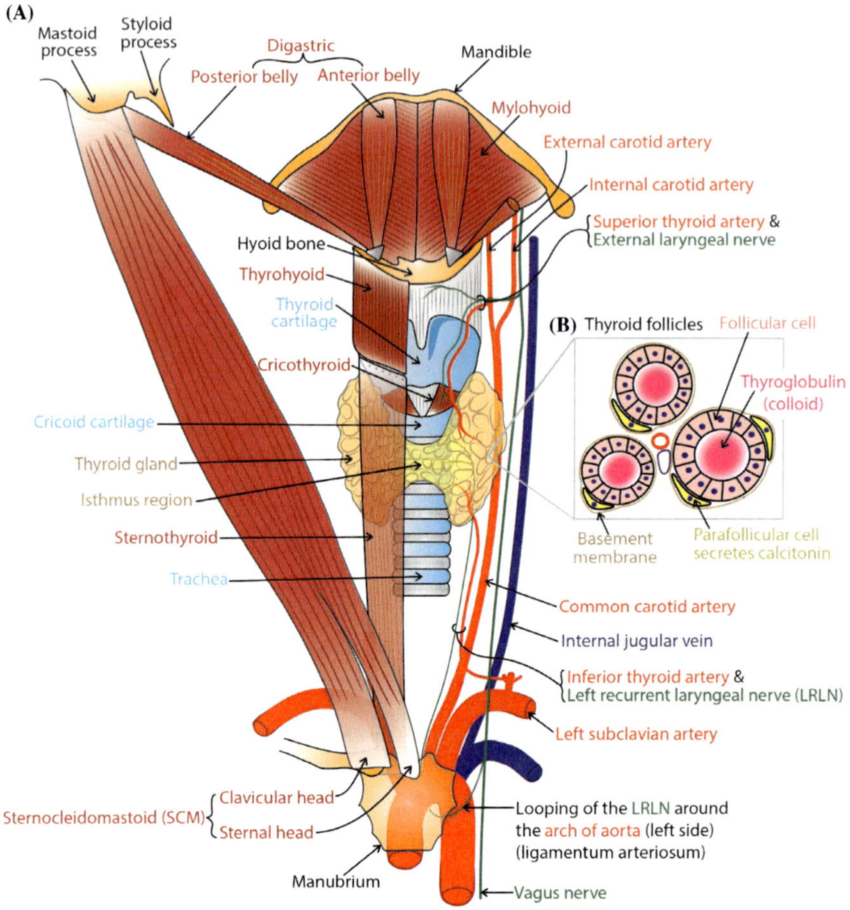

Figure 10.3. Neck. Anterior triangle. (A) The sternocleidomastoid muscle (SCM) separates the anterior triangle from the posterior triangle of the neck. It is attached above to the mastoid process; inferiorly, it is attached to the manubrium and the clavicle. Deep relations of the SCM are the common carotid artery, internal jugular vein (IJV), and vagus nerve (X). Posteromedially to the SCM are the thyroid gland and trachea/esophagus. The "strap muscles" (infrahyoid muscles) lie anterior to the trachea and the thyroid. **(B)** Thyroid follicles. The follicle is lined by simple cuboidal follicular cells, which secrete thyroglobulin. Associated with the follicular cells are calcitonin cells, which secrete calcitonin. ELN, external laryngeal nerve; RLN, recurrent laryngeal nerve (see **Fig. 10.4** for more details regarding the nerves).

4. *Thyroid gland* **(Fig. 10.3A)**
   a. Lobes: It has two lateral lobes interconnected by the isthmus. The superior pole of the lateral lobes extends up to the thyroid cartilage; the lower pole reaches the sixth tracheal cartilage ring. The isthmus overlies the second to fourth tracheal rings.
   b. *Arterial supply* **(Fig. 10.3A; Fig. 10.4)**:
      i. Superior thyroid artery: It is a branch of the external carotid artery. It is accompanied by the external laryngeal nerve (ELN), which innervates the cricothyroid muscle.
      ii. Inferior thyroid artery: It originates from the thyrocervical trunk (a branch of the subclavian artery). It is accompanied by the recurrent laryngeal nerve (RLN), which is a branch of the vagus nerve (CN X).
      iii. Thyroidea ima artery: It is a branch from the brachiocephalic trunk supplying the isthmus.
   c. *Histology* **(Fig. 10.3B)**: It is composed of many thyroid follicles whose lining follicular cells produce the pro-hormone, thyroglobulin. Thyroglobulin is stored in the follicular lumen. When required, it is internalized by the follicular cells and converted into thyroxine (T4) and triiodothyronine (T3) for metabolism. Besides T3 and T4, the thyroid gland also produces calcitonin (by the parafollicular cells, also called C-cells) (*For more details, refer to the chapter on the Endocrine System*).
   d. *Embryology*: The thyroid gland is derived from the proliferation of endodermal epithelial cells on the median surface of the developing pharyngeal floor. The site lies between the tuberculum impar and the copula and is known as the foramen cecum in the adult **(Fig. 10.5)**.
5. *Parathyroid glands*:
   a. The superior and inferior parathyroid glands (four of them) are embedded on the posterior aspect of the lateral lobes of the thyroid.
   b. *Histology*: The gland is composed mainly of chief cells with some oxyphil cells. The main function is the production of the parathyroid hormone, which stimulates osteoclasts and increases the serum calcium.
   c. *Embryology*: The superior parathyroids are derived from the fourth pharyngeal pouches, while the inferior parathyroids are from the third pharyngeal pouches.

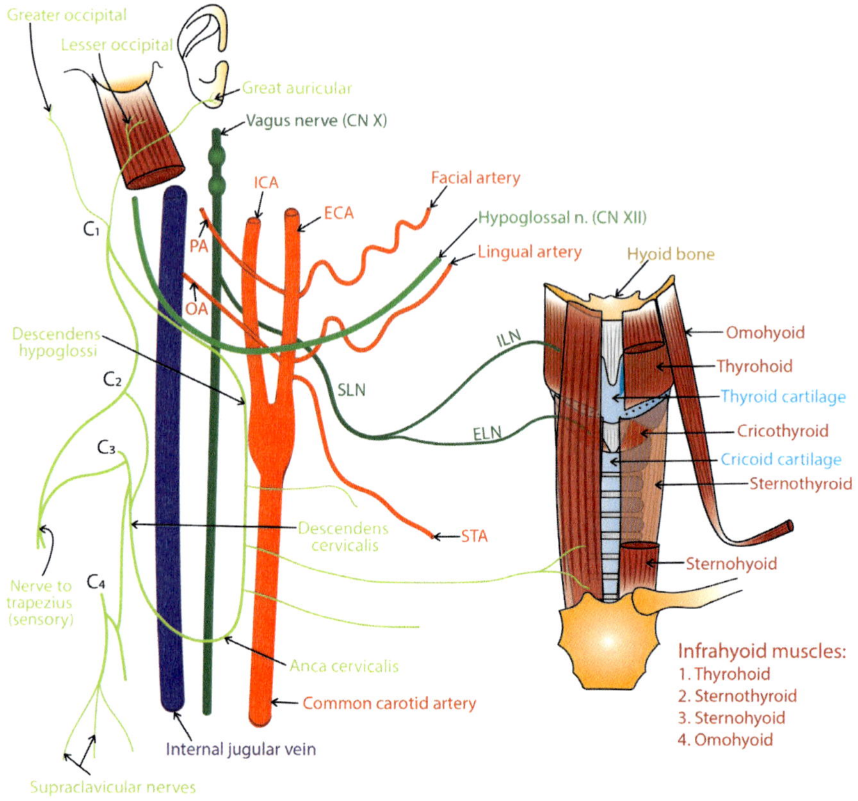

Figure 10.4. Cervical nerve plexus. The nerve plexus lies on the lateral aspect of the internal jugular vein (IJV). It is formed by C1–4. C1 hitch-hikes along the hypoglossal nerve (XII). It then descends as the descendens hypoglossi, which joins with the descendens cervicalis (C2, 3) to become the ansa cervicalis, supplying the infrahyoid muscles. The common carotid artery lies medial to the IJV. It terminates at the carotid sinus and gives rise to the internal carotid artery (ICA) and external carotid artery (ECA). The ECA gives rise to the superior thyroid artery (STA), lingual artery, facial artery, posterior auricular artery (PA), and occipital artery (OA). Between the ICA and IJV is the vagus nerve (X), which gives rise to the superior laryngeal nerve (SLN) and further into the internal laryngeal nerve (ILN) and external laryngeal nerve (ELN). Note that the ELN is closely related with the STA.

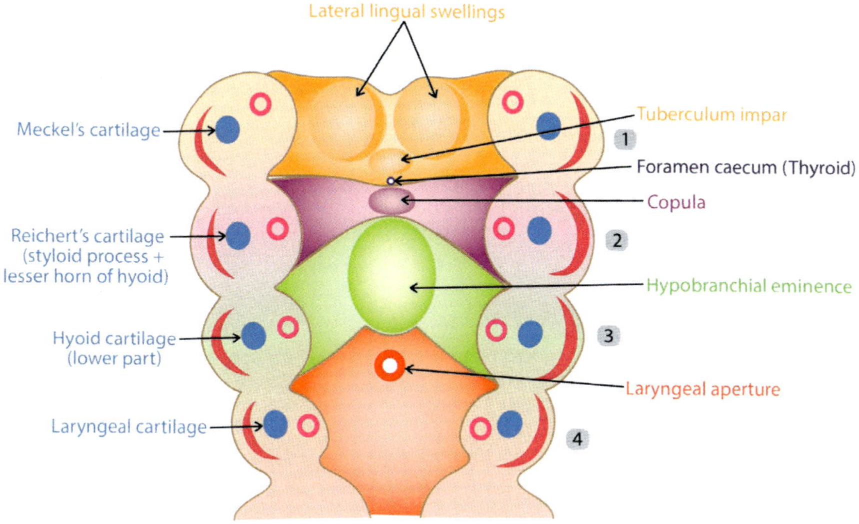

Figure 10.5. Development of the tongue. The anterior two-thirds of the tongue is developed from the first pharyngeal arch. It is derived from the lateral lingual swellings and tuberculum impar. The posterior part is developed from the hypobranchial eminence. Note the foramen caecum, which marks the site of development of the thyroid.

Applied anatomy

1. The anterior relation of the trachea is important because the incision is made through the skin for tracheostomy. The following structures are encountered during incision of the skin: skin, investing layer of the deep cervical fascia, anterior jugular veins, and transverse cervical nerves (a branch of the cervical plexus) **(Fig. 10.1; Fig. 10.4)**. The "strap muscles" anterior to the trachea and thyroid gland may be retracted to access the trachea.
2. Injury to the ELN or RLN during thyroid surgery (when ligation of thyroid arteries is necessary) may result in hoarseness of voice. Both nerves innervate the laryngeal muscles involved in phonation. Note that the superior thyroid artery is closely related to the ELN; the inferior thyroid artery is closely related to the RLN **(Fig. 10.3A)**. If the ELN is injured, the patient would not be able to produce sounds of high pitch, as the cricothyroid muscle is paralyzed.

Quiz 1: *What are the actions of calcitonin? What are the target cells of calcitonin?*

Quiz 2: *What is the embryological significance of aberrant thyroid tissues in the neck?*

Quiz 3: *What are goitres, and what are the common causes?*

Quiz 4: *What is hyperthyroidism or thyrotoxicosis?*

Carotid arteries **(Fig. 10.3A; Fig. 10.4)**

The right common carotid artery arises from the brachiocephalic trunk, while the left common carotid artery arises directly from the arch of the aorta. The common carotid artery ascends along the side of the trachea medial to the internal jugular vein. The vagus nerve lies posterior to it. The carotid sheath encloses the common carotid artery, internal jugular vein, and vagus nerve. At the superior border of the thyroid cartilage, the common carotid artery is bifurcated into the internal carotid artery and external carotid artery **(Fig. 10.4)**. Superior to the bifurcation, the internal carotid artery has a dilated region called the carotid sinus, which monitors changes in the blood pressure (baroreceptors). Associated with it at its origin is the carotid body, which is involved in chemoreception. The internal carotid artery mainly supplies the brain, and some of its branches supply the scalp and eye (retina). The external carotid artery mainly supplies structures outside of the skull, e.g., the neck, face, and scalp. Arterial anastomosis between the internal and external carotid arteries occurs at the medial angle of the eye and scalp (see **Fig. 10.6**). The external carotid artery gives rise to several branches: superior thyroid artery, lingual artery, ascending pharyngeal artery, facial artery, occipital artery, posterior auricular artery, maxillary artery, and superficial temporal artery.

Quiz 1: *Where is the site where the carotid pulse may be felt?*

Quiz 2: *What are the functions of the carotid sinus and carotid body? What is their innervation? How does the innervation to the carotid sinus help regulate the blood pressure?*

Quiz 3: *Clinically, it may be necessary to assess the possible fatty deposits (plaques) in the common carotid artery. What are the histological features of the common carotid artery?*

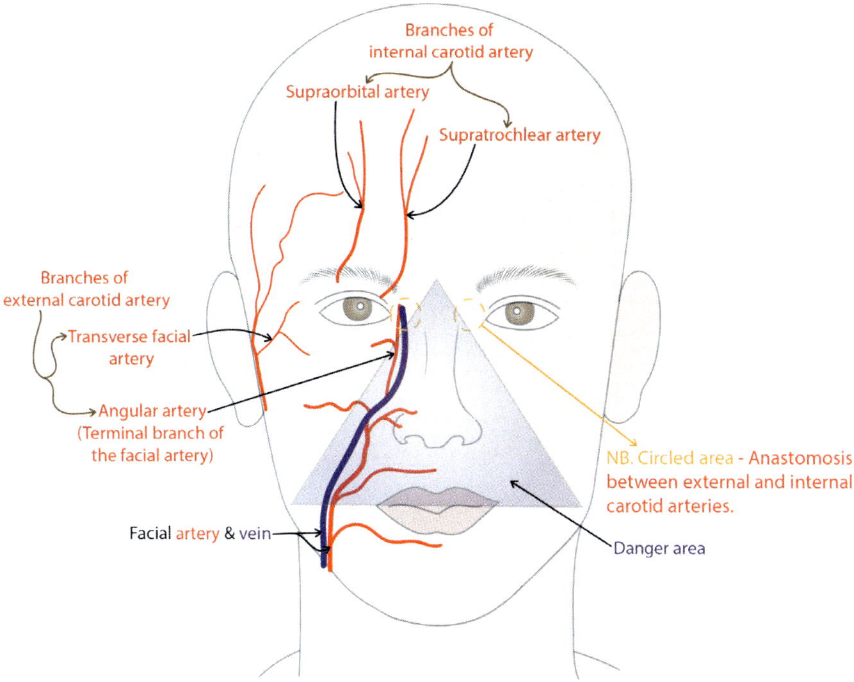

Facial vein drains into internal jugular vein in common with the anterior division of retromandibular vein

NB. Angular vein communicates with the cavernous sinus via the superior opthalamic veins. Infection from the face may be spread from the so-called "Danger area" of the face that can be demarcated by the two facial veins above the upper lip.

Figure 10.6. Face. Arterial supply and venous drainage. The arterial supply to the face is from three main sources: the facial artery (external carotid), the transverse facial artery (external carotid), and the supratrochlear and supraorbital arteries (internal carotid). The facial artery presents a tortuous course to terminate as the angular artery that anastomoses with the internal carotid artery (circled area). The facial vein presents a straight course posterior to the accompanying artery. Note the so-called "danger area" of the face where infection may be spread to the cavernous sinus via the superior ophthalmic vein.

Internal jugular vein **(Fig. 10.3A; Fig. 10.4)**

The internal jugular vein begins at the jugular foramen (base of the skull) from the sigmoid sinus (cranial cavity). It descends lateral to the carotid artery and the vagus nerve within the carotid sheath. It drains venous blood from the brain and the neck. At the root of the neck, it is joined by the subclavian vein to become the brachiocephalic vein. The right and left brachiocephalic veins join together to form the superior vena cava, which drains into the right atrium (heart).

Vagus nerve **(Fig. 10.3A; Fig. 10.4)** *(See also the section on Cranial Nerves)*

This is the tenth cranial nerve, which arises from the medulla (brainstem). It exits the cranial cavity through the jugular foramen along with the IX and XI cranial nerves. Details about this nerve will be described later. The vagus nerve descends into the neck. In the upper part of the neck, it lies posterior to the internal carotid artery. As it descends further, it lies posterior to the common carotid artery. It gives off the superior laryngeal nerve, which further divides into the internal laryngeal nerve (ILN) and external laryngeal nerve (ELN). The external laryngeal nerve is closely related to the superior thyroid artery. It innervates the cricothyroid muscle, a laryngeal muscle that tenses the vocal cord. Note that the close spatial relation between the ELN and the superior thyroid artery is of clinical significance.

Quiz: *What is the functional impairment if the ELN is damaged, e.g., accidentally ligated or damaged in thyroid surgery?*

Cervical nerve plexus **(Fig. 10.4)**

1. The cervical nerve plexus is formed by the cervical spinal nerves 1–4 (C1–4).
2. C1 "hitch-hikes" along the hypoglossal nerve (Xll) for a short distance and then descends lateral to the internal jugular vein as the "descendens hypoglossi."
3. C2 and C3 join to form the "descendens cervicalis," which forms a loop with the "descendens hypoglossi" called the "ansa cervicalis." Branches from the ansa provide motor innervation to the "strap muscles" (infrahyoid muscles).
4. Sensory nerves from the cervical nerve plexus innervate the skin of the neck, external ear, and occipital region. The sensory nerves, including the great auricular nerve, lesser occipital nerve, transverse cervical nerve, and supraclavicular nerve, emerge at the midpoint (Erb's point) on the posterior border of the sternocleidomastoid, a site where anesthetics may be administered to numb the skin in the neck region **(Fig. 10.2)**.

THE SCALP AND FACE

Before we learn about the soft tissues of the scalp and face, it is necessary to first consider the bones of the skull. The term "skull" refers to the entire skeletal framework that encloses the brain and the sense organs. The term "cranium" refers to the skull without the mandible. "Neurocranium" is the part of the cranium that protects the brain, while "viscerocranium" refers to the bones of the face (facial bones). The term "vertex" refers to the highest point of the skull. The top part of the neurocranium (superior parts of the frontal, parietal, and occipital bones) is the "calvaria" or "skull cap."

Skull Bones

The skull consists of 22 bones, some of which are paired and the rest are unpaired. The scalp includes the following bones: frontal (1), parietal (2), occipital (1), temporal (2), ethmoid (1), and sphenoid (1), where the numbers indicate whether the bones are paired or unpaired. The frontal, parietal, and occipital bones are connected by fibrous joints (or sutures), which allow no movement. There are three sutures in the skull: (a) coronal suture, which is a fibrous joint between the frontal and two paired parietal bones; (b) sagittal suture, which connects the parietal bones of both sides; (c) lambdoid suture, which lies between the two parietal bones and the occipital bone. The point where the coronal suture and sagittal suture intersect is the "bregma," whereas the junction between the sagittal and lambdoid suture is known as the "lambda." These bony landmarks are significant in neurosurgery as well as in experimental brain research.

Note that the frontal, parietal, and occipital bones are formed by "intramembranous ossification" without a pre-existing cartilage model; cartilage may be found in the base of the skull, e.g., sphenoid. (*Refer to the section on Bone Tissue in Foundation Topics in Human Anatomy.*)

Scalp

The scalp extends from the supraorbital margins anteriorly and to the superior nuchal line posteriorly. On both sides, the scalp extends to the zygomatic arch and to the external acoustic meatus. Therefore, the scalp covers the entire skull cap.

There are five layers of the scalp **(Fig. 10.7; Fig. 10.8)** as follows:

S – Skin: Histologically, it is a thin skin covering the entire scalp.
C – Subcutaneous tissue (loose connective tissue): It contains locules of fat.
A – Aponeurosis of the occipitofrontalis muscles.

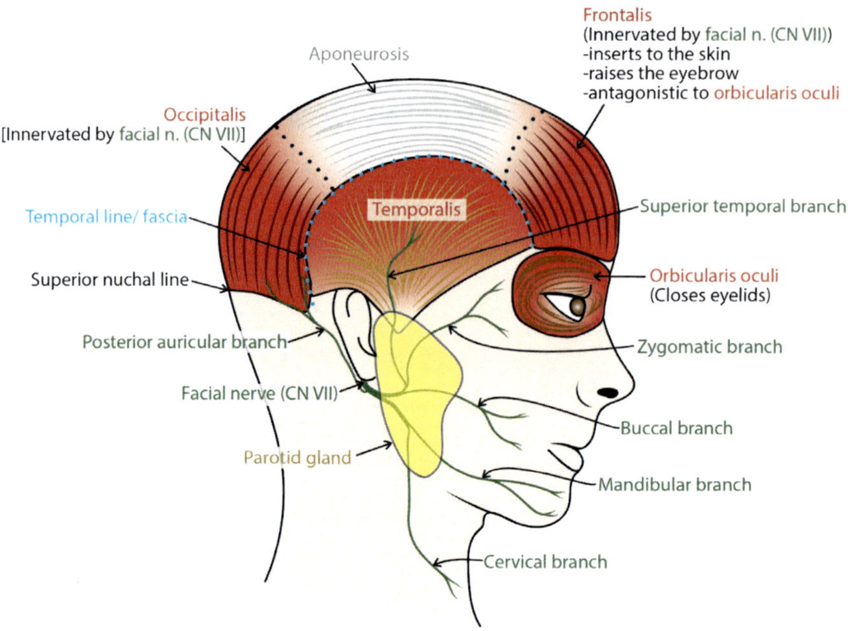

Figure 10.7. Scalp. The scalp extends from the supraorbital margin anteriorly to the superior nuchal line posteriorly. It is attached to the temporal lines on both sides. Showing the various branches of the facial nerve (T, temporal; Z, zygomatic; B, buccal; M, mandibular (marginal); C, cervical, PA, posterior auricular), of which the T and PA branches supply the frontalis and occipitalis, respectively.

The two muscle bellies of frontalis and the two bellies of occipitalis are connected by the galea (meaning: helmet) aponeurosis. The frontalis is attached to the eyebrows of the skin, while the occipitalis is attached to the superior nuchal lines of the occipital bone.

L – Loose connective tissue: Some veins from this layer communicate with the intracranial venous sinuses (e.g., superior sagittal sinus) via the emissary veins (diploic veins).

P – Periosteum or pericranium: This is continuous with the endocranium at the foramina.

Arteries supplying the scalp (Fig. 10.8)

1. Supratrochlear and supraorbital arteries (from the ophthalmic artery, which is a branch of the internal carotid artery)
2. Superficial temporal artery (from the external carotid artery)
3. Occipital artery (from the external carotid artery).

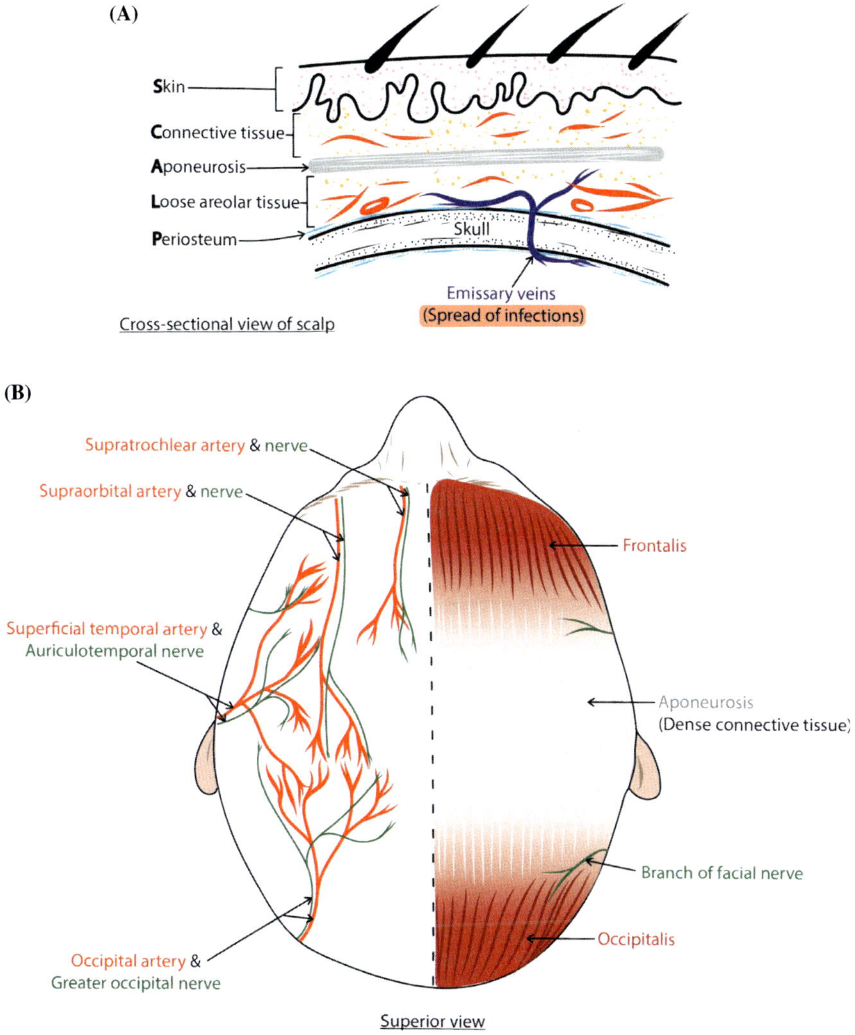

Figure 10.8. Scalp. (A) Layers of the scalp: S, skin; C, subcutaneous tissue; A, galea aponeurosis; L, loose connective tissue; P, pericranium (periosteum). **(B)** The aponeurosis connects the two bellies of the frontalis and occipitalis. The scalp is well vascularized with a rich arterial supply. It is also richly innervated by sensory nerves. The motor innervation of the occipito-frontalis muscle is by the facial nerve.

Innervation of the scalp (Fig. 10.8B)

1. Supratrochlear nerve (from the frontal nerve of the ophthalmic division of the trigeminal nerve, CN V1)
2. Supraorbital nerve (from the frontal nerve of the ophthalmic division of the trigeminal nerve, CN V1)

3. Zygomaticotemporal nerve (from the maxillary division, CN V2)
4. Auriculotemporal nerve (from the mandibular division, CN V3)
5. Greater occipital nerve (from the cervical nerve plexus).

Clinical considerations

1. The scalp is richly vascularized and bleeds profusely when lacerated. The walls of the arteries in the connective tissue layer are anchored to the surrounding fibrous tissues; therefore, the arteries do not constrict well when they are lacerated, resulting in profuse bleeding.
2. Infections involving the loose connective layer may spread inward via the emissary veins to the intracranial venous sinus, e.g., the superior sagittal sinus.
3. The occipitofrontalis muscle is innervated by the facial nerve. In a facial nerve injury, the patient is unable to raise the eyebrows on the affected side. This is because the frontalis acts to raise the skin of the forehead and eyebrows.

***Quiz**: Regarding the innervation of the scalp, where are the cell bodies of the following sensory nerves located: (1) the frontal nerve, (2) auriculotemporal nerve, and (3) greater occipital nerves?*

Face

The face consists of the following bones: frontal (1), maxilla (2), zygomatic (2), nasal (2), and mandible (1). (Numerals denote whether the bone is in a pair or single.)

- *Frontal bone* forms the supraorbital margin and supraorbital notch.
- *Maxilla* has a body, alveolar process, and infraorbital foramen.
- *Zygomatic bone (cheekbone)*: consists of the zygomatic foramen and zygomatic arch.
- *Mandible* has the condylar head, coronoid process, mandibular notch, ramus, angle, body, mental foramen, alveolar process, and inferior border. The medial surface of the mandible has the mandibular foramen, with a projection called the lingula, mylohyoid line, and submandibular and sublingual fossae.

Sensory innervation of the face (Fig. 10.9)

The face is developed from three main processes during the embryonic stage: (1) frontonasal process (over the forehead), (2) maxillary process (upper jaw), and (3) mandibular process (lower jaw). The sensory innervation to the three areas is by

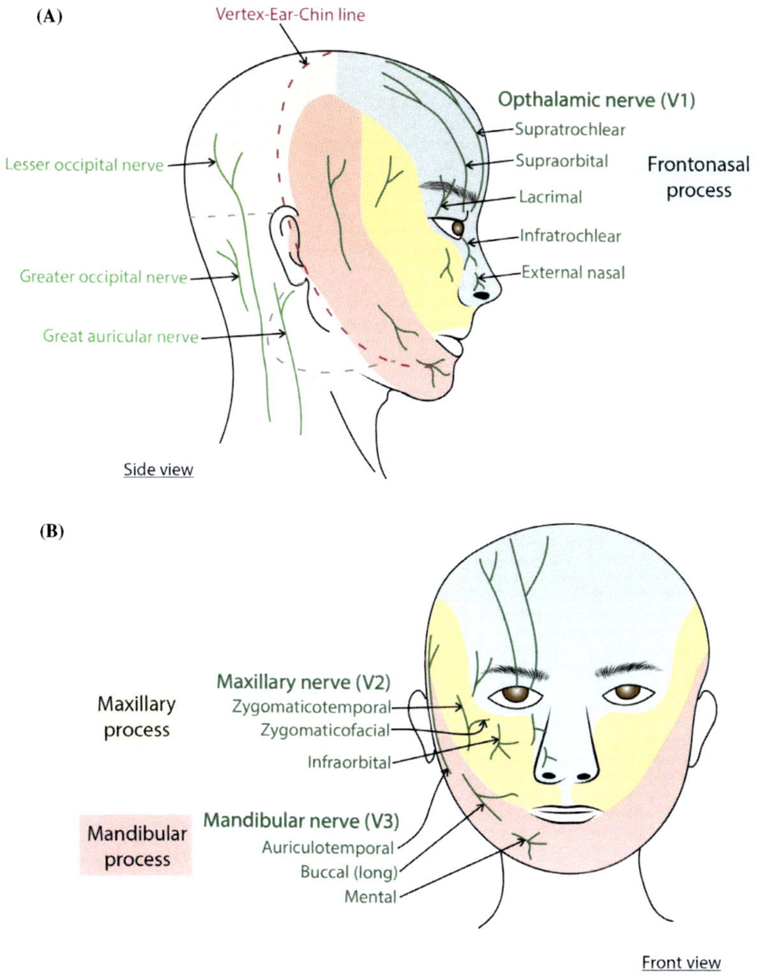

Figure 10.9. Face-sensory innervation. (A, B) The face is developed from three main processes, of which sensory innervation is by the trigeminal nerve (V). The frontonasal process is supplied by the ophthalmic nerve (V1), the maxillary process by the maxillary nerve (V2), and the mandibular process by the mandibular nerve (V3). Posterior to the vertex-ear-chin line (see A), the sensory innervation is by the cervical nerve plexus.

the ophthalmic division (V1), maxillary division (V2), and mandibular division (V3) of the trigeminal nerve (V), respectively. The three trigeminal divisions and their branches supply the facial skin anterior to the "vertex-ear-chin" line. Posterior to the line, the sensory innervation is by the cervical nerve plexus.

Trigeminal nerve and its divisions and branches:

1. *Ophthalmic division* includes supratrochlear, supraorbital, and infratrochlear, lacrimal, and external nasal nerves.
2. *Maxillary division* includes infraorbital, zygomaticofacial, and zygomaticotemporal nerves.
3. *Mandibular division* includes buccal (long buccal), auriculotemporal, and mental nerves.

Applied anatomy

Trigeminal neuralgia: This is a type of severe, excruciating pain affecting the face. This may involve one or more areas innervated by the three divisions of the trigeminal nerve.

***Quiz**: Describe the pain pathway from a lesion of the lower lip to the brain.*

Arterial supply of the face (Fig. 10.6)

1. Supratrochlear artery (from the internal carotid)
2. Supraorbital artery (from the internal carotid)
3. Facial artery and angular artery (from the external carotid)
4. Transverse facial artery (from the external carotid)

An arterial anastomosis is established between the internal and external carotid arteries at the medial angle of the eye **(Fig. 10.6)**.

***Quiz**: Why do you think the facial artery presents a tortuous course as it ascends to supply the face?*

Venous drainage of the face (Fig. 10.6)

The facial vein, traveling posterior to the facial artery, drains into the internal jugular vein after confluency with the anterior division of the retromandibular vein.

Applied anatomy

The angular vein (at the medial angle of the eye) communicates with the cavernous sinus (CS) via the superior ophthalmic vein (SOV). Thus, there is a potential risk of the spread of infections from the so-called "danger area of the face" demarcated by the two facial veins above the lips into the CS ("cavernous sinus thrombosis").

***Quiz**: Describe the sympathetic innervation of the facial artery (vascular smooth muscles) and the sweat glands of the face. Where do the sympathetic nerve fibers originate?*

Muscles of the face (Fig. 10.10)

The muscles of the face are developed embryologically from the second pharyngeal (branchial) arch. They are supplied by the nerve to the second arch, the facial nerve (VII), which arises from the brainstem (pons). The muscles of the face are attached to the bones of the face on the one hand and to the skin on

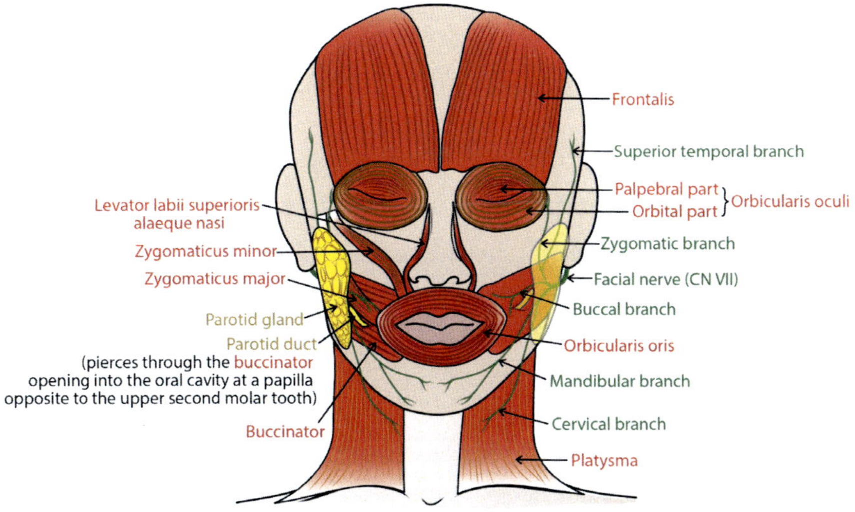

Figure 10.10. Muscles of the face. The muscles of the face are derived from the second branchial (pharyngeal) arch. They help raise the eyebrows (frontalis), the angle of the mouth, e.g., smiling (zygomaticus major and minor), the upper lip (levator labii superioris alaeque nasi), closing the eye (orbicularis oculi), the mouth (orbicularis oris), or keeping food in the mouth during chewing (buccinator). They are supplied by the branches of the facial nerve (VII) (T, temporal; Z, zygomatic; B, buccal; M, mandibular; C, cervical) after passing through the parotid gland.

the other. They are often regarded as the "muscles of facial expression." The facial muscles act on the orifices (openings) of the head region, either as a "dilator" or a "sphincter," including the mouth, eye, nose, etc.

1. *Orbit*: Orbicularis oculi (closing the eye) and frontalis (raising the eyebrows, opening the eye).
2. *Oral*: Zygomaticus major and minor, levator labii superioris alaeque nasi (opening the mouth), buccinator (blowing, "bugler muscle"; helps keep foods in the mouth), risorius ("smiling muscle"), levator labii superioris, and orbicularis oris (closing the mouth, "kissing muscle")
3. *Others*: Platysma ("shaving muscle"), procerus, and corrugator (frowning).

Innervation of facial muscles **(Fig. 10.10)**

All muscles of facial expression are innervated by the facial nerve (CN VII). The facial nerve gives rise to five terminal branches anteriorly: temporal, zygomatic, buccal, mandibular, and cervical, which emerge anteriorly from the parotid gland to innervate the facial muscles.

More specifically, the temporal branch innervates the frontalis, the zygomatic branch innervates the orbicularis oculi, the buccal branch innervates the buccinator, the mandibular branch innervates the orbicularis oris, and the cervical branch innervates the platysma. (Other branches from the facial nerve are described separately.)

Facial nerve: its origin, course, and distribution **(Fig. 10.11)**

The facial nerve innervates the facial muscles through a two-neuronal motor pathway. The upper motor neurons are localized in the motor cortex in the precentral gyrus (frontal lobe). From the upper motor neurons, the descending axons synapse either with (a) the lower motor neurons in the ipsilateral facial motor nucleus (FMN) in the pons or (b) cross over to synapse with the lower motor neurons in the FMN on the contralateral side. The axons of the lower motor neurons from the ipsilateral FMN supply the muscles of the ipsilateral upper quadrant of the face, whereas the crossed fibers (axons) supply the muscles of both the upper and lower quadrants of the face on the contralateral side. Overall, the facial nerve contains axons from both the ipsilateral and contralateral FMN. Facial nerve lesion may occur in the upper motor neuron (e.g., cerebral stroke) or in the lower motor neuron (Bell's palsy). The upper motor neuron lesion may be caused

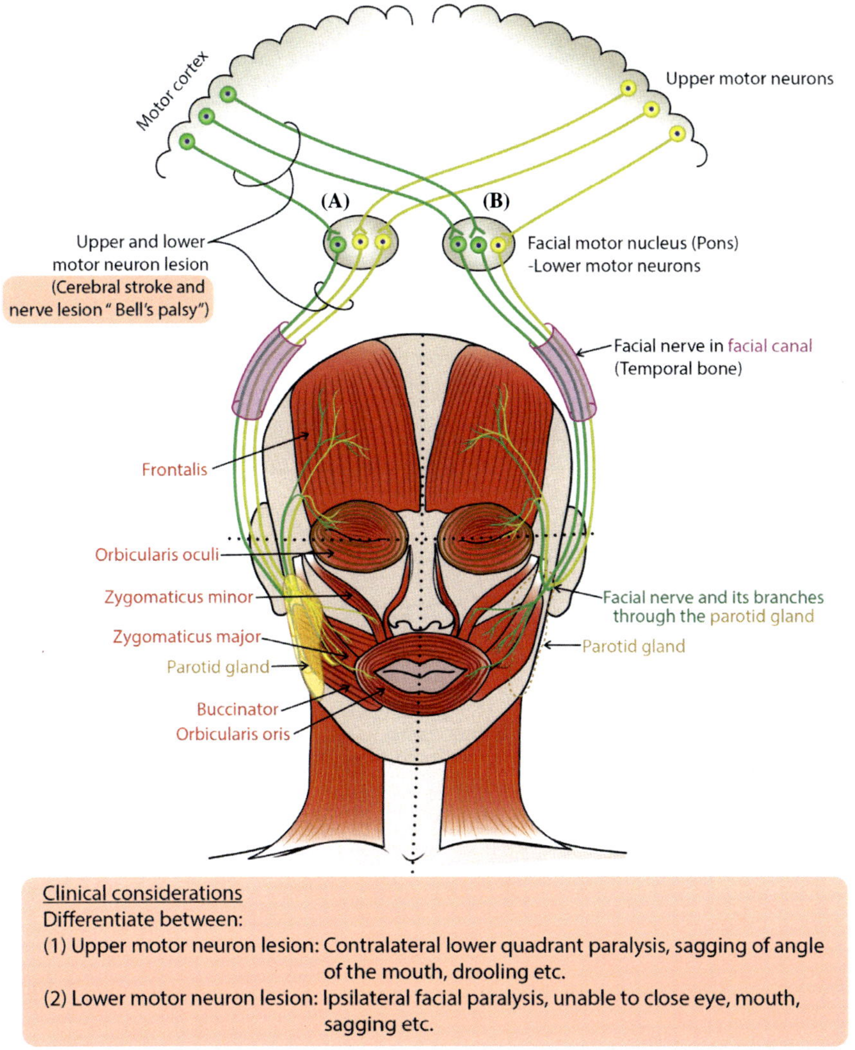

Figure 10.11. Facial nerve and its innervation of the facial muscles. The facial nerve supplies the facial muscles through a two-neuronal pathway: the upper and lower motor neurons. The upper motor neurons are localized in the motor cortex in the frontal lobe. They send their descending axons to synapse either with **(A)** the lower motor neurons in the ipsilateral facial motor nucleus (FMN), or with **(B)** the lower motor neurons of the contralateral FMN. In **(A)**, the axons from the lower motor neurons of the ipsilateral FMN travel in the facial nerve to supply the muscles in the ipsilateral upper quadrant of the face. In **(B)**, the axons from the lower motor neurons of the contralateral FMN supply the muscles in the contralateral upper and lower quadrants. In other words, the facial nerve is composed of axons from the bilateral FMN. Injury to the axons in **(A)** and **(B)** is called the upper and lower motor neuron injury of the facial nerve, respectively.

by a cerebral stroke affecting the descending axons in the cerebrum (corticobulbar fibers), thereby resulting in paralysis of facial muscles (i.e., orbicularis oris) in the lower quadrant of the contralateral side of the face. In Bell's palsy, all the muscles of facial expression on the ipsilateral side of the face are paralyzed. It may be caused by several factors, including tumors of the parotid gland, surgical procedures within the middle ear or mastoid process, and a viral infection. On the affected side, the patient is unable to raise his eyebrow, close his eye, smile, and purse the oral cavity (drooling of saliva may occur).

N.B. The facial nerve takes a long course from its origin to innervate its target tissues. It leaves the cranial fossa through the internal acoustic meatus, passes through the inner ear (within the facial canal), and descends on the posterior wall of the middle ear (tympanum). The nerve exits the skull through the stylomastoid foramen. It traverses through the parotid gland lateral to the external carotid artery and retromandibular vein and gives rise to the five terminal motor nerve branches mentioned above. More details regarding the course and distribution of the facial nerve are described elsewhere. (*See the section on Cranial Nerves.*)

Applied anatomy

1. How do you differentiate the upper motor neuron lesion from the lower motor neuron lesion of the facial nerve?

Answer:

- Upper motor neuron lesion: contralateral lower quadrant muscle paralysis, sagging of the angle of the mouth, drooling, etc.
- Lower motor neuron lesion: ipsilateral facial paralysis, unable to close the eye, sagging of the mandibular division (V3) of the mouth.

2. Test for facial nerve lesion
   » Ask the patient to raise his/her eyebrows — testing the frontalis (there may be drooping of the eyelid)
   » Ask the patient to close his/her eyes — testing the orbicularis oris muscle
   » Ask the patient to smile and show his/her teeth — testing the zygomaticus major/minor, risorius muscles
   » Ask the patient to blow — testing the buccinator, the "bugler muscle."

Quiz 1: *What might be the cause of cerebral ischemia and/or infarct? What are the pathological features to be expected at the site of a cerebral infarct?*

Quiz 2: *In parotid gland surgery, the facial nerve branches may be damaged, e.g., the zygomatic branch. In the latter, would it be a lower or upper motor neuron lesion of the facial nerve? Which muscle is likely to be paralyzed? What would be the functional loss?*

Parotid gland (Fig. 10.12)

1. *Relations*: The parotid gland is the largest salivary gland, located on both sides of the face. It is related to the sternocleidomastoid, posteriorly; anteriorly, it overlies the masseter muscle.
2. The parotid duct courses forward, pierces the buccinator, and opens into the vestibule opposite to the upper second molar tooth.
3. In a horizontal plane, the gland is wedge-shaped.
   Anterior: It is related to the ramus of the mandible, masseter, and medial pterygoid.
   Posterior: Posterior belly of the digastric muscle and sternocleidomastoid.
4. It is pierced by the terminal branches of the facial nerve that lie superficial to the external carotid artery and retromandibular vein. The nerve "separates" the gland into superficial and deep parts.
5. Posteromedial to the gland are the styloid process and associated muscles (styloglossus, stylopharyngeus, and stylohyoid), pharynx, and internal carotid artery/internal jugular vein.
6. *Histology*: It is exclusively a serous gland. The surface is invested by a layer of capsule, which sends in a septum dividing the parenchyma into many lobules. The serous acinus is capped by myoepithelial cells. The intercalated duct begins at the acinus, which leads to the striated duct, interlobular duct, and the main parotid duct. Serous secretions or saliva contain electrolytes, amylase, IgA, etc. (*Refer also to the chapter on the Digestive System*).
7. *Secretomotor innervation*: It is innervated by the glossopharyngeal nerve (CN IX), which originates from the inferior salivatory nucleus in the medulla. The nerve exits through the jugular foramen, gives off a recurrent tympanic branch, and forms the tympanic nerve plexus over the promontory

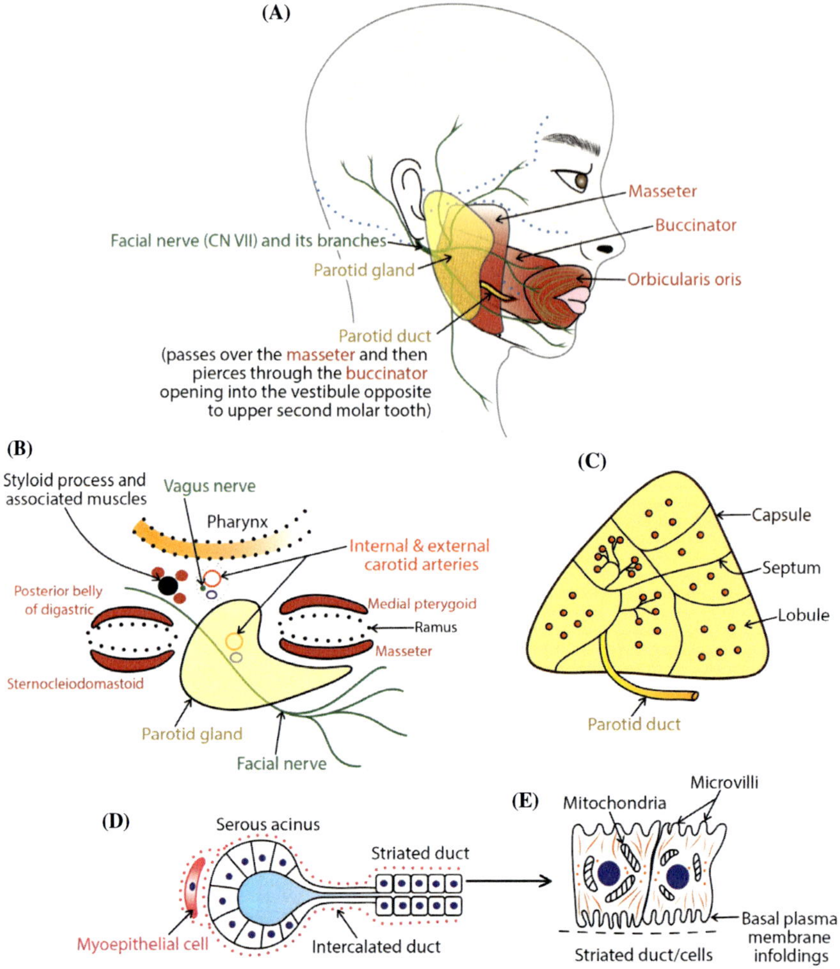

Figure 10.12. Parotid gland. **(A)** The gland lies by the side of the ear overlying the masseter. It is pierced by the facial nerve. Posteriorly, it is limited by the sternocleidomastoid. Anteriorly, it "overflows" over the masseter. **(B)** In a horizontal section, the wedge-shaped parotid is related anteriorly to the ramus of the mandible, to which are attached the medial pterygoid and masseter muscles. Posteriorly, it is related to the sternocleidomastoid muscles and the posterior belly of the digastric. Postero-medially is the styloid process and the muscles attached to it. Medially is the pharynx, internal carotid, and internal jugular vein. **(C)** The parotid has a capsule and septa that divide the gland into many lobules. **(D)** It is composed mainly of serous acinus, which leads to the intercalated duct and striated duct **(E)**. The main parotid duct runs forward, pierces the buccinator, and opens into the vestibule opposite to the upper second molar tooth.

in the middle ear (tympanum). These nerve fibers continue forward as the lesser petrosal nerve (LPN). The LPN exits through the foramen ovale and enters the infratemporal fossa. The nerves containing preganglionic parasympathetic fibers synapse with the postganglionic parasympathetic ganglion cells in the otic ganglion (a parasympathetic ganglion suspended to the nerve to medial pterygoid). The postganglionic parasympathetic fibers "hitch-hike" along the auriculotemporal nerve (V3) to innervate the parotid gland. (*See below the section on Cranial Nerves.*)

CRANIAL CAVITY AND THE BRAIN

The brain is located at the base of the skull in the cranial fossae: anterior, middle, and posterior. It is covered by three meningeal layers, including the dura (outermost), arachnoid (middle layer), and pia mater (innermost). The floor of the cranial fossae has many openings or foramina, allowing the exit of 12 cranial nerves and the entry of arteries (internal carotid and vertebral); hence, in the event of a skull base fracture, the neurovascular structures may be lesioned or traumatized.

Cranial Fossae (Fig. 10.13)

1. **Anterior cranial fossa**: The floor is formed by the orbital plate of the frontal bone, cribriform plate, and crista galli of the ethmoid. The posterior limit is defined by the lesser wing of the sphenoid, the anterior clinoid process, and the jugum sphenoidale (chiasmatic sulcus).
2. **Middle cranial fossa**: The floor is formed by the greater wing and body of the sphenoid. The posterior limit is defined by the petrous part of the temporal bone, the posterior clinoid process, and the dorsum sellae.
3. **Posterior cranial fossa**: Its floor is formed by the occipital bone.

Anterior Cranial Fossa (Fig. 10.13)

It houses the frontal lobe and olfactory bulb/tract. The cribriform plate has multiple foramina that transmit olfactory nerves (CN I), which are sensory fibers from the olfactory mucosa over the superior nasal concha.

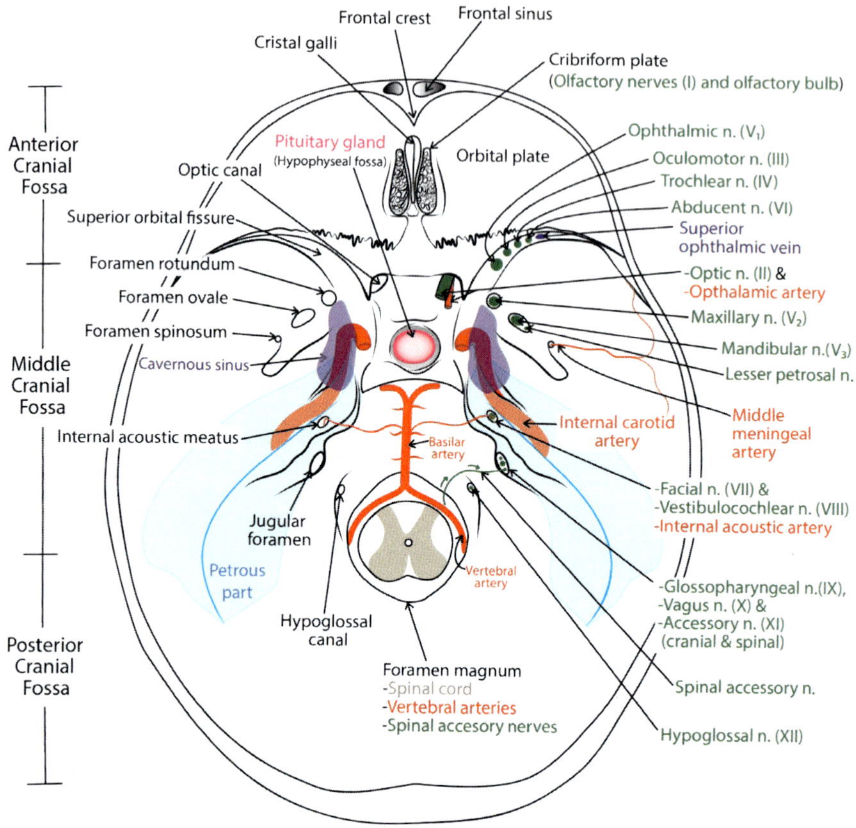

Figure 10.13. Cranial cavity. The floor of the cranial cavity is divided into three cranial fossae: anterior, middle, and posterior. The left half of the figure shows the three fossae and various foramina (for details, refer to the text). The right half of the figure shows structures (nerves, arteries, and veins) passing through them, respectively.

Middle Cranial Fossa (Fig. 10.13)

It accommodates the temporal lobes. In the center is the hypophyseal fossa on the body of the sphenoid (sella turcica), in which the pituitary gland (hypophysis) is lodged.

There are many foramina and openings in the middle cranial fossa for the passage of cranial nerves and blood vessels:

1. Optic canal transmits the optic nerve (CN II) and ophthalmic artery.
2. Superior orbital fissure transmits the oculomotor nerve (CN III), trochlear nerve (CN IV), ophthalmic nerve (CN V_1) (nasociliary nerve, frontal nerve,

and lacrimal nerve), abducent nerve (CN VI), and superior ophthalmic vein (SOV).

3. Foramen rotundum transmits the maxillary nerve (V_2) (It leads to the pterygopalatine fossa).
4. Foramen ovale transmits the mandibular nerve (V_3) and lesser petrosal nerve (a branch of the CN IX) (It leads to the infratemporal fossa inferiorly).
5. Foramen spinosum transmits the middle meningeal artery, which is a branch of the maxillary artery.
6. Foramen lacerum (upper part only) is continuous with the carotid canal for the passage of the internal carotid artery. Some emissary veins may pass through it.

Posterior Cranial Fossa (Fig. 10.13)

It houses the cerebellum and the brainstem, lying on the "clivus" — the sloping bony surface in the middle down to the basiocciput.

1. Internal acoustic foramen (meatus) transmits the facial nerve (CN VII), vestibulocochlear nerve (CN VIII), and internal acoustic artery (labyrinthine artery).
2. Jugular foramen transmits the glossopharyngeal nerve (CN IX), vagus nerve (CN X), accessory nerve (CN XI), and inferior petrosal sinus (beginning of the internal jugular vein).
3. Foramen magnum transmits the spinal accessory nerve (CN XI) and vertebral arteries and marks the beginning of the spinal cord.
4. Hypoglossal canal transmits the hypoglossal nerve (CN XII).

Meninges (Fig. 10.14; Fig. 10.15)

The meninges are the protective coverings of the brain. They also enclose dural venous sinuses that drain the brain and bone tissues:

1. **Dura mater**: This has two sublayers: the outer endosteal dura (endocranium) and the inner meningeal or fibrous dura. External to the endosteal dura is the extradural space. The subdural space lies between the dura mater and the arachnoid mater. Some cerebral veins from the cerebrum drain into the dural sinuses.

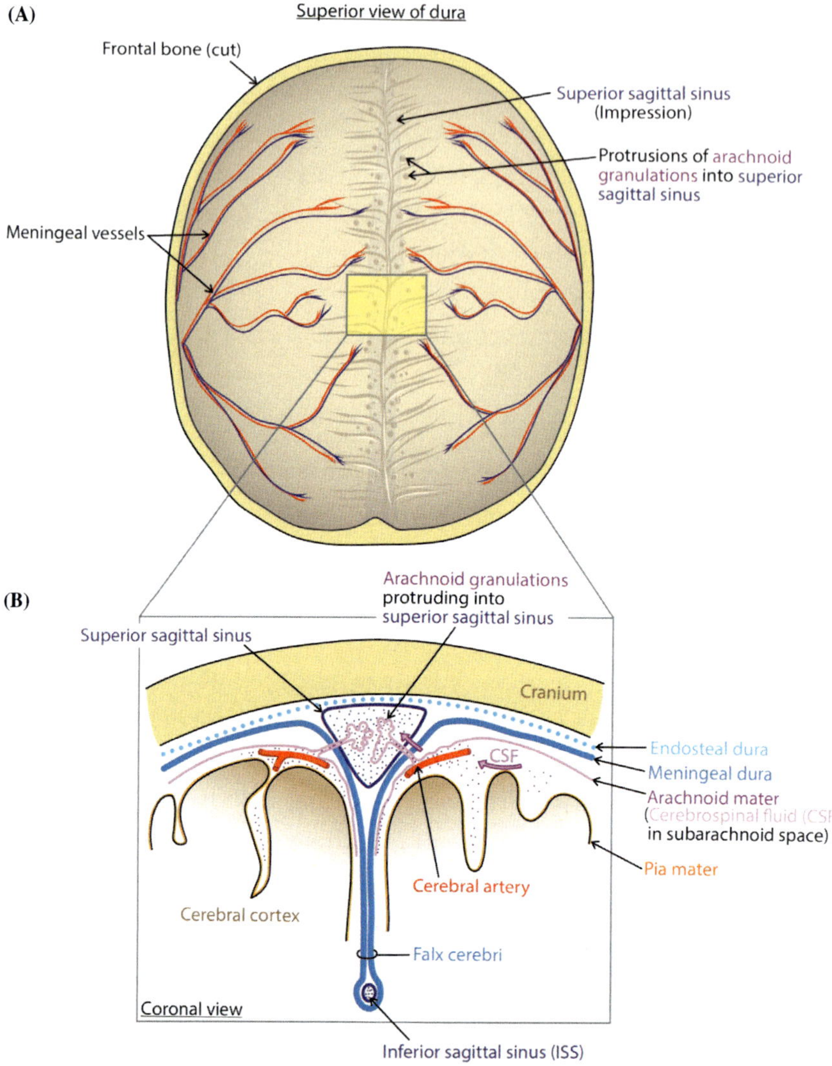

Figure 10.14. Meninges. (A) Surface view of the dura following the removal *of* the calvaria. The dura is composed of the outer endosteal dura (endocranium) and the inner meningeal dura (See B). Over the surface along the midline are irregular "bumps," which represent the underlying "arachnoid granulations." **(B)** This is a coronal section of the skull and brain. Note the three layers of meninges: dura, arachnoid, and pia mater. In the midline, the meningeal dura doubles back to form the falx cerebri, enclosing the superior sagittal sinus (SSS) and inferior sagittal sinus (ISS). The cerebrospinal fluid (CSF) in the subarachnoid space is drained (purple arrow) by the arachnoid granulations into the SSS. The subarachnoid space also contains the cerebral arteries. Deep to the arachnoid is the pia mater, which lines the immediate surface of the brain.

(A)

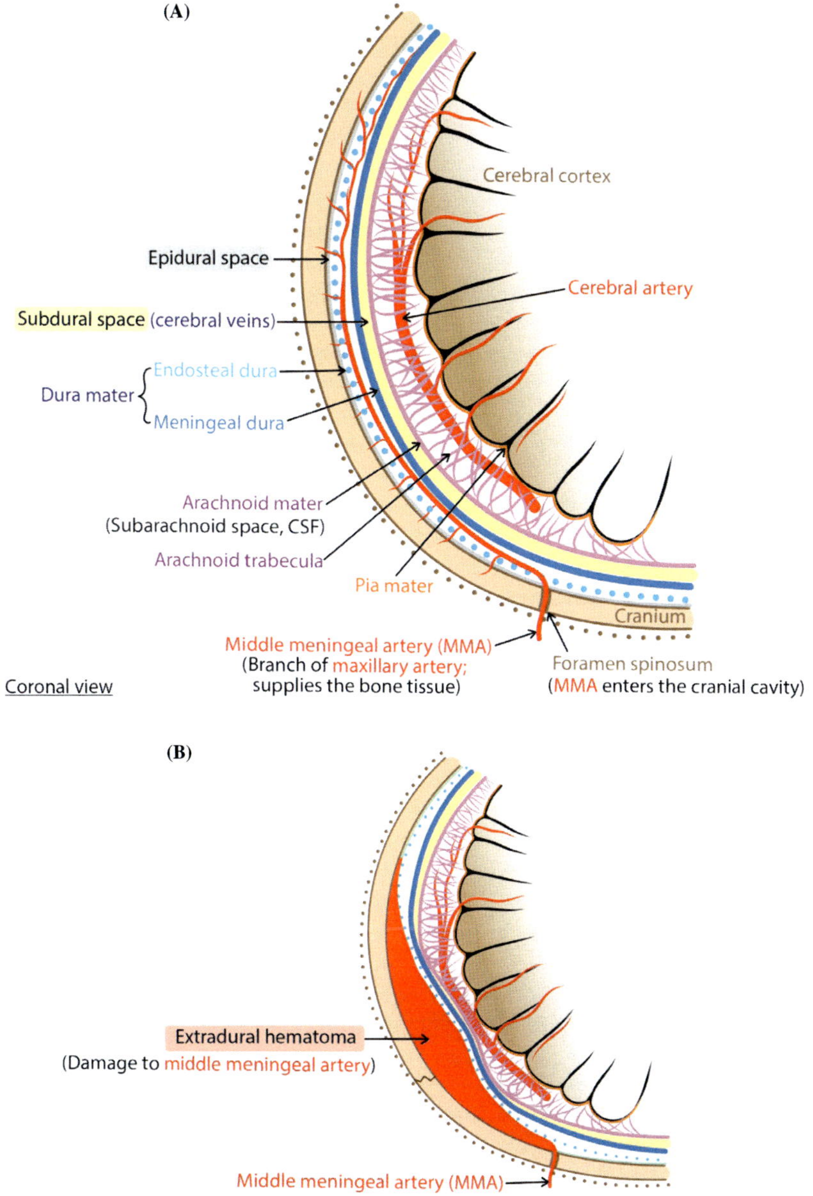

Figure 10.15. Meninges. (A) They are composed of three main layers: Dura mater (outer endosteal layer and the inner meningeal layer), arachnoid mater (spider-web-like), and the pia mater that covers the immediate brain surface. The space external to the dura is the extradural space, and the space deep to it is the subdural space containing the superficial cerebral veins. Between them is the middle meningeal artery (MMA). The space deep to the arachnoid is the subarachnoid space, filled with cerebrospinal fluid (CSF). The cerebral arteries course along this space. **(B)** Damage to the middle meningeal artery can lead to extradural hematoma, in which the endosteal dura is lifted due to the collection of blood.

2. **Arachnoid mater**: It is spider-web-like. The subarachnoid space contains cerebrospinal fluid (CSF) and cerebral arteries. Arachnoid granulations **(Fig. 10.15)** invaginate into the superior sagittal sinus (SSS). Arachnoid granulations facilitate CSF absorption into the SSS.
3. **Pia mater**: It is the innermost layer of the meninges, covering the gyri (gyrus) and sulci (sulcus) of the brain.

Dural Septa and Dural Venous Sinuses (Fig. 10.16)

1. The dural septum (pl. septa) is formed by a double-layered meningeal dura. The sickle-shaped falx cerebri is the main dural septum, which is attached anteriorly to the crista galli and frontal crest. Its superior border is attached to the calvaria, while it has a free inferior border. Posteriorly, the falx cerebri anchors on the superior surface of the tentorium cerebelli that overlies the two cerebellar hemispheres. The occipital lobes rest on the tentorium cerebelli, which is also formed by a double-layered meningeal dura.
2. The main function of the dural septa, falx cerebri, and tentorium cerebelli is to prevent the displacement of the brain.
3. The dural septum carries the venous sinuses, which receive drainage from the superficial cerebral vein as well as the CSF, e.g., the superior sagittal sinus.

The following are some of the endothelium-lined dural venous sinuses associated with the falx cerebri and tentorium cerebelli:

1. **Superior sagittal sinus (SSS)**: It runs along the superior border of the falx cerebri.
2. **Inferior sagittal sinus (ISS)**: It runs along the free inferior border of the falx cerebri.
3. **Cavernous sinus (CS)**: It lies on both sides of the hypophyseal fossa.
4. **Straight sinus (CS)**: It is at the junction between the falx cerebri and the tentorium cerebelli.
5. **Transverse sinus (TS)**: It is attached to the margins of the tentorium cerebelli.
6. **Sigmoid sinus (SS)**: It receives drainage from the cavernous sinus through the superior petrosal sinus (SPS).

Note that the drainage from all the dural sinuses is ultimately to the internal jugular vein (IJV). The inferior petrosal sinus (IPS) drains directly to the IJV.

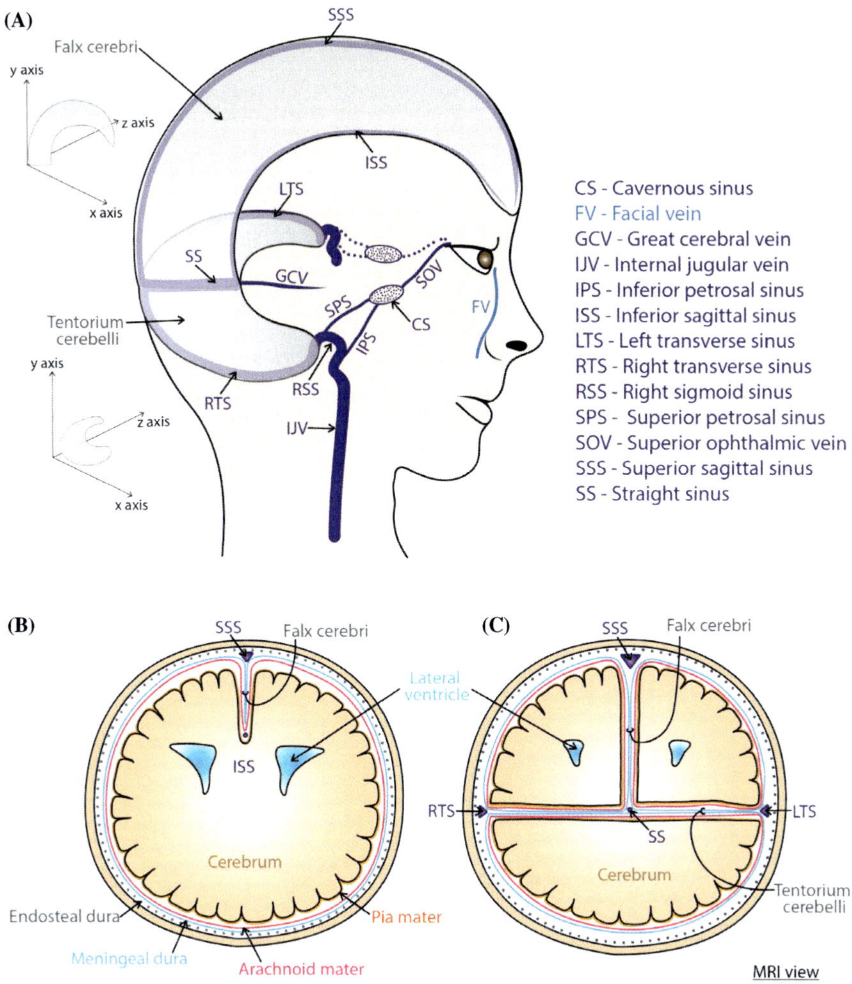

Figure 10.16. Dural septa (sing. septum). (A) The dural septum is formed by a double-layered meningeal dura. The falx cerebri is a sickle-shaped dural septum, which is attached anteriorly to the frontal crest and crista galli. It is attached superiorly to the skull bones and encloses the superior sagittal sinus (SSS). Its free inferior border encloses the inferior sagittal sinus (ISS). The ISS is joined by the great cerebral vein (GCV), forming the straight sinus (SS). Note that the falx cerebri is attached to the upper surface of the tentorium cerebelli, which is also formed by a double-layered meningeal dura. The SS joins with the right or left transverse sinus (RTS/LTS), continues as the right or left sigmoid sinus (RSS/LSS), and then continues inferiorly as the internal jugular vein (IJV). The cavernous sinus drains into the RTS/LTS via the superior and inferior petrosal sinuses (SPS/IPS). **(B)** and **(C)** are coronal sectional views of the dural septa.

Cavernous Sinus (Fig. 10.17)

1. The cavernous sinus (CS) lies lateral to the pituitary gland (hypophysis) in the hypophyseal fossa of the sphenoid (body) on both the sides.
2. It extends anteriorly from the superior orbital fissure to the petrous temporal bone and foramen lacerum, posteriorly.
3. The internal carotid artery and abducens nerve pass through the CS containing the venous plexuses.
4. It receives venous drainage from the facial vein via the SOV, hypophyseal vein, and sphenoparietal sinus. It drains into the SS posteriorly via the SPS and IPS.
5. The CN III, CN IV, CN V_1, and CN V_2 nerves traverse along the lateral wall of the CS.

Brain — A Brief Overview

It comprises the cerebrum (including the cerebral cortex and diencephalon), midbrain, cerebellum, and brainstem.

1. **Cerebral cortex (Fig. 10.18)**: The surface of the cerebrum appears highly convoluted with many gyri (singular: gyrus) and sulci (singular: sulcus). It is described that the convoluted configurations may increase the neuronal population for the complex neural circuitry. Superolaterally, the cerebral hemisphere has a deep groove or sulcus, the central sulcus (sulcus of Rolando), demarcating the boundaries between the frontal lobe and the parietal lobe anteroposteriorly. Anterior to the central sulcus is the precentral gyrus, the primary motor cortex (frontal lobe); lying posteriorly to the central sulcus is the postcentral gyrus, the primary somatosensory cortex (parietal lobe). The lateral sulcus (Sylvian fissure) demarcates the temporal lobe from the frontal and the parietal lobes above.
   The occipital lobe is at the posterior pole of the brain, demarcated by the occipitoparietal sulcus.

   <u>Frontal lobe **(Fig. 10.18)**</u>: It has the superior, middle, and inferior gyri. Broca's motor speech area is localized in the inferior frontal gyrus. Prefrontal cortex — this is the area for higher intellect, decision making, personality, and emotion. The precentral gyrus is the primary motor cortex.

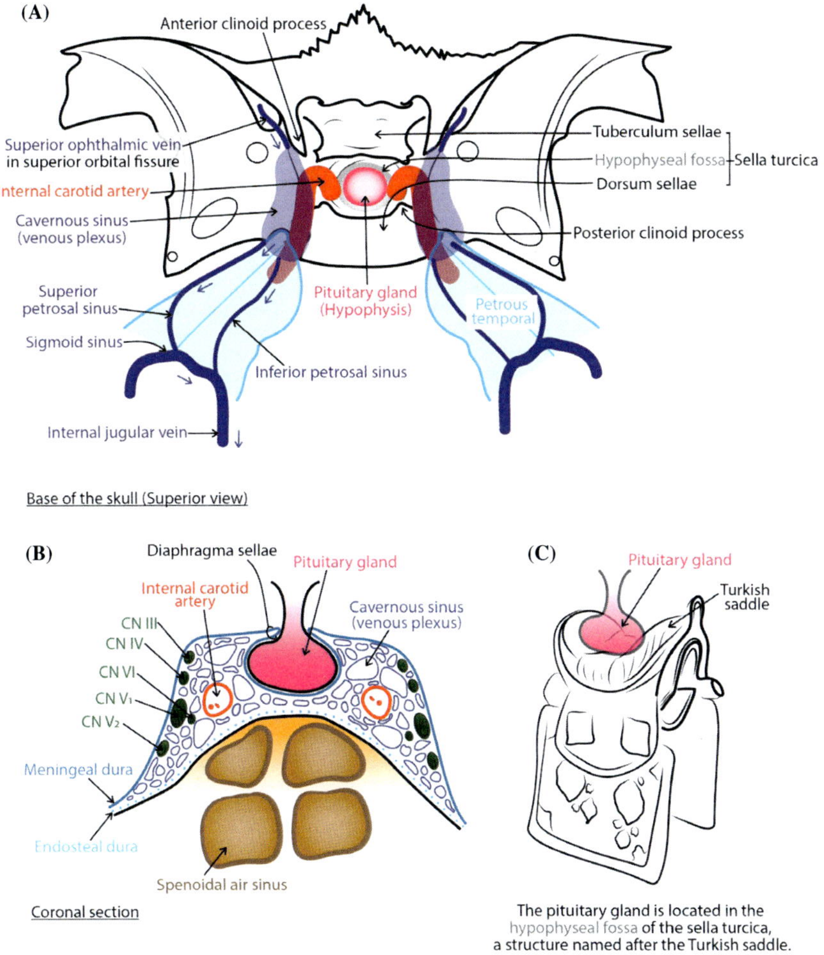

Figure 10.17. Cavernous sinus. (A) The bilateral cavernous sinus lies lateral to the hypophysis (pituitary). It extends from the superior orbital fissure to the posterior clinoid process and foramen lacerum. Anteriorly, it receives the drainage from the superior ophthalmic vein. Posteriorly, the sinus drains into the sigmoid sinus (SS) via the superior and inferior petrosal sinuses (SPS, IPS). **(B)** In a coronal section, the sinus lies between the two layers of meningeal dura. The internal carotid artery, surrounded by the venous plexus along with the VI nerve, traverses through it. The lateral wall is related to the III, IV, V_1, and V_2 nerves.

Definition: "Homunculus" is a neurological map of the areas and proportions of the cerebral cortex responsible for processing or integrating motor or sensory functions from different parts of the body **(Fig. 10.19)**.

<u>Parietal lobe **(Fig. 10.18)**</u>: It consists of the postcentral gyrus, which is the primary somatosensory cortex.

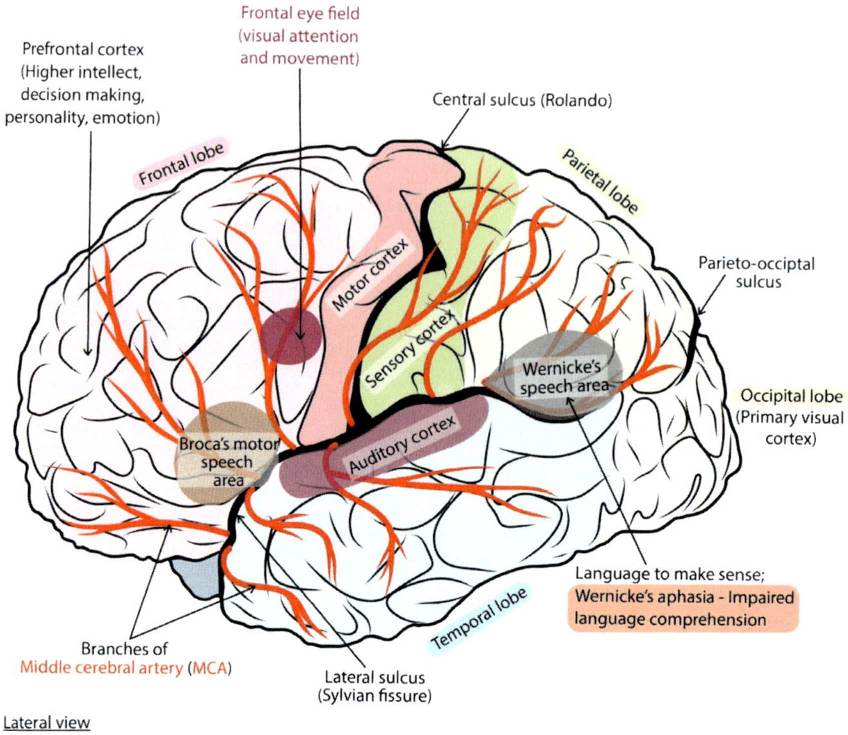

Figure 10.18. Cerebrum — cerebral cortex. Lateral view of the left cerebral hemisphere. The central sulcus (of Rolando) separates the frontal lobe from the parietal lobe. The lateral sulcus (Sylvian fissure) separates the temporal lobe from the frontal/parietal and occipital lobes. The parieto-occipital sulcus demarcates the occipital lobe. Refer to the text for a more detailed description of the different areas of the cerebral cortex and their functions. Note the middle cerebral artery (MCA) supplies most of the cerebral cortex: pre- and postcentral gyri, Broca's motor speech area, frontal cortex, superior temporal gyrus (Wernicke's area), etc.

Temporal lobe **(Fig. 10.20)**: It has three gyri — superior, middle, and posterior. Wernicke's speech area (sensory) is localized in the posterior part of the superior temporal gyrus. Lesion of this area leads to impaired language comprehension — "Wernicke's aphasia." The superior temporal gyrus is the primary auditory cortex. The temporal lobe also contains the "limbic system," comprising the hippocampus, which is involved in learning, memory, cognition, etc. Degenerative changes of neurons in the limbic system are associated with Alzheimer's disease. Anterior to the hippocampus is the amygdaloid nucleus, which is related to fear, anxiety, and depression functions.

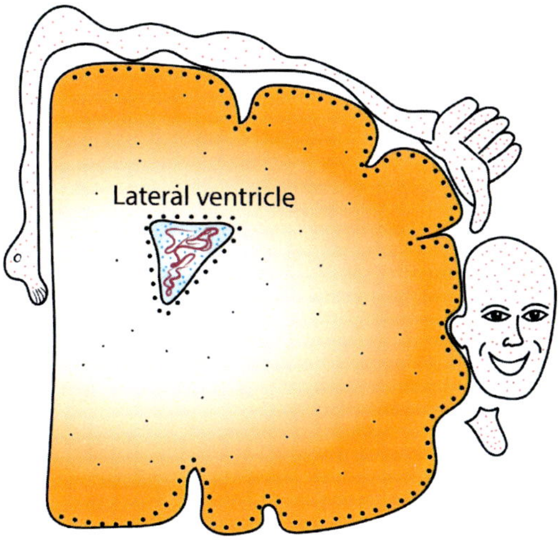

Figure 10.19. Cerebral cortex — Homunculus. The "cartoon figure" is based on a neurological map of the areas and proportions of the brain dedicated to processing the sensory and motor functions from different parts of the body.

Occipital lobe (**Fig. 10.18; Fig. 10.20; Fig. 10.21**): On its medial side is the calcarine sulcus (calcarine means "spur" in Latin), responsible for visual function (visual cortex). Above the calcarine sulcus is the cuneus gyrus; below it is the lingual gyrus.

2. **Diencephalon (Fig. 10.21)**: It consists of the thalamus, hypothalamus, epithalamus, and subthalamus. The thalamus, with its many subnuclei, is a relay station for ascending and descending nerve fibers (tracts). The hypothalamus regulates the autonomic nervous system, involved in many functions: sleep, hunger sensation, emotion, homeostasis, etc.

   The epithalamus lies at the roof of the third ventricle and is related to the pineal gland. The pineal gland produces the hormone melatonin, involved in diurnal rhythm and sleep. The subthalamus nucleus is part of the basal ganglia.
3. **Midbrain (superior and inferior colliculi)**: It contains the superior and inferior colliculi, which act as reflex centers for visual and auditory functions, respectively.
4. **Cerebellum (Fig. 10.21)**: The two cerebellar hemispheres show many folia. There are several afferent pathways. The main efferent pathway is the

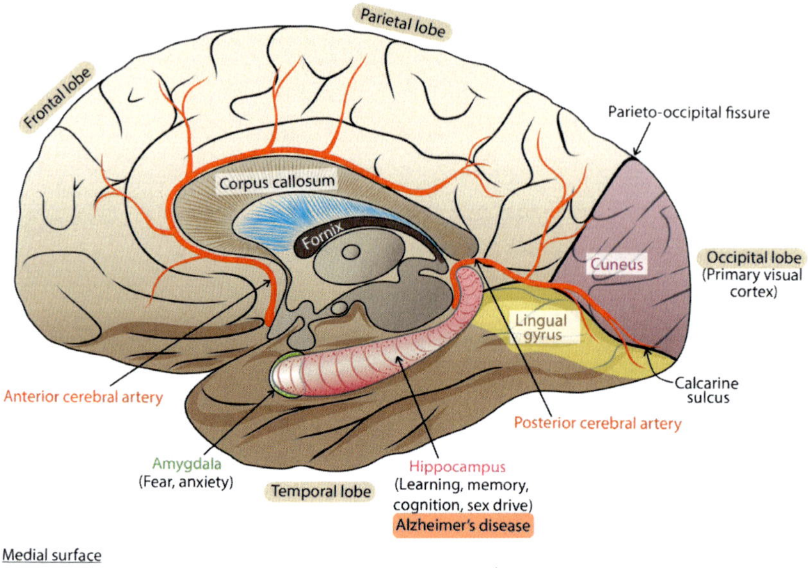

Figure 10.20. Cerebral cortex. Medial surface of the right cerebral hemisphere. Posteriorly is the occipital lobe showing the calcarine sulcus and its adjacent cuneus and lingual gyri. This subserves the visual function (visual cortex). The anterior cerebral artery supplies most of the medial surface of the frontal and parietal lobes. Note that the visual cortex is supplied by the posterior cerebral artery (PCA). The temporal lobe is the site for the primary auditory function. It houses the limbic system structures, including the hippocampus (learning, memory, cognition, and sex drive). At the tip of it is the almond-shaped amygdala (fear conditioning, anxiety, hormone secretions).

dentato- rubrospinal tract being regulated by the Purkinje neurons in the cerebellar cortex. The cerebellum subserves motor coordination, balance, muscle tone, synergy, etc.

5. **Brainstem (Fig. 10.21)**: It consists of the midbrain, pons, and medulla oblongata. It has CVS (cardiovascular system) and RS (respiratory system) regulatory centers. Most of the 12 cranial nerves (except for I and II) arise from the brainstem.

Arterial Supply of the Brain

It is supplied by the Circle of Willis, which is formed by the internal carotid arteries and the vertebral arteries. (Details for this will be covered separately in neuroanatomy.)

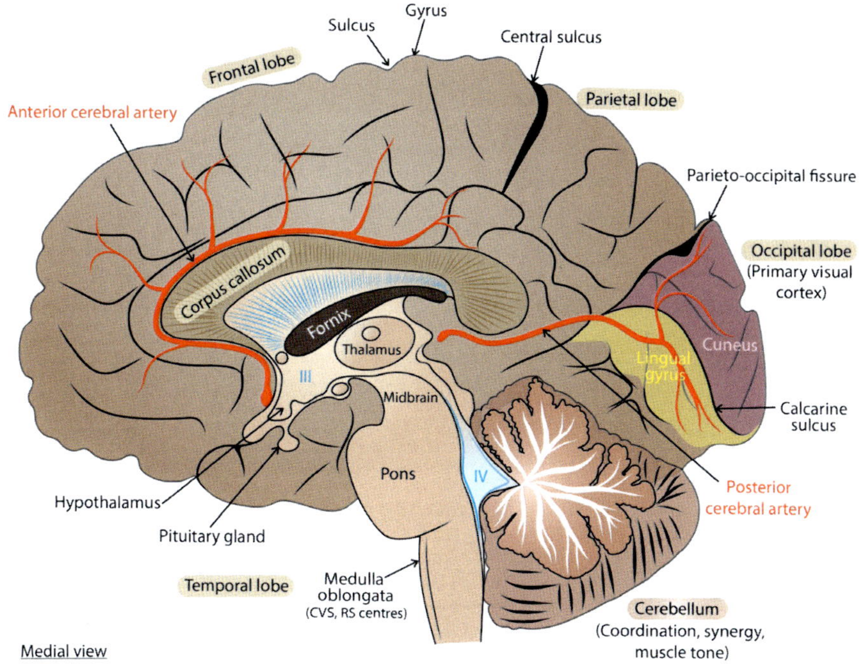

Figure 10.21. Cerebrum (cerebral cortex). Medial view of the right cerebral hemisphere. The surface of the cerebral cortex shows many sulci (grooves) and gyri (elevations). The two cerebral hemispheres are interconnected by the white matter — corpus callosum. On the medial surface of the occipital lobe is the calcarine sulcus. The thalamus lies below the fornix. Below the thalamus are the hypothalamus, brainstem, and cerebellum. Refer to the text for a more detailed description of different areas of the cerebral cortex and their functions. Note that the anterior cerebral artery (ACA) supplies most areas of the medial aspect of the cerebral hemisphere. The posterior cerebral artery (PCA) supplies the visual cortex.

1. **Anterior cerebral artery (ACA) (Fig. 10.18; Fig. 10.20; Fig. 10.21)**: It supplies the medial side of the cerebral cortex (controlling lower limb area) above the corpus callosum and cingulate gyrus.
2. **Middle cerebral artery (MCA) (Fig. 10.18; Fig. 10.20; Fig. 10.21)**: It supplies the pre- and postcentral gyrus (primary motor and sensory cortex) and the temporal lobe (primary auditory cortex).
3. **Posterior cerebral artery (PCA) (Fig. 10.18; Fig. 10.20; Fig. 10.21)**: It supplies the occipital lobe (visual cortex).

Applied anatomy

1. The CS receives venous drainage from the facial (angular) vein via the SOV **(Fig. 10.17)**. Infection from the "danger area" of the face may be spread to the CS. Cavernous sinus thrombosis may result from an infection of the face (i.e., *Staphylococcus*).
2. Different types of intracranial hemorrhages may be associated with the meninges:
   a. *Extradural hemorrhage* ***(Fig. 10.15)***: Rupture of the middle meningeal artery due to the impact at the pterion (meeting point of the greater wing of the sphenoid, squamous temporal, frontal, parietal). The pterion can be surface marked as follows: one finger breadth from the orbital margin and two finger breadths above the zygomatic arch. A hematoma may compress the motor cortex, leading to contralateral muscle weakness (paralysis).
   b. *Subdural hemorrhage* ***(Fig. 10.15)***: Damage to the superior/superficial cerebral veins crossing the subdural space may lead to hematoma formation, often in the elderly following a fall with head injury.
   c. *Subarachnoid hemorrhage* ***(Fig. 10.15)***: This is caused by rupture of an arterial aneurysm. Blood-stained CSF may be detected.
   d. *Intracerebral hemorrhage*: Cerebral ischemia or infarct due to a rupture of an aneurysm, or thrombosis.

ORBIT AND THE EYE

The orbit contains the eyeball and extraocular muscles that move the eyeball **(Fig. 10.22)**, cranial nerves, arteries and veins, and the adipose tissue. The superolateral part of the orbit contains the lacrimal fossa, which houses the lacrimal gland.

The bony orbit is pyramidal shaped, with an apex, four walls, and a base. The roof is formed by the orbital plate of the frontal bone; the floor by the maxilla; the medial wall by the ethmoid bone, and the lateral wall by the zygomatic bone. The base forms the orbital margin with a supraorbital notch, while the apex contains the optic canal and superior orbital fissure opening into the middle cranial fossa. The inferior orbital fissure lies between the sphenoid and maxilla,

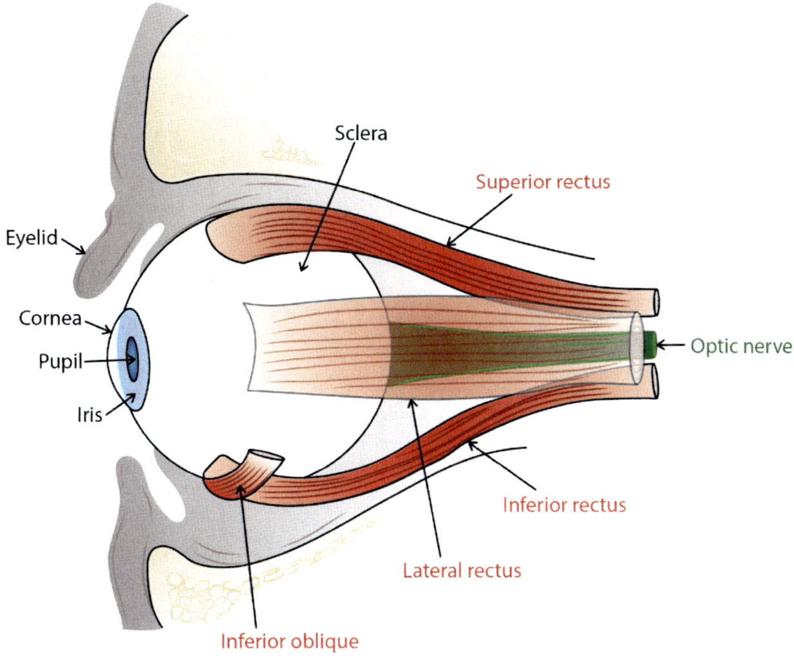

Figure 10.22. Eyeball. The eyeball is housed in the pyramidal-shaped bony orbit formed by the frontal (orbital plate), lacrimal, zygomatic, maxilla, sphenoid, and ethmoid. The outermost layer of the eyeball includes the cornea and the sclera. The extraocular muscles, which move the eyeball, are attached to the eyeball behind the corneoscleral junction (limbus). The optic nerve from the posterior aspect of the eyeball transmits the electrical signal to the brain.

and it continues anteriorly into the infraorbital groove and canal, which opens at the infraorbital foramen to transmit the infraorbital nerve. The apex provides the passage for the cranial nerves and blood vessels that supply the contents of the orbit. In the living, the surface of the body orbit is lined by a layer of periosteum, periorbita.

Extraocular Muscles (Fig. 10.23; Fig. 10.24)

- There are four rectus and two oblique muscles attached to the eyeball.
- All four rectus muscles arise from the "common tendinous ring" at the apex of the orbit. They are inserted into the ocular surface posterior to the "limbus" (corneoscleral junction).

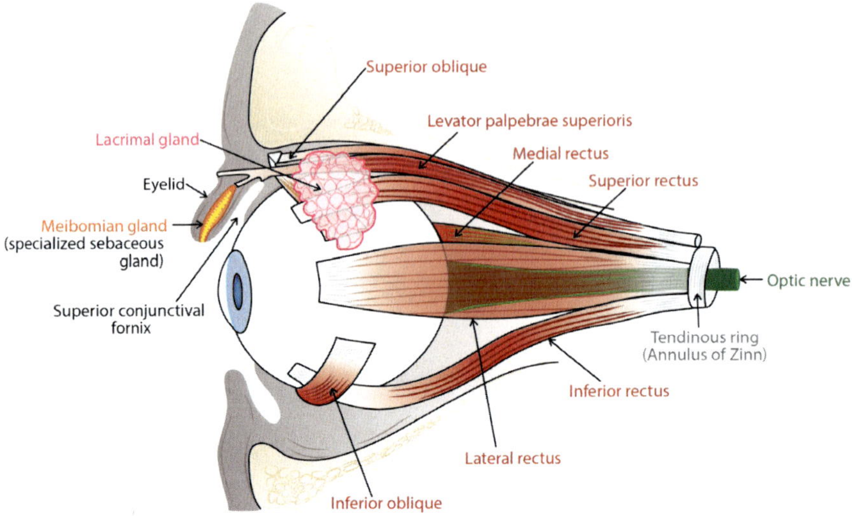

Figure 10.23. Extraocular muscles. The four rectus muscles (superior rectus, lateral rectus, medial rectus, and inferior rectus) arise from the tendinous ring at the apex of the orbit. They are inserted into the eyeball posterior to the corneoscleral junction (limbus). The levator palpebrae superioris muscle arises above the superior rectus; it is inserted into the upper eyelid (containing the tarsal plate and the meibomian gland) and the eyebrow. The lacrimal gland is located superolateral to the eyeball; its tiny ducts open into the superior conjunctival fornix. The optic nerve passes through the optic canal within the tendinous ring.

- The superior oblique muscle arises posteriorly from the sphenoid bone near the medial orbital wall and runs forward along that wall. At the medial orbital margin, its tendon passes through the trochlea (a fibrocartilaginous pulley) and then inserts onto the postero-supero-lateral quadrant of the eyeball.
- The inferior oblique arises from the floor of the orbit medially and is inserted into the postero-infero-lateral quadrant of the eyeball.
- In addition is the levator palpebrae superioris, which is inserted into the upper eyelid.

Tendinous Ring (Fig. 10.25)

The "tendinous ring" is a thickened ring of periorbita (periosteum) encircling the optic canal and the medial part of the superior orbital fissure. It provides attachment for the four rectus muscles.

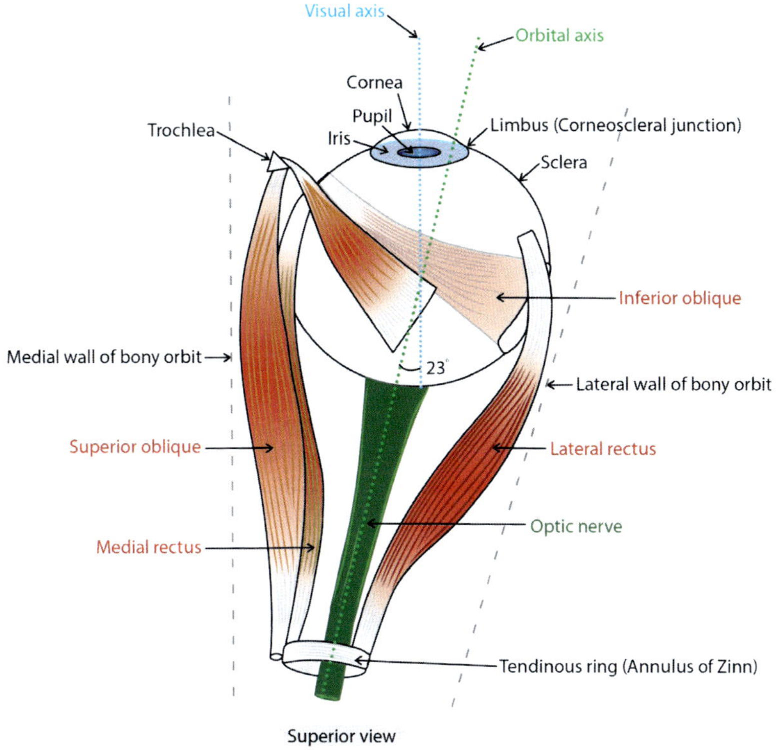

Figure 10.24. Extraocular muscles (superior view). The superior oblique muscle arises from the medial wall of the bony orbit posteriorly. It runs forward with its tendon hooking around the trochlea. It angulates back and is inserted into the postero-superolateral quadrant of the eyeball. The inferior oblique muscle arises from the floor of the body orbit medially. It is inserted into the postero-inferolateral quadrant of the eyeball.

Structures pass through the apex within the tendinous ring:

1. **<u>Optic canal</u>**: Optic nerve (CN II) and ophthalmic artery, which gives rise to the central artery supplying the retina.
2. **<u>Superior orbital fissure</u>**: Oculomotor nerve (CN III) (upper and lower divisions), nasociliary nerve (from CN V_1), and abducent nerve (CN VI).

Structures pass through the superior orbital fissure outside of the tendinous ring:

1. Frontal nerve (F) and lacrimal nerve (L) — CN V_1
2. Trochlear nerve (CN IV)
3. Superior ophthalmic vein (SOV)

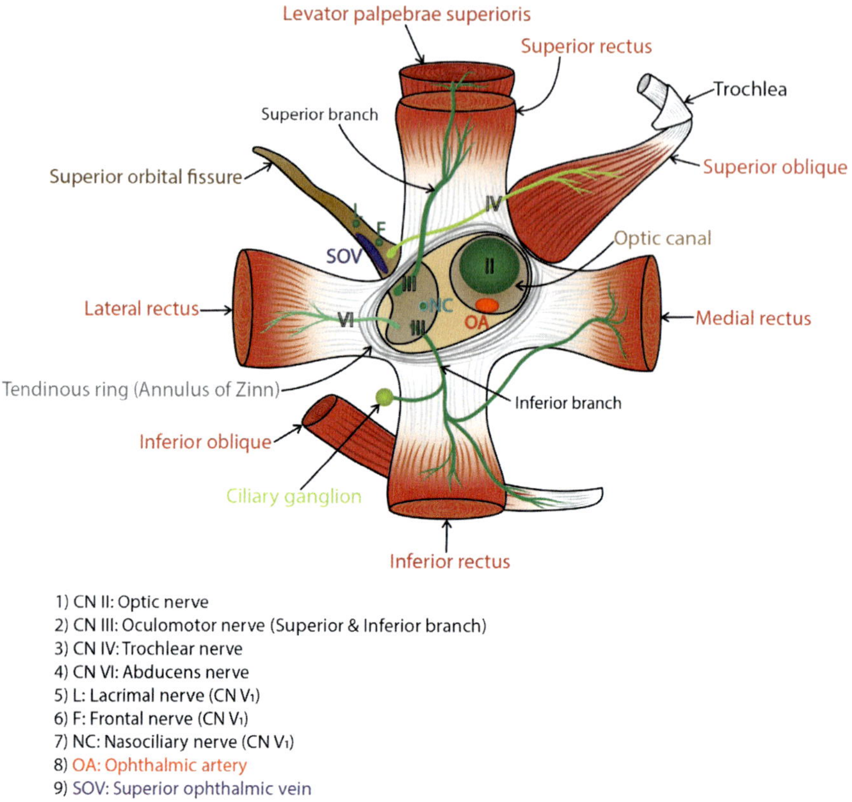

Figure 10.25. Extraocular muscles — attachment and innervation. This is an antero-posterior view of the apex of the right orbit showing the "tendinous ring," which covers the medial part of the superior orbital fissure. It encircles the entire optic canal, which transmits the optic nerve (II) and central artery. Note that the four recti arise from the tendinous ring. Passing through the superior orbital fissure within the tendinous ring are the III, VI, and nasociliary (NC) nerves. Passing through the orbital fissure outside of the tendinous ring include the lacrimal (L), frontal (F), and IV nerves and superior ophthalmic vein (SOV).

Actions of extraocular muscles

The eyeball moves around three axes: horizontal, vertical, and anteroposterior:

1. Horizontal axis: Elevation and depression
2. Vertical axis: Medial rotation (adduction) and lateral rotation (abduction)
3. Anteroposterior axis: Intorsion and extorsion. This axis allows intorsion and extorsion. In intorsion, the 12 o'clock position of the eye rotates medially; in extorsion, it rotates laterally.

Movements and innervation

1. Superior rectus: Elevation, adduction (medial rotation), intorsion — CN III nerve
2. Inferior rectus: Depression, adduction (medial rotation), extorsion — CN III nerve
3. Medial rectus: Adduction (medial rotation) — CN III nerve
4. Lateral (external) rectus: Abduction (lateral rotation) — CN VI nerve
5. Superior oblique: Depression, intorsion (looking down and laterally); abduction (lateral rotation) — CN IV nerve.
6. Inferior oblique: Elevation, extorsion (looking up and laterally); abduction (lateral rotation) — CN III nerve.

Eye

The eyeball has three main layers: sclera, choroid, and retina **(Fig. 10.26)**.

1. **Sclera**: It is a fibrous coat forming the "white part" of the eye and continues as the transparent cornea anteriorly at the corneoscleral junction "limbus."
2. **Choroid**: It is a well-vascularized layer with some pigment-containing cells. Anteriorly, the choroid is widened as the ciliary body, bearing finger-like projections, the ciliary processes that are connected to the lens via the suspensory ligaments.
   a. The ciliary body contains the ciliary muscles (radial, meridional, and circular), which regulate the shape of the lens for far and near focusing ("accommodation"). For instance, when the ciliary muscles contract, the suspensory ligaments are lax, and the lens becomes more rounded for short distance focusing (e.g., when reading). The ciliary muscles relax when one looks at an object at a distance (e.g., viewing a flying kite). When traced further anteriorly, the choroid continues as the iris with a central aperture, "pupil."
   b. The iris has radial (dilator pupillae) and circular (sphincter pupillae) muscles, which regulate the size of the pupil in bright or dark conditions. The dilator pupillae muscle is supplied by postganglionic sympathetic fibers that originate from the superior cervical ganglion (SCG) (*see the section on Sympathetic Innervation of the Head and Neck*). The sphincter pupillae is innervated by parasympathetic fibers originating from the

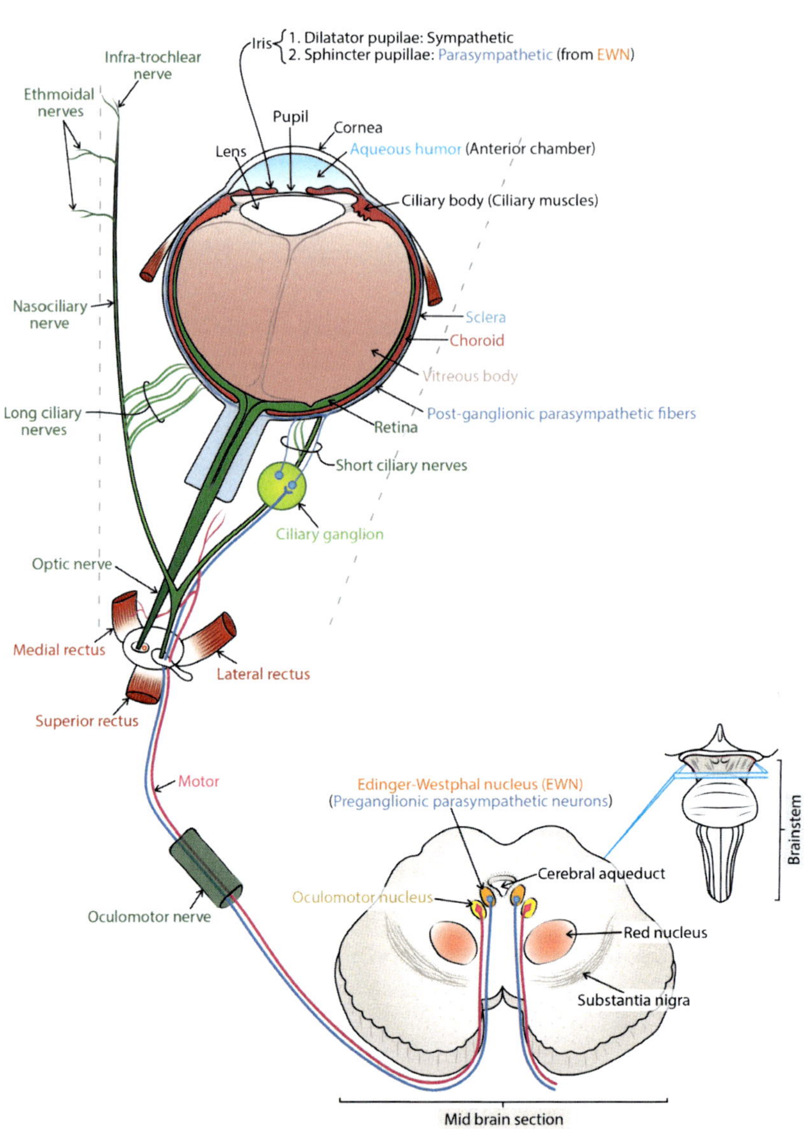

Figure 10.26. Eye and its innervation. A horizontal section of the right eyeball showing its three layers: cornea/sclera, choroid, and retina. The choroid is expanded anteriorly as the ciliary body, containing the ciliary muscles; anteriorly, it continues as the iris, containing the dilator pupillae and sphincter pupillae. The innermost layer is the retina, whose retinal ganglion cells give rise to the optic nerve. The eyeball is filled up anteriorly by the aqueous humor, and posteriorly, it is occupied by the vitreous body. The ciliary muscles are supplied by the Edinger–Westphal nucleus (EWN), localized in the midbrain (superior colliculus). The preganglionic parasympathetic nerve fibers (axons) are conveyed by the oculomotor nerve and synapse in the ciliary ganglion. The postganglionic parasympathetic nerve fibers also supply the sphincter pupillae. The dilator pupillae is supplied by the sympathetic nerve fibers from the cervical sympathetic ganglion.

Edinger–Westphal nucleus (EWN) in the midbrain at the level of the superior colliculus. Preganglionic parasympathetic fibers from the EWN travel with the oculomotor nerve (CN III) and synapse in the ciliary ganglion. Postganglionic parasympathetic fibers then pass through the short ciliary nerves to innervate the ciliary muscle and, more anteriorly, the sphincter pupillae, which encircles the pupil.

3. **Retina**: This is the neural layer of the eye, which contains the photoreceptors: rods and cones. The rods containing the visual pigment, rhodopsin, are sensitive to light intensity. The cones contain iodopsin and are sensitive to colors. The macula lutea is the site of the retina (central area) containing exclusively cone cells. Transduction of photoenergy to electrical energy occurs in the photoreceptors, whose electrical impulse is transmitted via bipolar neurons and later via the retinal ganglion cells. The axons of the retinal ganglion cells converge to form the optic nerve (CN II), which conveys the nerve impulse to the lateral geniculate body of the thalamus. The impulse is then relayed to the superior colliculus (or pretectal area), and/or ultimately to the visual cortex (adjacent areas of the calcarine sulcus of the occipital lobe).
4. **Aqueous and vitreous body**: The aqueous humor fills the space between the cornea and lens. The iris divides the space into the anterior and posterior chambers. The fluid is produced by the ciliary processes. It circulates through the posterior chamber, pupil, and anterior chamber to be absorbed by the sinus sclerae (canal of Schlemm) at the corneoscleral junction **(Fig. 10.26)**. The vitreous body fills up the entire space between the lens and the retina.

It is normal to see some "floaters," named "flying mosquitoes" in Chinese, in the body (cellular or fibrous debris).

Quiz 1: *What is a pupillary reflex? Describe the neural pathway involved in the reflex.*

Quiz 2: *What is an accommodation reflex? Describe the neural pathway involved in the reflex.*

Quiz 3: *What is a corneal reflex? Describe the neural pathway involved in the reflex.*

Quiz 4: *What is the so-called "blind spot" of the eye?*

Quiz 5: *What would be the functional loss if the oculomotor nerve is lesioned?*

Hints: divergent squint, diplopia, loss of accommodation, dilation of the pupil, and ptosis (drooping of the upper eyelid). Explain the causes for these conditions.

Applied anatomy and clinical considerations

1. *Cornea*: It is lined by the stratified squamous epithelium. It is avascular; hence, it is suitable for corneal transplant. It is richly innervated by ophthalmic division (V_1) of the trigeminal nerve.
2. *Glaucoma*: It is caused by an increase in intraocular pressure (IOP) due to a blockage of aqueous humor drainage. Glaucoma, either acute or chronic, may lead to a loss of peripheral vision (death of retinal ganglion cells) or even total blindness. "Cupping of the optic disc" indicates optic nerve damage, which is commonly seen in glaucoma.
3. *Lens*: The increase in opacity due to aging or other causes can lead to a "cataract," causing blurred vision. This can be corrected with an artificial lens implant.
4. *Retinal detachment or tear*: Clinical signs include "sudden increase in massive floaters," flashes of light, loss of visual field, etc.
5. *Age-related macular degeneration (ARMD)*: Loss of central vision.

Lacrimal gland and its drainage apparatus (Fig.10.23)

The lacrimal gland lies in the superolateral part of the orbit. It consists of the orbital and palpebral parts. It is histologically a serous gland and has 10–12 ducts opening into the superior conjunctival fornix. By capillary action, the lacrimal fluid flows over the cornea to the lacus lacrimalis. From here, the lacrimal fluid is drained through the puncta into the lacrimal canaliculi and then into the nasolacrimal duct, which opens into the inferior meatus of the nasal cavity. The secretomotor innervation of the lacrimal gland is by the facial nerve (CN VII) via the greater petrosal nerve and pteryopalatine ganglion (*see the section on Cranial Nerves*).

Dry eyes: This may be due to many reasons. It may be attributed to changes in one of the three compositions of the tear film: mucus, aqueous fluid, and fatty oils.

NASAL CAVITY

1. The two nasal cavities, separated by the nasal septum, begin at the nostrils (openings of the vestibule) and end at the choanae (the two openings leading into the nasopharynx).

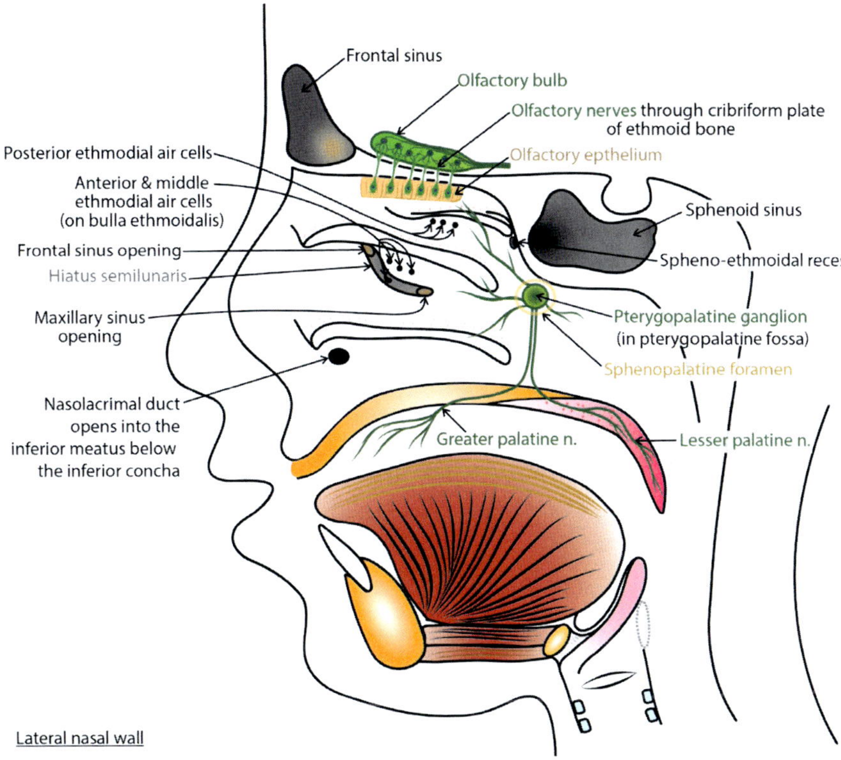

Figure 10.27. **Nasal cavity.** Lateral wall of the right nasal cavity (sagittal section). Three shelf-like projections: superior, middle, and inferior nasal concha(e) hang from the lateral wall. Beneath each concha are the superior, middle, and inferior meatuses, respectively. Over the superior nasal concha is the olfactory epithelium, which sends the olfactory nerves through the cribriform plate to the olfactory bulb. In the middle meatus is the hiatus semilunaris, which receives the openings of the anterior ethmoidal air cells and the frontal sinus. Posteriorly, the hiatus receives the opening of the maxillary sinus. The nasolacrimal duct opens into the inferior meatus. Note that the pterygopalatine ganglion lies lateral to the sphenopalatine foramen at the level of the middle nasal concha. It is housed in the pterygopalatine fossa. The ganglion sends nasal branches supplying the nasal mucosa; other branches of the pterygopalatine ganglion include the greater and lesser palatine nerves supplying the hard and soft palate, respectively.

2. The nasal cavity functions to moisturize and warm the air; also, it helps to filter dust particles. It is also involved in olfaction.
3. At the vestibule, it is lined by the skin, which is a keratinized, stratified squamous epithelium; over the superior concha (see below), it is lined by the olfactory epithelium (smell). The remainder of the nasal cavity is lined by the respiratory epithelium (ciliated pseudostratified columnar epithelium).
4. Three shelf-like projections hang from the lateral wall: superior, middle, and inferior concha (or turbinate) **(Fig. 10.27)**. The superior and middle conchae are parts of the ethmoid bone, whereas the inferior concha is a bone by itself.
5. Beneath the superior, middle, and inferior concha are the superior, middle, and inferior meatus, respectively.
6. Above the superior concha is the sphenoethmoidal recess, which receives the opening of the sphenoidal sinus.
7. **Inferior meatus**: The nasolacrimal duct opens into it **(Fig. 10.27)**.
8. **Superior meatus**: Openings of the posterior ethmoidal air cells.
9. **Middle meatus**: Hiatus semilunaris is a semicircular opening or gap in the middle meatus **(Fig. 10.27)**. Above the hiatus is the bulla ethmoidalis. Opening into the hiatus anteriorly are the frontal sinus/anterior ethmoid air cells. Opening into the hiatus posteriorly is the maxillary sinus. On the bulla are the openings of the middle ethmoidal air cells.
10. **Innervation of the nasal cavity**: The olfactory nerves supply the area over the superior concha; the remaining area is innervated by the nasal branches of the pterygopalatine ganglion, which is housed in the pterygopalatine fossa lateral to the sphenopalatine foramen at the level of the middle concha **(Fig. 10.27)**. (*Details regarding the connections of the ganglion are to be described later.*)

Nasal Septum (Fig. 10.28)

1. The nasal septum separates the two nasal cavities. It is formed by the (a) perpendicular plate of ethmoid, (b) septal cartilage, (c) vomer, and (d) maxilla/palatine.
2. It is lined by the respiratory epithelium, except for over the roof area, which is olfactory.
3. **Arterial supply**: Anterior and posterior ethmoidal arteries (from the internal carotid artery), sphenopalatine artery (maxillary artery), greater

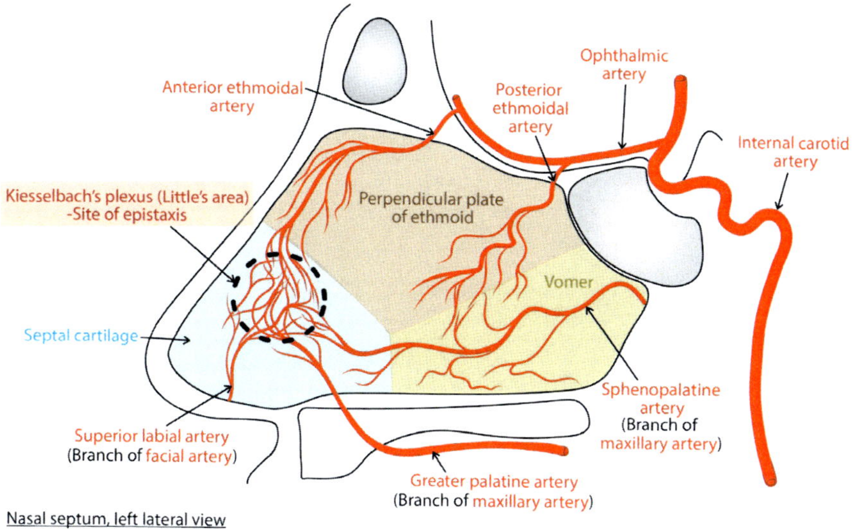

Figure 10.28. Nasal septum. It is made up of the perpendicular plate of the ethmoid, vomer, and septal cartilage. The mucous membrane is lined mainly by the respiratory epithelium. The arteries supplying the septum include the anterior and posterior ethmoidal arteries (from the internal ophthalmic artery), sphenopalatine artery (from the maxillary artery through the sphenopalatine foramen), greater palatine artery, and the superior labial artery (from the facial artery). They form an arterial anastomosis at the antero-inferior area of the septum — Little's area (Kisselbach's plexus). This is the site of nose bleeding — epistaxis.

palatine artery (maxillary artery), and superior labial artery (from the facial artery). These arteries form an arterial anastomosis (Kisselbach's plexus) at the anteroinferior area of the nasal septum, "Little's area," which is the common site of nose bleeding (epistaxis).

4. **Innervation**: Nasopalatine nerve from the pterygopalatine ganglion (maxillary nerve, V_2). Anterior and posterior ethmoidal nerves; also, the olfactory nerves.

Maxillary Sinus

It is an air-filled sinus that opens into the posterior part of the hiatus semilunaris **(Fig. 10.27)**. It is lined by the respiratory epithelium. Infection of the nasal cavity may spread to the sinus-sinusitis. The maxillary sinus is related medially to the nasal cavity. The floor is related to the upper premolars and the first molar tooth. It is supplied by branches of the maxillary nerve and the pterygopalatine ganglion **(Fig. 10.29)**.

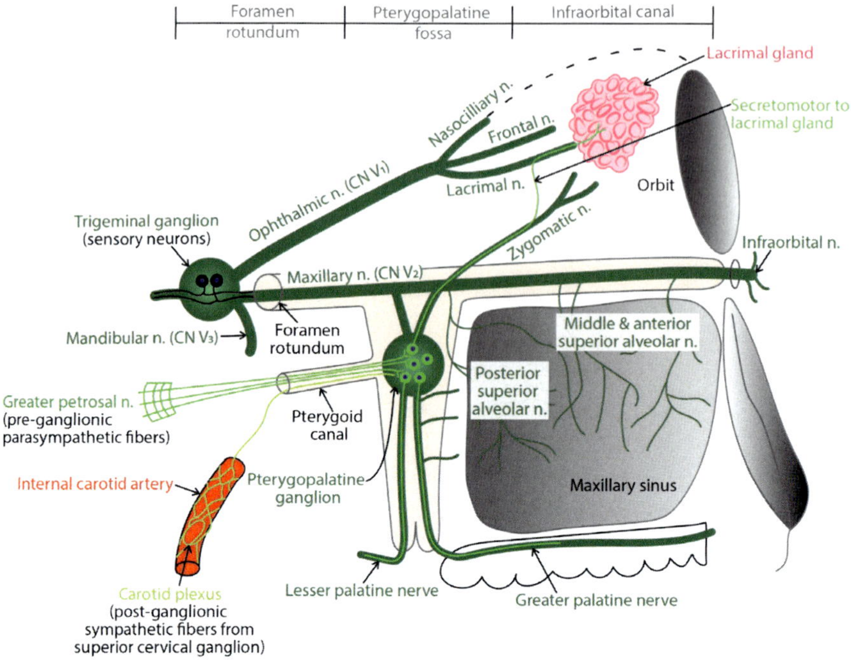

Figure 10.29. Maxillary nerve: Its origin, course, and distribution. It is one of the three divisions of the trigeminal nerve attached to the pons. From the trigeminal ganglion, it leaves the cranial fossa through the foramen rotundum. The ganglion contains the sensory trigeminal ganglion cells. For convenience of description, the nerve may be divided into three parts: the foramen rotundum, the pterygopalatine fossa, and the infraorbital canal. It gives rise to three branches: zygomatic nerve, infraorbital nerve, and posterior superior alveolar nerves. The infraorbital nerve gives rise to the anterior and middle superior alveolar nerves supplying the teeth of the upper jaw and the maxillary sinus. The pterygopalatine ganglion is suspended to the maxillary nerve in the pterygopalatine fossa. The ganglion receives preganglionic parasympathetic fibers from the greater petrosal nerve (a branch of the facial nerve). The postganglionic parasympathetic (neurons) fibers travel along the zygomatic nerve and then the lacrimal nerve to supply the lacrimal gland. The deep petrosal nerve fibers are distributed as the carotid nerve plexus (postganglionic sympathetic fibers). They pass through the pterygoid canal and enter the pterygopalatine ganglion without making any synaptic contacts. Together with the parasympathetic fibers, they supply the glands in the hard and soft palate via the greater and lesser palatine nerves, as well as the glands in the nasal cavity.

Maxillary Nerve (Fig. 10.29)

It is one of the three divisions of the trigeminal nerve (V): (1) Ophthalmic (V_1), (2) Maxillary (V_2), and (3) Mandibular division (V_3). It is exclusively sensory, supplying the structures in the upper jaw, including the maxilla, maxillary sinus, upper teeth, hard and soft palate, and face (the trigeminal nerve arises from the pons). The trigeminal ganglion (also called the Gasserian ganglion or semilunar ganglion) contains the sensory neurons (pseudounipolar neurons) (first-order neurons), which receive all sensory inputs (pain, temperature, and touch) from all three divisions. The afferents terminate either in the chief (simple touch) or spinal nucleus of V (pain), where they make synaptic contacts with the second-order neurons. The axons from the second-order neurons cross over and ascend to the thalamus nucleus (VPM) via the trigeminothalamic tract. They synapse with the third-order neurons in the VPM. The axons from the third-order neurons project to the primary somatosensory cortex in the postcentral gyrus (facial area). (*The descriptions of the ophthalmic and mandibular nerves are under separate sections.*)

Course of the maxillary nerve (Fig. 10.29)

1. The long course of the maxillary nerve may be divided into three parts: foramen rotundum, pterygopalatine fossa, and infraorbital canal.
2. It leaves the middle cranial fossa via the foramen rotundum and enters the pterygopalatine fossa (medial to the pterygomaxillary fissure, lateral to the sphenopalatine foramen). The pterygopalatine ganglion (a parasympathetic ganglion) is suspended to the maxillary nerve within the fossa.
3. In the pterygopalatine fossa, the maxillary nerve gives rise to three terminal branches: zygomatic nerve, infraorbital nerve, and posterior superior alveolar nerves (PSAN, see figure).
4. The infraorbital nerve terminates and emerges at the infraorbital foramen, supplying the lower eyelid, external nose, and upper lip. Along its course, it also gives rise to anterior and middle superior alveolar nerves supplying the maxillary sinus and upper teeth.

Pterygopalatine Ganglion (Fig. 10.29)

The pterygopalatine ganglion is suspended to the maxillary nerve in the pterygopalatine fossa. It receives the preganglionic parasympathetic fibers from the greater petrosal nerve (a branch of the facial nerve). After synapsing with the postganglionic neurons in the ganglion, the postganglionic nerve fibers (axons) travel along the zygomatic nerve and then "hitch-hike" along the lacrimal nerve to supply the lacrimal gland.

The pterygopalatine ganglion also gives rise to greater and lesser palatine nerves, which supply the hard and soft palate, respectively. The greater and lesser palatine nerves carry sensory as well as secretomotor fibers. It also gives rise to nasal branches and the nasopalatine nerve that supply the nasal cavities and maxillary sinus (other minor branches are excluded).

The pterygopalatine ganglion also receives the deep petrosal nerve containing the postganglionic sympathetic nerve fibers that originate from the SCG. They travel along the internal carotid artery as the internal carotid plexus. The sympathetic fibers merely traverse through the ganglion without making any synaptic contacts. They are distributed by the ganglionic branches mainly to supply the seromucous glands or blood vessels.

N.B. The so-called "nerve of the pterygoid canal" refers to the deep petrosal nerve and greater petrosal nerve in the pterygoid canal (sphenoid bone) that communicates with the pterygopalatine fossa.

***Quiz**: The pterygopalatine ganglion has been called by some as the "ganglion of hay fever." Why? (Hints: Runny nose, sneezing, and lacrimation).*

ORAL CAVITY

The oral cavity has two parts: the vestibule (the space between the cheek and the teeth) and the oral cavity proper (from the inner aspect of the teeth to the palatoglossal folds that guard the oropharyngeal isthmus), leading into the oropharynx. The roof of the oral cavity is formed by the hard palate (maxilla and palatine bones), the floor is formed by the tongue, and the lateral walls are formed by the cheeks (buccal mucosa). The parotid duct opens into the vestibule opposite the upper second molar tooth. The submandibular duct opens onto the floor of the mouth at the sublingual papilla, located on either side of the lingual frenulum.

The oral mucosa is lined by a stratified squamous epithelium (non-keratinized). Equipped with teeth, the tongue, and salivary glands, the mechanical and chemical breakdown of food occurs in the oral cavity. The saliva contains enzymes such as amylase that start the digestion of carbohydrates in the oral cavity. The muscles of mastication and the temporomandibular joint play a vital role in the digestion process.

Because the mandible is the "key bone" involved in mastication (chewing movements), the mandible and its parts are examined first, followed by the temporomandibular joint and the muscles that move the mandible during mastication (muscles of mastication).

Mandible (Fig. 10.30)

1. The mandible is the largest bone in the skull. It articulates with the glenoid (mandibular) fossa of the temporal bone, forming the "temporomandibular joint."
2. **Parts of the mandible**: Head (condylar head), coronoid process, mandibular notch, neck, ramus, body, angle, alveolar process (the part that bears the lower teeth), mandibular foramen, lingula, mental foramen, mylohyoid line, submandibular fossa, and sublingual fossa.

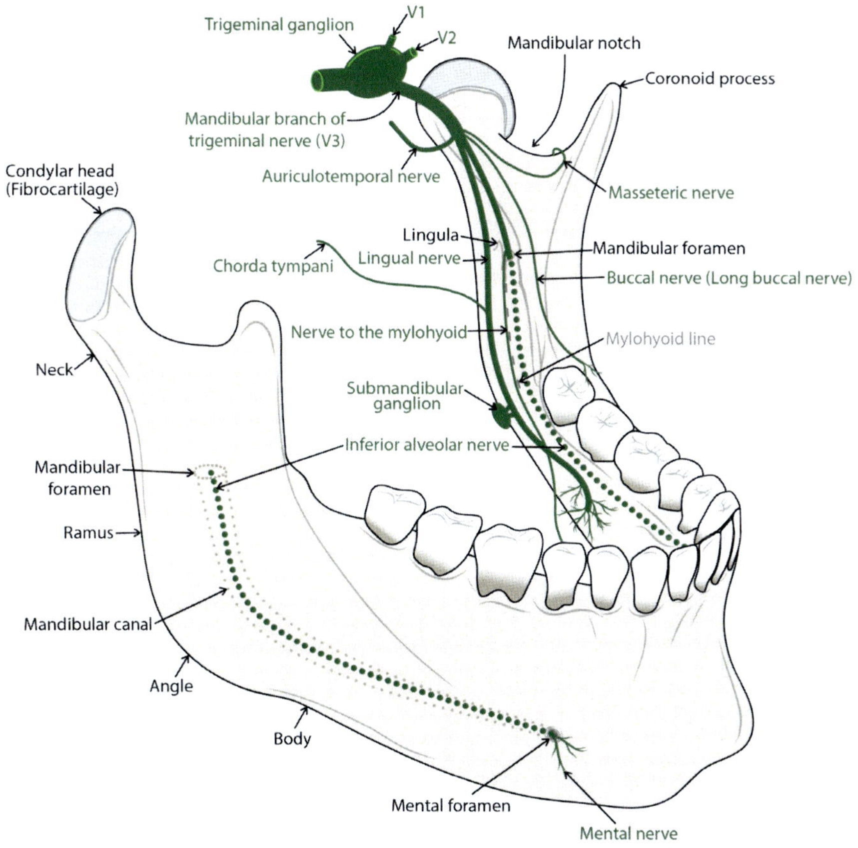

Figure 10.30. Mandible. Its parts include the condylar head, neck, coronoid process, mandibular notch, ramus, body, and mental foramen. On the medial surface of the ramus are the mandibular foramen, lingula, and the mylohyoid groove. The following are nerves that are closely related to the mandible: (1) lingual nerve, (2) nerve to the mylohyoid, (3) auriculotemporal nerve, (4) masseteric nerve, (5) mental nerve, and (6) inferior alveolar nerve.

3. **Ossification and development**: The mandible is primarily formed by intramembranous ossification. It develops from the first pharyngeal arch and is closely associated with Meckel's cartilage, although this cartilage does not contribute directly to mandibular bone formation. Secondary bone formation occurs at the condylar head, coronoid process, and symphyseal menti, where ossification proceeds by an endochondral mechanism.
4. The following nerves are closely related to the mandible; hence, they may be damaged in the fracture of the bone:
   a. Lingual nerve: It is closely related to the mandibular third molar (last molar) region.
   b. Nerve to mylohyoid: It lies in the mylohyoid groove.
   c. Auriculotemporal nerve: It lies medial to the neck of the mandible.
   d. Masseteric nerve: It crosses the mandibular notch.
   e. Mental nerve: It emerges at the mental foramen.
   f. Inferior alveolar nerve: It enters the mandibular foramen, runs within the mandibular canal, and terminates by dividing into the mental and incisive nerves (the mental nerve exits via the mental foramen).

Temporomandibular joint (Fig. 10.31)

1. Articulations: It occurs between the head of the mandible and the mandibular fossa/articular tubercle of the temporal bone above.
2. It is a synovial joint whose cavity is separated into the upper and lower compartments by an intraarticular disc. The articular surfaces and articular disc are fibrocartilage.
3. The articular disc divides the synovial cavity into upper and lower compartments. The upper allows protraction and retraction, while the lower compartment allows rotation (elevation/depression) for opening and closing of the mouth.
4. Ligaments:
   a. *Lateral ligament*: It strengthens the lateral aspect of the joint.
   b. *Stylomandibular ligament*: This is a thickened band of the deep cervical fascia (investing layer). It extends from the styloid process to the angle of the mandible.
   c. *Sphenomandibular ligament*: This extends from the spine of the sphenoid to the lingula. It is derived from Meckel's cartilage sheath. It serves as a swing ligament.
5. Innervation: Masseteric nerve and auriculotemporal nerve (Branch of V_3).

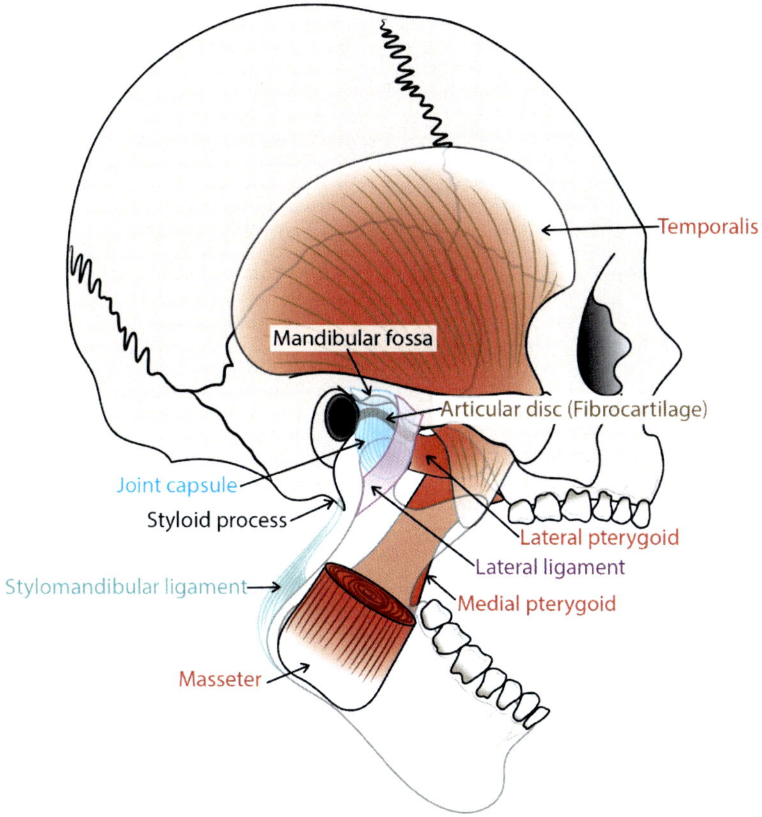

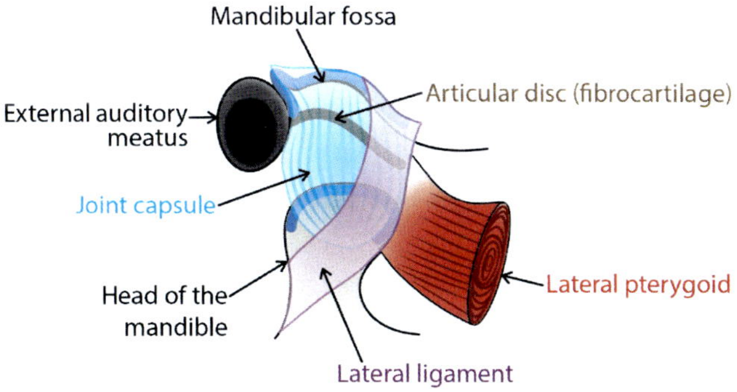

Figure 10.31. Temporomandibular joint. It is a synovial joint whose articulations are between the head of the mandible and the mandibular fossa and the articular tubercle above (temporal bone). The articular surfaces are lined with fibrocartilage. The synovial cavity is divided into the upper and lower compartments by an intraarticular disc (fibrocartilage). The joint is reinforced laterally by the lateral ligament. Two accessory ligaments, the stylomandibular ligament and sphenomandibular ligament, contribute to stabilizing the joint. All four muscles of mastication move the joint: the temporalis, lateral pterygoid, medial pterygoid, and masseter.

6. Clinical anatomy: Dislocation of the joint tends to be anterior below the articular tubercle.

Muscles of mastication and actions on the mandible (Fig. 10.32)

1. Masseter: Elevation
2. Temporalis: Elevation and retraction (horizontal fibers)
3. Medial pterygoid: Elevation (upward and medially) and protraction

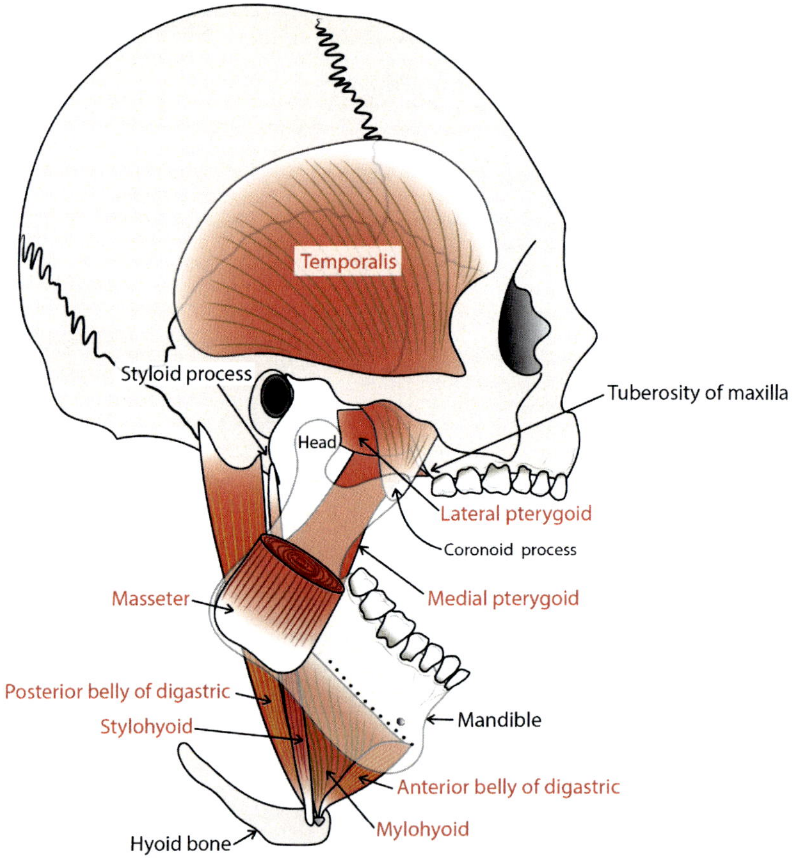

Figure 10.32. Muscles of mastication. (1) Temporalis — arises above from the squamous temporal and inserts into the coronoid process. (2) Lateral pterygoid — arises from the lateral surface of the lateral pterygoid plate, and inserts into the neck of the mandible, capsule, and intra-articular disc. (3) Medial pterygoid — arises from the medial surface of the lateral pterygoid plate and maxillary tuberosity and inserts into the medial surface of the angle of the mandible. (4) Masseter — arises from the zygomatic arch and inserts into the lateral surface of the ramus.

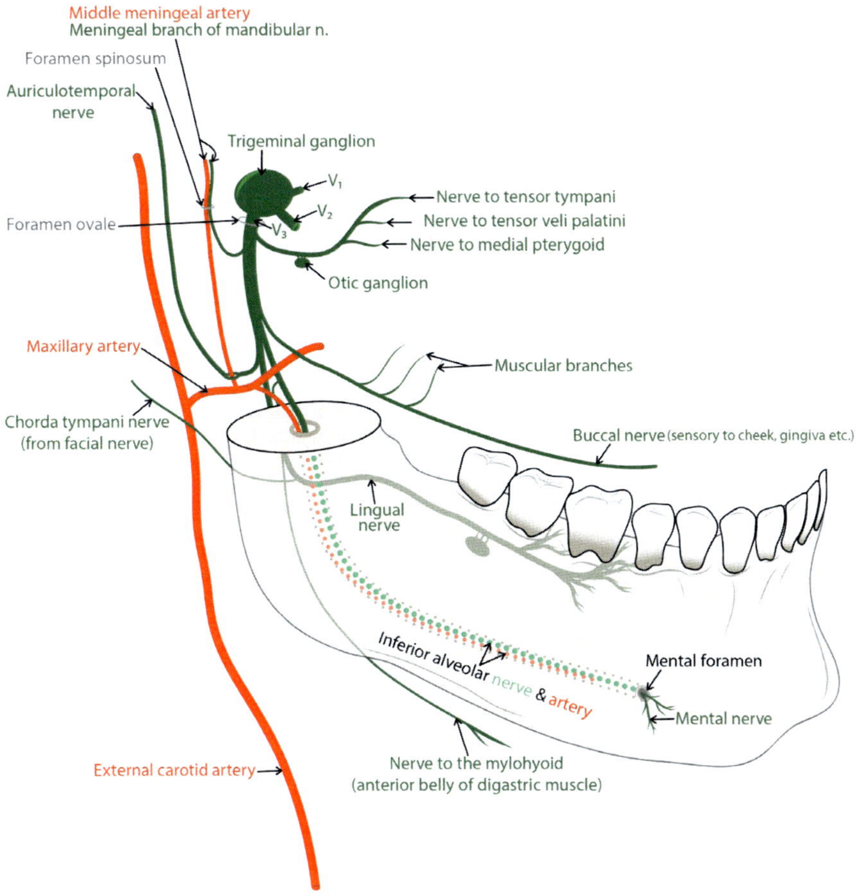

Figure 10.33. Mandibular nerve (V_3): its course and distribution. It leaves the middle cranial fossa through the foramen ovale. Both the sensory and motor roots join to form the trunk below the foramen ovale. The trunk gives rise to the nerve to the medial pterygoid, which also supplies the tensor tympani and tensor palatini. The otic ganglion is suspended to the nerve to the medial pterygoid. The meningeal branch ascends through the foramen spinosum, accompanied by the middle meningeal artery. The trunk gives rise to anterior and posterior divisions. The anterior division is mainly a motor supplying the muscles of mastication and the buccal nerve. The posterior division gives rise to the auriculotemporal nerve, lingual nerve, and inferior alveolar nerve. The nerve to the mylohyoid arises from the posterior division. Note that the chorda tympani nerve joins with the lingual nerve.

4. Lateral pterygoid: Protraction, which helps in opening the mouth.
5. Pterygoids acting together: Side-to-side chewing movement.
6. They are innervated by the mandibular nerve (V_3). They all act on the temporomandibular joint.

Mandibular nerve — its origin, course, and distribution (Fig. 10.33)

1. Mandibular nerve is the third division (V_3) of the trigeminal nerve emerging from the pons.
2. It is referred to as the nerve of the first pharyngeal arch, as it innervates structures derived from the first pharyngeal arch.
3. It is composed of both sensory and motor fibers.
4. <u>Course and branches</u>:
   a. It leaves the middle cranial fossa through the foramen ovale and enters the infratemporal fossa containing the muscles of mastication, maxillary artery, and pterygoid venous plexus.
   b. Below the foramen ovale, the sensory root (larger) is joined by the motor root (smaller) to form the trunk.
   c. From the main trunk of the mandibular nerve arise the meningeal branch and the nerve to the medial pterygoid. The otic ganglion is suspended from the nerve to the medial pterygoid, which also supplies motor fibers to the tensor veli palatini and tensor tympani muscles.
   d. The trunk gives rise to the anterior and posterior divisions:
      - *Anterior division*: This is mainly motor that innervates the masseter, lateral pterygoid, and temporalis. Its sensory branch is the buccal nerve, which innervates the buccal mucosa and adjacent gingiva.
      - *Posterior division*: It gives rise to the auriculotemporal nerve, which also carries the postganglionic parasympathetic fibers from the otic ganglion to provide secretomotor innervation to the parotid gland.
   e. The mandibular nerve gives rise to the lingual nerve, which is joined by the chorda tympani, a branch of the facial nerve (CN VII). The lingual nerve provides general sensory innervation to the anterior two-thirds of the tongue.
   f. The chorda tympani carries taste fibers (special sensory) from the anterior two-thirds of the tongue and preganglionic parasympathetic fibers to the submandibular ganglion. The postganglionic fibers from the submandibular ganglion provide secretomotor innervation to both the submandibular and sublingual glands.

g. Note that the lingual nerve is closely related medially to the lower last molar tooth. The nerve may be damaged during an extraction of the "wisdom tooth."

   Quiz: *What would be the functional deficits if the lingual nerve is damaged at this site?*

h. Furthermore, it also gives rise to the inferior alveolar nerve innervating the lower teeth and gums. The terminal branch is the mental nerve that emerges at the mental foramen innervating the adjacent skin areas.

i. Before the inferior alveolar nerve enters the mandibular foramen, it gives rise to the nerve to the mylohyoid, which innervates the mylohyoid and the anterior belly of the digastric muscle.

Submandibular Gland (Relations, Histology, and Secretomotor Innervation (Fig. 10.34)

1. The submandibular gland lies in the submandibular region, bounded by the anterior and posterior bellies of the digastric muscle.
2. Laterally, the gland is related to the body of the mandible (submandibular fossa), skin, investing layer of the deep cervical fascia, and submandibular lymph nodes.
3. The mandibular branch of the facial nerve is also related to it laterally.
4. Medially, the submandibular gland lies on the mylohyoid muscle and the hyoglossus muscle.
5. Crossing from the posterior to the superolateral aspect of the gland is the facial artery.
6. The gland has superficial and deep parts, which are continuous around the posterior border of the mylohyoid muscle.
7. The deep part of the gland lies on the hyoglossus muscle.
8. The submandibular duct arises from the deep part of the submandibular gland, courses forward in the floor of the mouth, and opens at the sublingual caruncle on either side of the lingual frenulum.
9. The lingual nerve hooks around the submandibular duct.
10. The submandibular ganglion is suspended from the lingual nerve and lies on the hyoglossus.
11. The hypoglossal nerve (CN XII) also lies on the hyoglossus.

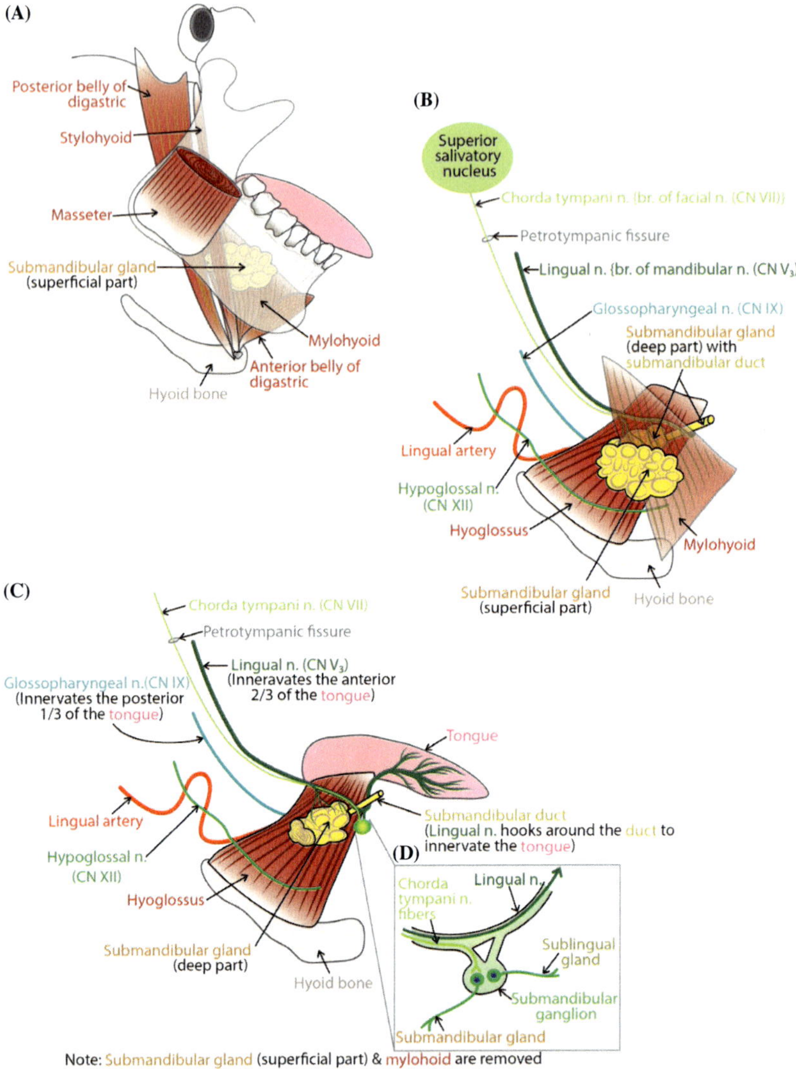

Figure 10.34. Submandibular gland. **(A)** The submandibular gland lies in the submandibular region, bounded by the anterior and posterior bellies of the digastric muscle. **(B)** The floor is formed by the mylohyoid and hyoglossus. **(C)** Lying on the hyoglossus from above downward are the submandibular duct, lingual nerve (hooks around the submandibular duct), submandibular ganglion (suspended to the lingual nerve), and the hypoglossal nerve (XII). Deep to the hyoglossus are the glossopharyngeal nerve (IX) and the lingual artery. **(D)** Submandibular ganglion is attached to the lingual nerve. Note that the ganglion receives the preganglionic parasympathetic fibers via the chorda tympani (B), which synapse with the postganglionic parasympathetic neurons. The latter sends their fibers (axons) to supply the submandibular gland (acini) or travel along the lingual nerve to supply the sublingual gland. The chorda tympani carries preganglionic parasympathetic fibers from the superior salivatory nucleus.

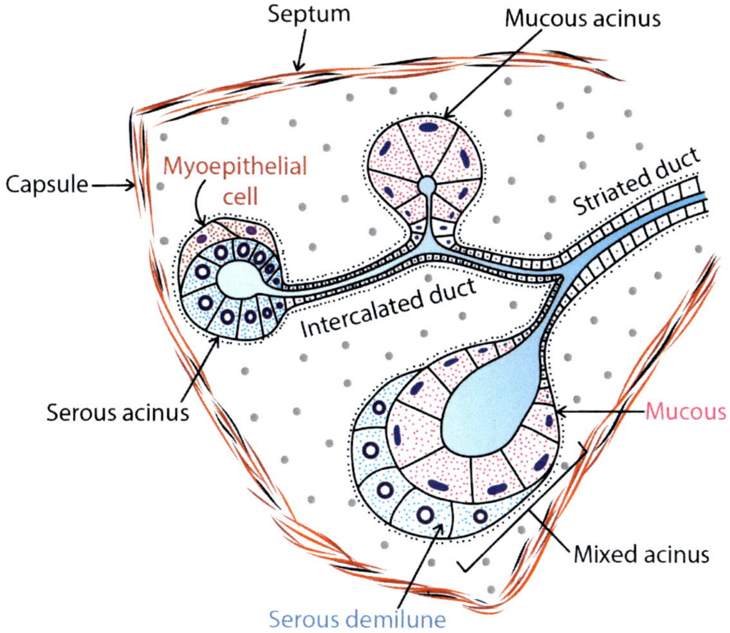

Figure 10.35. Submandibular gland — a lobule. It is covered on its surface by a layer of capsule. Many septa (singular "septum") extend from the capsule into the parenchyma, dividing the gland into many lobules. The gland has three types of acini: mucous acinus, serous acinus, and mixed acinus. Myoepithelial cells cap the acinus. In a mixed acinus, the serous demilune caps the mucous acinus. From the acinus, the secretions are poured into the intercalated duct, striated duct, and interlobular duct.

12. Deep to the hyoglossus are the glossopharyngeal nerve (CN IX) and lingual artery (branch of the external carotid).
13. Histologically, the submandibular gland is a mixed salivary gland composed of both serous and mucous acini, with a predominance of serous units. Mixed acini are also present, in which mucous acini are capped by serous demilunes. Myoepithelial cells surround the acini and aid in secretion by contracting to expel the acinar contents **(Fig. 10.35)**.
14. The submandibular gland has a layer of covering capsule **(Fig. 10.35)**, which sends septa (fibrous partitions) dividing the gland into many lobules. Secretions (saliva) from the acini are discharged into the acinus lumen and then into the intercalated duct, striated duct, interlobular duct, and the main duct.

15. Innervation: It is innervated by the facial nerve via the chorda tympani branch. The preganglionic parasympathetic fibers originating from the superior salivatory nucleus synapse with the postganglionic neurons in the submandibular ganglion, from which the postganglionic fibers innervate the acini, including those of the sublingual gland **(Fig. 10.34)**.

Applied anatomy

1. The submandibular duct (Wharton's duct) runs forward and opens at the sublingual caruncle at the floor of the oral cavity. The duct may be blocked by a stone.
2. In a surgical procedure involving the submandibular gland, care should be taken to protect the nerves that are closely associated with it. These nerves include the marginal mandibular branch of the facial nerve, lingual nerve, and hypoglossal nerve. Note that the facial artery is also closely related to the gland.

Tongue

Development (Fig. 10.35)

1. The anterior 2/3 of the tongue is developed from the first pharyngeal arch and is derived from two lateral lingual swellings and the tuberculum impar.
2. The posterior 1/3 of the tongue develops from the hypobranchial eminence, which is derived predominantly from the third and fourth pharyngeal arches.
3. Involvement of the copula (second arch) in its development is not clear.

Surface features of the tongue (Fig. 10.36)

1. The tongue is divided into the anterior two-thirds and posterior one-third by the sulcus terminalis, like an inverted "V."
2. At the apex of the sulcus terminalis is the foramen caecum, which marks the site of origin of the thyroid gland.
3. The tongue surface is lined by a non-keratinized stratified squamous epithelium and has many surface projections, the lingual papillae: filiform papilla, fungiform papilla, and circumvallate papilla.
4. Both the filiform and fungiform papillae are distributed over the anterior two-thirds of the tongue.

(A)

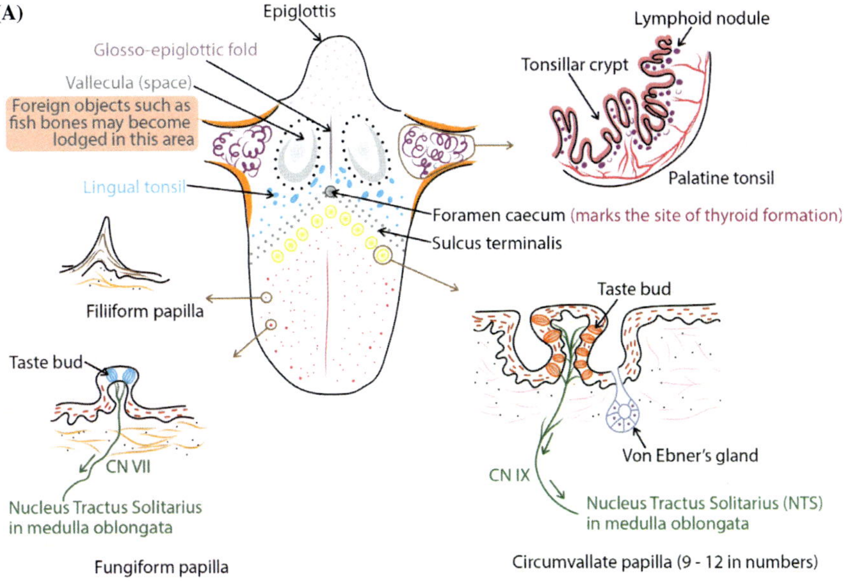

(B)

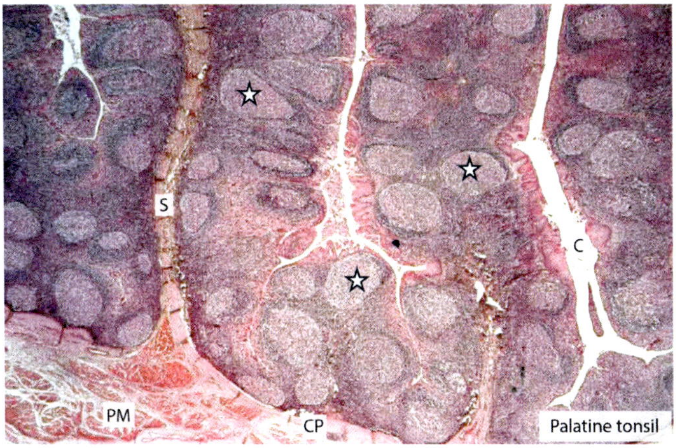

Figure 10.36. Tongue — surface features. (A) The tongue is divided into the anterior two-thirds and posterior one-third by the inverted "V" sulcus terminalis. The foramen caecum is at the apex of the sulcus terminalis. Filiform and fungiform papillae are mainly distributed over the anterior two-thirds. The taste buds on the fungiform papillae are supplied by the VII nerve via the chorda tympani. Anterior to the sulcus are 9–12 circumvallate papillae, whose taste buds are localized at the sides. Von Ebner's glands open into the groove surrounding the papilla. The taste buds are supplied by the IX nerve. Over the dorsal surface of the posterior one-third are lingual tonsils. On both sides are the palatoglossal and palatopharyngeal folds. Between the folds ("pillars") is the palatine tonsil, lined by the stratified squamous epithelium. **(B)** C, tonsillar crypt; S, septum; CP, capsule; PM, pharyngeal muscles; white star, lymphatic follicles (nodule). (H & E stain).

5. The filiform papillae, which lack taste buds, aid in gripping and moving food.
6. The fungiform papillae have taste buds.
7. The circumvallate papillae are 10–12 in number and lie anterior to the sulcus terminalis.
8. In histological sections, circumvallate papillae appear mushroom-shaped and are surrounded by a trench (moat). Some serous glands, known as von Ebner's glands, open into the trench. Taste buds containing sensory and supporting cells are located on the lateral walls of the papilla.
9. Sensory innervation of the tongue:
   a. The anterior two-thirds of the tongue receive the special sensory innervation (taste fibers) from the facial nerve (CN VII) via chorda tympani. The general sensation is by the lingual nerve, which is a branch of the mandibular division of the trigeminal nerve (CN V_3).
   b. *The posterior one-third* of the tongue, including the circumvallate papillae, receives the special (taste) and the general sensory innervation by the glossopharyngeal nerve (CN IX).
   c. All taste sensations are transmitted to the nucleus of the tractus solitarius (NTS) in the medulla of the brainstem. General sensations (pain, temperature, and touch) from the tongue are transmitted centrally to the sensory nucleus of the trigeminal nerve (nucleus of V).
10. The tongue is supplied by the lingual artery, which is a branch of the external carotid artery.

Muscles of the tongue (Fig. 10.37)

The tongue consists of intrinsic and extrinsic muscles.

1. Intrinsic muscles: They are arranged into the superior, longitudinal, vertical, and horizontal bundles, which help in changing the shape of the tongue.
2. Extrinsic muscles:
   a. They take origin from the outside of the tongue and are involved in movement and positioning the tongue.
   b. The genioglossus muscle originates from the mental spine of the mandible and is responsible for the protrusion of the tongue (protraction).
   c. The hyoglossus muscle, originating from the hyoid bone, depresses the back of the tongue to accommodate more food bolus.

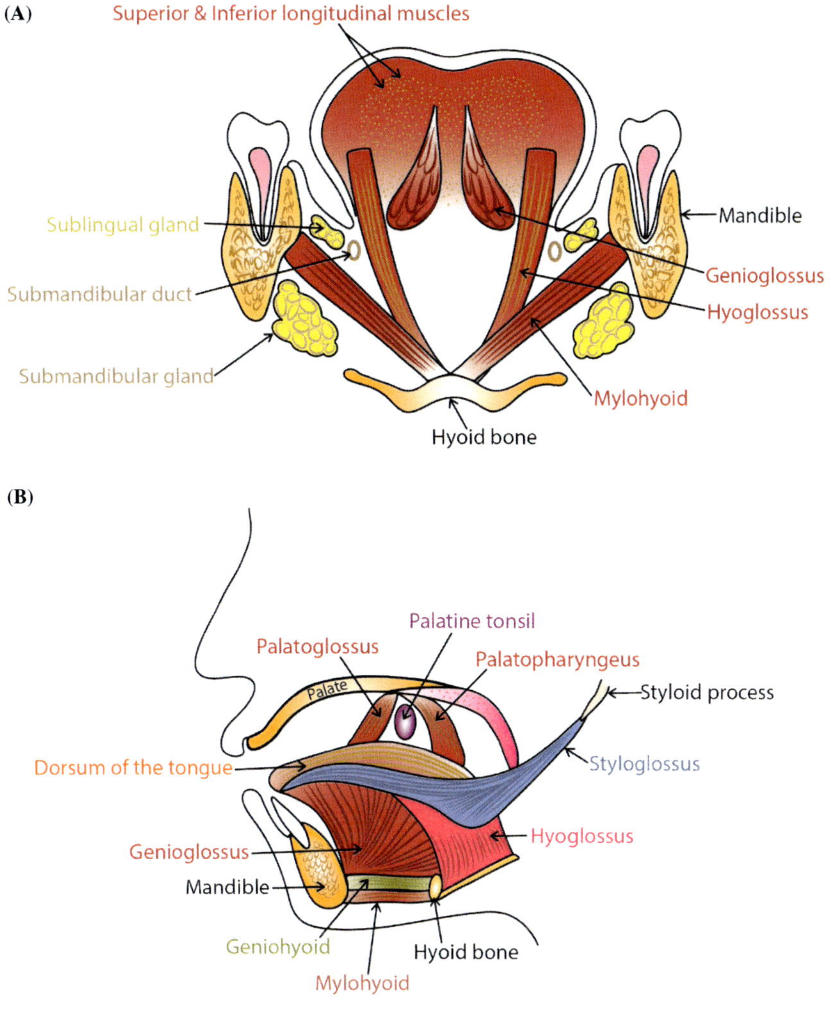

Figure 10.37. Muscles of the tongue. (A) Intrinsic muscles. They are composed of superior and inferior longitudinal, transverse, and vertical muscle bundles. They change the shape of the tongue: **(B)** Extrinsic muscles: genioglossus, hyoglossus, palatoglossus, and styloglossus. They take origin from the outside of the tongue and move the tongue.

d. *The styloglossus muscle, originating from the styloid process of the temporal bone*, retracts or elevates the posterior part of the tongue.

e. *The palatoglossus muscles of both* sides act as a sphincter, squeezing the food bolus through the oropharyngeal isthmus (fauces) into the oropharynx.

3. <u>Innervation</u>: All intrinsic and extrinsic muscles are innervated by the hypoglossal nerve (CN XII), which arises from the medulla, except for the

palatoglossus muscle, which is innervated by the vagus nerve via the pharyngeal nerve plexus with motor fibers originating from the nucleus ambiguus.

4. Applied anatomy: Test for a XII nerve lesion. The tongue deviates to the lesion side on protrusion.

Soft palate (Fig. 10.38)

1. It is a fibromuscular partition that separates the oropharynx from the nasopharynx.
2. It forms the roof of the oropharynx and the floor of the nasopharynx.
3. It is involved in deglutition (swallowing), respiration, and phonation.
4. During swallowing, it shuts the pharyngeal isthmus (passage between the nasopharynx and oropharynx).
5. Muscles associated with the soft palate:
   a. *Palatoglossus*: The bilateral muscles act like a sphincter guarding the oropharyngeal isthmus (fauces), squeezing the food bolus into the oropharynx. It is innervated by the vagus nerve via the pharyngeal nerve plexus, with motor fibers originating from the nucleus ambiguus.
   b. *Palatopharyngeus*: Longitudinal muscle of the pharynx. It helps pull the pharynx up and moves the food bolus down. Innervation is by the pharyngeal nerve plexus.
   c. *Tensor veli palatini*: Tensing the soft palate. Innervation is by the nerve to the medial pterygoid.
   d. *Levator palatini*: Elevating the soft palate. Innervation is by the pharyngeal nerve plexus.
   e. *Musculi uvuli*: Draws up the soft palate. Innervation is by the pharyngeal nerve plexus.
6. Histology:
   a. Its superior surface is lined by the respiratory epithelium.
   b. The inferior or oral surface is lined by a non-keratinized stratified squamous epithelium.
   c. The core of the soft palate is occupied by the mucous glands and muscle fibers mentioned above.

***Quiz**: How would you test the lesion of the vagus nerve?*

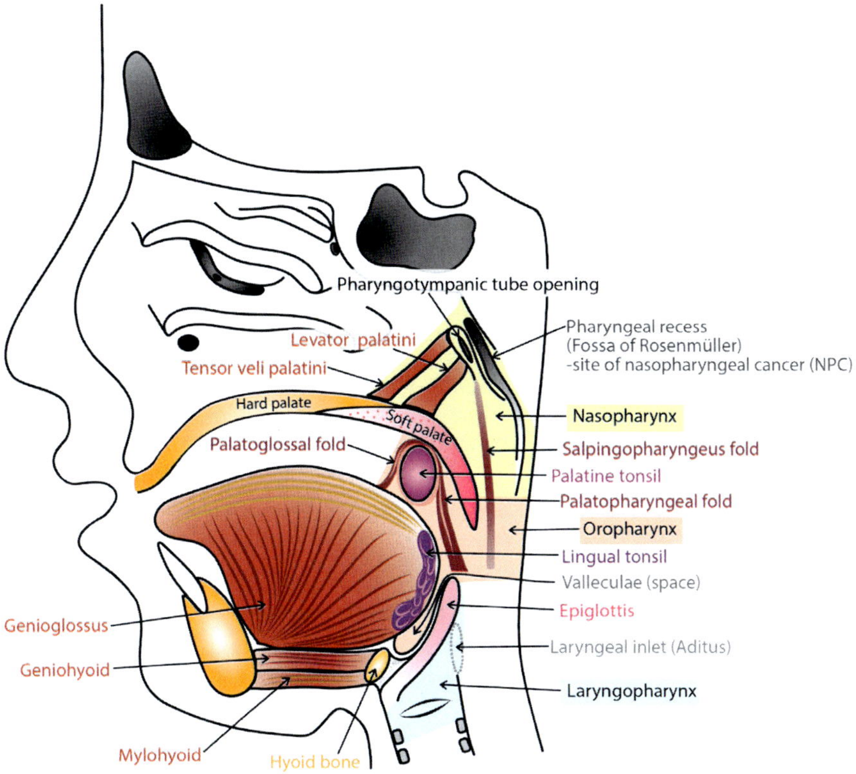

Figure 10.38. Soft palate and pharynx (sagittal section). The soft palate forms the roof of the oropharynx. The following muscles are associated with the soft palate: tensor palatini, levator palatini, palatoglossus, palatopharyngeus, and musculi uvuli. The pharynx is divided into three parts: (1) nasopharynx, (2) oropharynx, and (3) laryngopharynx. The nasopharynx lies posterior to the nasal cavity. It receives the opening of the choanae (posterior nasal openings). The oropharynx lies posterior to the oral cavity (posterior to the oropharyngeal isthmus, fauces). The laryngopharynx lies posterior to the laryngeal inlet (aditus). PG, palatoglossus; PP, palatopharyngeus.

PHARYNX

The pharynx is divided into three parts: the nasopharynx, oropharynx, and laryngopharynx **(Fig. 10.38)**.

1. **Nasopharynx**: It lies posterior to the nasal cavity, behind the two nasal openings known as choanae, which form the anterior border of the nasopharynx. The mucosa is lined by the respiratory epithelium. The lateral wall shows the opening of the pharyngotympanic tube (Eustachian tube), which communicates laterally with the middle ear (tympanum). Associated

with the tubal opening are the tensor palatini and levator palatini muscles, which tense or elevate the soft palate, respectively. Contraction of these muscles helps equalize the pressure between the nasopharynx and the middle ear at a high altitude.

Skirting the opening of the auditory tube is the tubal elevation. The salpingopharyngeal fold with the underlying salpingopharyngeus muscle extends from the opening downward into the pharyngeal wall (longitudinal muscle). Posterior to the salpingopharyngeal fold lies the pharyngeal recess, "fossa Rosenmüller," a common site of nasopharyngeal carcinoma (NPC). The tubal tonsil is located on the tubal elevation, while the pharyngeal tonsil is situated on the posterior wall of the nasopharynx. In children, the pharyngeal tonsil may enlarge abnormally, forming adenoids, which can obstruct the nasal passage and interfere with normal respiration.

2. **Oropharynx**: It lies posterior to the palatoglossal folds guarding the oropharyngeal isthmus. On the lateral walls are the palatoglossal and palatopharyngeal folds with the underlying palatoglossus and palatopharyngeus muscles, respectively. The palatine tonsil lies between these two folds or "pillars." The posterior part of the tongue with the lingual tonsil forms the floor of the oropharynx. The roof is formed by the soft palate.

   Inflammation of the mucosa of the oropharynx is common in conditions such as influenza and pharyngitis, commonly referred to as a sore throat. Sensory innervation of the oropharynx is provided by the glossopharyngeal nerve (CN IX), which mediates the pain associated with a sore throat. The mucosa of the oropharynx is lined by non-keratinized stratified squamous epithelium.
3. **Laryngopharynx**: It faces the laryngeal inlet or aditus, anteriorly. On both sides of the aditus is the "piriform fossa," a site where a fish bone or foreign object may be lodged. Innervation of the laryngopharynx is by the internal laryngeal nerve, a branch of the superior laryngeal nerve from the vagus nerve (CN X). The mucosa is lined by the stratified squamous epithelium.

Muscles of the Pharynx

The pharynx is composed of an outer layer of circular (constrictor) muscles and an inner layer of longitudinal muscles. Although these muscles are skeletal (striated), their function is under involuntary (reflex) control during swallowing and speech.

Motor innervation is provided primarily by the pharyngeal plexus, chiefly via the pharyngeal branch of the vagus nerve (CN X). The motor neurons originate from the nucleus ambiguus (NA) in the medulla. Their efferent fibers travel briefly with the cranial root of the accessory nerve (CN XI) and then join the vagus nerve (CN X) to reach the pharyngeal muscles through the pharyngeal plexus.

The circular muscles serve mainly as the constrictors:

1. Superior constrictor
2. Middle constrictor
3. Inferior constrictor

The longitudinal muscles are "elevators" as they lift the pharyngeal walls up. They are:

1. Stylopharyngeus
2. Palatopharyngeus
3. Salpingopharyngeus

N.B. The muscles play important roles in swallowing or deglutition.

Quiz 1: *Describe the mechanism of deglutition.*

Quiz 2: *Where is the central projection of pain fibers from the mucous membrane of the pharynx? (In other words, which brainstem nucleus receives the sensory projections?) Where are the cell bodies of the sensory neurons located?*

Quiz 3: *What is the "gag reflex"? What are the neural pathways involved in this reflex?*

LARYNX

General organization and features:

1. It serves as an air passage and is involved in phonation.
2. The structural framework of the larynx includes the hyoid bone and cartilages, such as the thyroid, epiglottis, cricoid, and arytenoid (**Fig. 10.39**).
   a. The hyoid bone lies at the level of C3, thyroid cartilage at the level of the C4/C5 level, and cricoid cartilage at the C6 level.

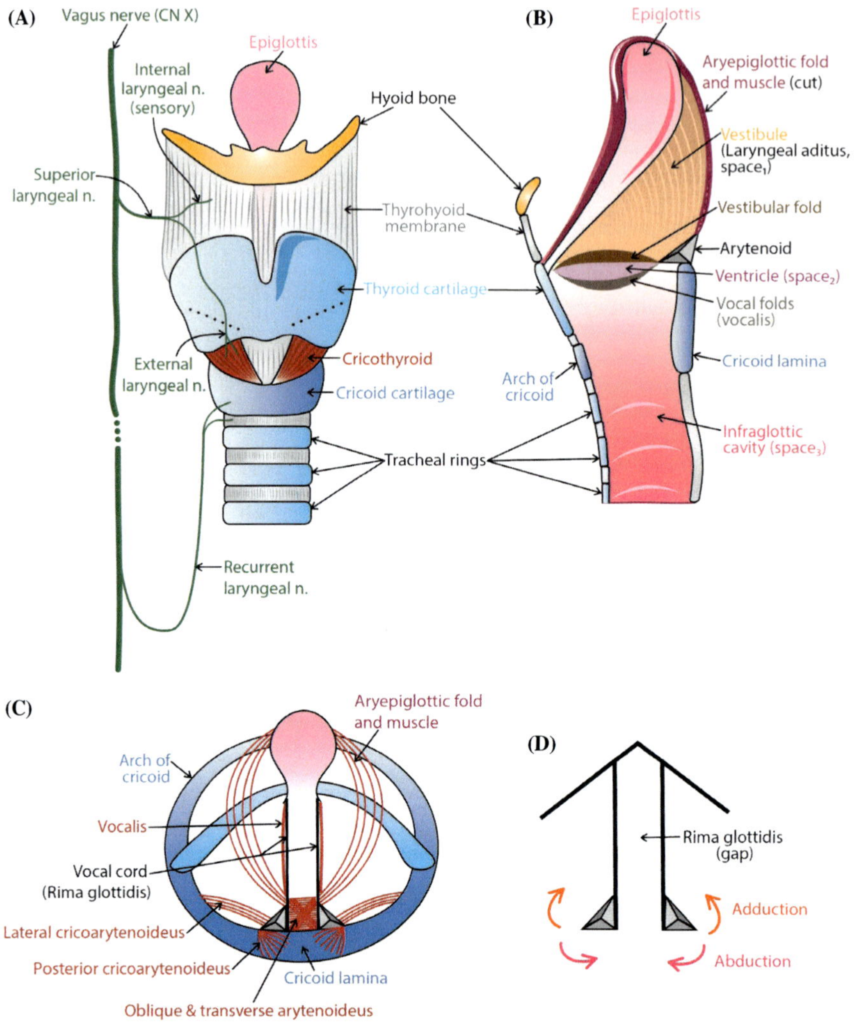

Figure 10.39. Larynx. (A) Anterior view showing the epiglottis, thyroid, and cricoid cartilages. The hyoid bone is also included. The thyrohyoid membrane is pierced by the internal laryngeal nerve (ILN). Extending between the thyroid and cricoid is the cricothyroid muscle, innervated by the external laryngeal nerve (ELN). **(B)** In a sagittal section, the laryngeal cavity is divided into three parts: vestibule, ventricle, and infraglottic cavity. They are separated by the vestibular folds and the vocal folds. Identify the aryepiglottic muscle (sphincter of the aditus) and the vocalis muscle (deep to the vocal folds). **(C)** Superior view showing the aryepiglottic fold and its underlying muscle, the aryepiglottic muscle. Between the cricoid and arytenoid are the posterior cricoarytenoideus and lateral cricoarytenoideus, which act as abductors and adductors of the vocal folds, respectively **(D)**.

b. The thyroid cartilage consists of two thyroid laminae that form the thyroid prominence, also known as the Adam's apple. The thyroid notch, a midline indentation, is palpable along the superior border of the cartilage.
c. Cricoid cartilage is a signet ring-shaped with an anterior arch and posterior lamina. This forms the complete ring in the airway at the level of C6.
d. The arytenoid cartilage is pyramidal-shaped and sits on the posterior lamina of the cricoid cartilage. Its apex points upward, supporting the corniculate cartilage, and its muscular process projects laterally, providing attachment for intrinsic laryngeal muscles. The vocal process projects anteriorly for attachment of the vocal cord. Movements of the arytenoid cartilages by the posterior and lateral cricoarytenoid muscles cause abduction and adduction of the vocal cords, respectively.

3. **Anterior view (Fig. 10.39)**: When viewed from the front, the following structures can be identified: thyrohyoid membrane, cricothyroid membrane, and the cricothyroid muscle extending between the cricoid and thyroid cartilages. The thyrohyoid membrane is pierced by the internal laryngeal nerve, which is from the superior laryngeal nerve, a branch of the vagus nerve (CN X).
4. **Superior view (Fig. 10.39)**: When looking into the laryngeal inlet or the "aditus" with a laryngoscope, the following structures can be identified: vestibular folds and vocal folds (vocal cords). The space between the vocal folds is "rima glottidis," while the space between the vestibular folds (false vocal cord) is "rima vestibuli." Vibration of the vocal folds produces sound and changes the tone of voice.
5. In a hemisection of the larynx, the larynx is divided into three parts **(Fig. 10.39)**:
   a) Vestibule — from the laryngeal inlet "aditus" till the vestibular folds;
   b) Ventricle — between the vestibular folds and vocal folds; and
   c) Infraglottic cavity — below the vocal folds.

<u>Sensory innervation</u>

- The recurrent laryngeal nerve provides sensory innervation to the mucous membrane of the larynx below the level of the vocal folds.
- The internal laryngeal nerve provides sensory innervation to the mucous membrane of the larynx above the level of the vocal folds.

Histology

Most of the laryngeal cavity is lined by the respiratory epithelium (pseudostratified ciliated columnar epithelium), whereas the vocal folds are lined by the stratified squamous epithelium.

Applied anatomy

1. Injury to the ELN or RLN may result in paralysis of the laryngeal muscles, causing "hoarseness of voice."
2. As the ELN and RLN are closely associated with the superior thyroid artery and inferior thyroid artery, respectively, they are at risk of injury during thyroid surgery, including partial or total thyroidectomy.
3. Laryngeal papilloma is a benign, wart-like tumor of the larynx, caused by infection with the human papilloma virus (HPV).

EAR

The ear is divided into three parts: the external ear, the middle ear, and the inner ear.

1. External Ear (Fig. 10.40)

The outer one-third of the external auditory canal is cartilaginous, while the inner two-thirds is osseous (bony). The junction between the cartilaginous and bony parts of the external auditory canal is narrowed and concave anteriorly. It is lined by the skin, which contains ceruminous glands that

Table 10.1. Muscles of larynx — actions and innervation.

S. no.	Muscles (intrinsic) of the larynx	Actions	Innervation
1	Posterior cricoarytenoideus	Abductor of vocal cords	RLN
2	Lateral cricoarytenoideus - Interarytenoideus	Adductors	RLN
3	Aryepiglottis - Thyroepiglottis - Oblique arytenoideus	Sphincters of aditus	RLN
4	Cricothyroid	Tensor of vocal cords	ELN
5	Vocalis	Varying the tension of vocal cord	RLN
6	Thyroarytenoideus	Varying the tension of vestibular folds	RLN

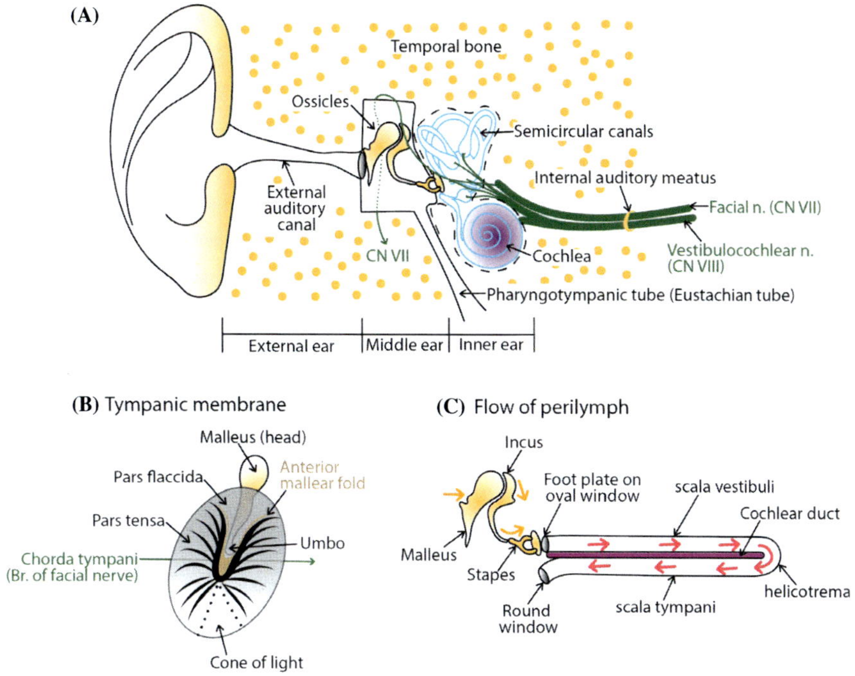

Figure 10.40. External, middle, and inner ear. (A) The external ear extends from the external auditory canal to the tympanic membrane. The middle ear (tympanum) houses the ossicles. The inner ear contains the semicircular canals and cochlea/saccule/utricle. Note that the middle ear communicates with the nasopharynx via the pharyngotympanic tube. The middle ear is housed in the temporal bone and is closely related to the facial nerve. **(B)** Tympanic membrane as viewed laterally. It has two main parts: pars tensa and pars flaccida. It is related medially to the handle of the malleus and the chorda tympani nerve. **(C)** Transmission of sound waves from the ossicles (malleus, incus, stapes) — scala vestibuli — helicotrema — scala tympani containing the perilymph. This causes vibration of the cochlear duct and its sensory receptor, the organ of Corti, in the endolymph. The sound signal is then transmitted to the brainstem nuclei via the vestibulocochlear nerves [VIII] (see A).

are modified sweat glands. Secretions from these glands form earwax. The medial end of the external auditory tube is closed by the tympanic membrane, which consists of two parts: pars tensa and pars flaccida. The pars flaccida is bounded by the anterior and posterior mallear folds. The lateral (outer) surface of the tympanic membrane is concave, referred to as the "umbo." Attached to the medial (inner) surface of the tympanic membrane is the handle of the malleus. The chorda tympani nerve, a branch of the facial nerve, runs across the medial aspect of the tympanic membrane, close to the handle of the malleus.

2. **Middle Ear (Fig. 10.40; Fig. 10.41)**

The middle ear consists of four walls, a roof, and a floor. It houses the auditory ossicles, namely, the malleus, incus, and stapes, which help in the conduction of sound from the external ear to the inner ear.

The following are relations of the four walls of the middle ear:

a. **Anterior wall (carotid wall)**: It is related to the pharyngotympanic (auditory or eustachian) tube, internal carotid artery, and tensor tympani (whose tendon is attached to the handle of the malleus). The tensor tympani muscle dampens the vibration of the tympanic membrane.

b. **Posterior wall (mastoid wall)**: It is related to the aditus leading to the mastoid antrum. A pyramid eminence containing the stapedius muscle is present on the posterior wall, and the tendon of the stapedius emerges from it to attach to the neck of the stapes. The stapedius dampens the vibration of the oval window membrane. It is innervated by the facial nerve (CN VII).

c. **Roof (tegmental)**: The roof of the middle ear is formed by the tegmen tympani, which separates it from and is related superiorly to the temporal lobe of the brain.

d. **Floor (jugular)**: It is related to the internal jugular vein.

e. **Lateral wall (tympanic)**: It is related to the tympanic membrane and chorda tympani nerve.

f. **Medial wall (labyrinthine wall)**: It is related to the promontory (formed by the basal turn of the cochlea), tympanic nerve plexus lying on the promontory, oval window (sealed by the footplate of stapes), and round window (sealed by a fibrous membrane).

The tympanic nerve plexus is derived from the glossopharyngeal nerve (CN IX) and gives rise to the lesser petrosal nerve, which passes anteriorly to synapse in the otic ganglion in the infratemporal fossa. Postganglionic parasympathetic fibers from the otic ganglion run along the auriculotemporal nerve and provide secretomotor innervation to the parotid gland. (*See the section on the Parotid Gland.*)

3. **Inner Ear**

It consists of two main parts: the cochlea (for hearing) and the semicircular canals (for balance). They are supplied by the vestibulocochlear nerves (CN VIII). The vestibular apparatus contains the saccule and utricle, which are connected by the utriculo-saccular duct. The ductus reuniens joins the saccule with the cochlear duct.

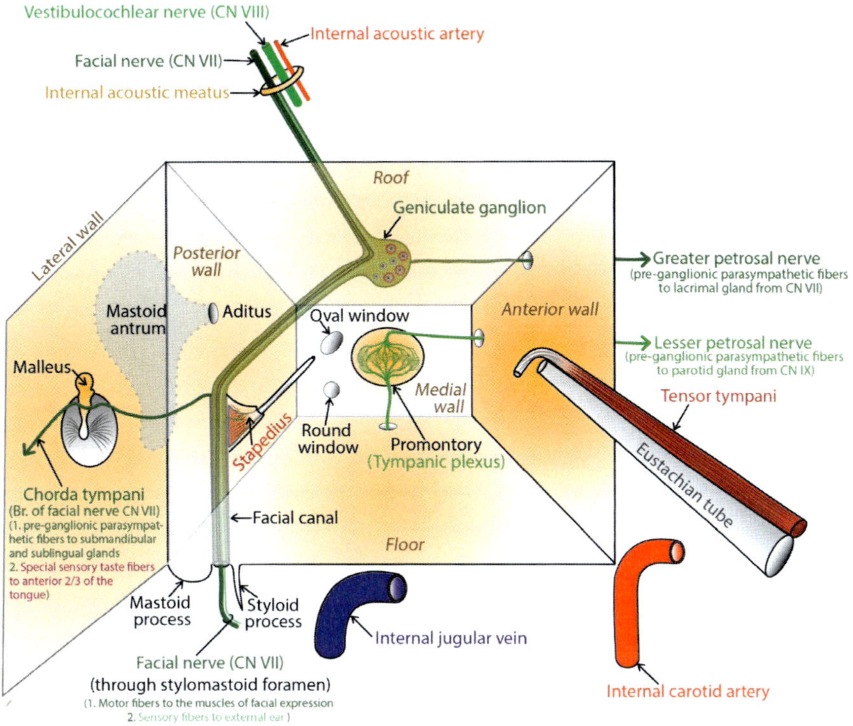

Figure 10.41. Middle ear (tympanum) — its relations. Lateral wall: The lateral wall is flipped over to the left, showing its medial surface, which is related to the tympanic membrane, handle of the malleus, and chorda tympani nerve. Anterior wall: opening of the pharyngotympanic tube, and above it is the tensor tympani muscle. Related anteriorly is also the internal carotid artery. Posterior wall: aditus, pyramid, which houses the stapedius, and the facial nerve. Floor: internal jugular vein. Roof: temporal lobe. Medial wall: promontory (basal turn of the cochlea), tympanic nerve plexus, oval window, and round window. Note that the lesser petrosal nerve arises from the tympanic nerve plexus. It runs forward. The greater petrosal nerve originates from the geniculate ganglion (of the facial nerve). Note the course of the facial nerve: through the internal acoustic meatus, roof (geniculate ganglion), posterior wall, and then exits through the stylomastoid foramen.

a. Cochlea: Sound is detected by the organ of Corti, where sensory hair cells convert it into neural signals. These signals travel via the spiral ganglion to the cochlear nerve, which then transmits them to the cochlear nucleus in the brainstem **(Fig. 10.42)**.
b. Semicircular canals **(Fig. 10.40)**: The anterior, posterior, and lateral semicircular canals detect angular (rotational) acceleration of the head and help maintain balance. They are filled with endolymph and contain sensory receptors in the ampullae. Sensory information from

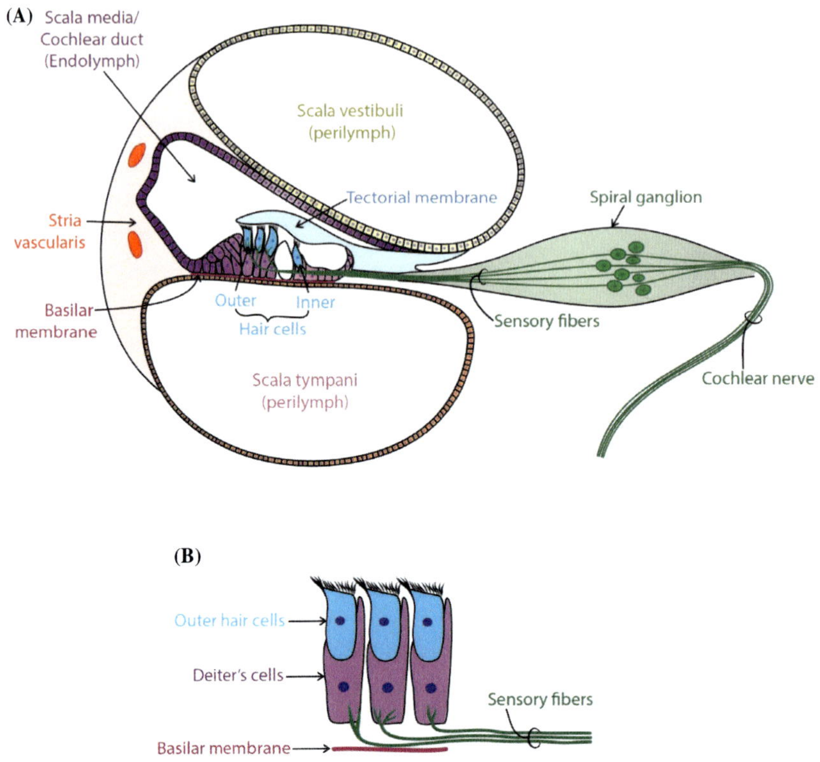

Figure 10.42. Organ of Corti — inner ear. The organ of Corti lies within the cochlear duct, filled with endolymph. It is composed of outer and inner hair cells resting on the basilar membrane. Circulation of the perilymph (in the scala vestibuli and scala tympani) causes vibration of the basilar membrane and the tectorial membrane over the hair cells supported by the Deiters' cells. This stimulates the nerve fibers of the spiral ganglion cells in the cochlea and triggers the electrical impulse that is conducted to the cochlear nucleus (in the brainstem) by the cochlear nerve.

the semicircular canals is carried by the vestibular division of the vestibulocochlear nerve (CN VIII).

c. Vestibular organs: The utricle and saccule detect linear acceleration. Their sensory receptors respond to the movement of otoliths. Impulses are carried by the vestibular nerve to the vestibular nuclei in the brainstem.

4. **Sound Transmission Pathway (Fig. 10.40)**

Sound waves → external auditory meatus (canal) → tympanic membrane → malleus → incus → stapes → oval window → scala vestibuli (cochlea) → vibration of cochlear fluids → organ of Corti (located in the cochlear duct and bathed in endolymph) → scala tympani → round window.

Applied anatomy

1. *Conductive hearing loss*: Due to infections of the middle ear (otitis media) and damage to the ossicles.
2. *Sensorineural hearing loss*: Nerve damage or lesion, e.g., acoustic neuroma.
3. Discuss how a facial nerve lesion might affect hearing if the lesion occurs: (a) at the internal acoustic meatus, or (b) at the stylomastoid foramen.
4. *Vertigo*: It may be caused by the overstimulation of sensory receptors, among others, in the semicircular canals and vestibular organs (due to the movements of otoliths) — labyrinthitis.
5. *Cochlea implant*: This is implanted behind the ear (processor) and at the base of the cochlea (receiver). It helps stimulate the auditory nerve. The signals are eventually interpreted as sounds by the brain.

BACK OF THE NECK AND SUBOCCIPITAL REGION

General Features

1. The back of the neck and suboccipital region are involved in flexion, extension, lateral flexion, and rotation.
2. There are seven cervical vertebrae. The atypical vertebrae are C1 (atlas), C2 (axis), and C7 (vertebra prominens), while C3–6 are typical cervical vertebrae.
   (a) Atlas: It consists of anterior and posterior arches connected by lateral masses. It has transverse processes containing the foramen transversarium and superior articular facets that articulate with the occipital condyles. The body and spinous process, present in the typical cervical vertebrae, are absent.
   (b) Axis: Its distinctive feature is the presence of the odontoid process. It also has the body, transverse process, and foramen transversarium.
   (c) Typical cervical vertebrae include the body, transverse process, foramen transversarium, and the bifid spinous process, which is the characteristic feature of these vertebrae.
3. **Ligamentum nuchae**: This is a fibrous band (elastic tissue) over the spine of the cervical vertebrae. It provides attachment of muscles and deep cervical fascia.
4. **Occipital bone**: Posteriorly, the neck extends up to the superior nuchal line and external occipital protuberance (inion). The inferior nuchal line,

occipital condyles, and foramen magnum are features of the occipital bone. The brainstem passes through the foramen magnum, where the medulla oblongata of the brainstem continues as the spinal cord.

5. **Atlanto-occipital joint**: The synovial joint occurs between the superior articular facets of the atlas and the two occipital condyles. The atlanto-occipital membranes (anterior and posterior) bridge the articular margins. The joint allows anterior, posterior, and lateral flexion.
6. **Atlanto-axial joint**: It is a synovial pivot type of joint between the odontoid process of the axis and the anterior arch of the atlas. It allows rotation.
7. **Vertebral artery**: The paired artery arises from the first part of the subclavian artery. It enters the foramen transversarium at the level of C6 and ascends through the foramina transversaria of C5, C4, C3, C2, and C1 to reach the suboccipital region (**Fig. 10.43**). At the level of the foramen magnum, the right and left vertebral arteries enter the cranial cavity and unite at the junction of the pons and medulla to form the basilar artery (at the base of the skull).

Suboccipital Triangle (Fig. 10.43)

The suboccipital triangle is bounded by the following muscles:

1. **Rectus capitis posterior major**: Superiorly, it is attached to the lateral part of the area below the inferior nuchal line, while inferiorly, it is attached to the axis.
2. **Rectus capitis posterior minor**: Superiorly, it is attached to the medial part of the area below the inferior nuchal line, while inferiorly, it is attached to the atlas.
3. **Obliquus capitis superior (Superior oblique)**: Superiorly, it is attached to the occipital bone between the superior and inferior nuchal lines, lateral to the rectus capitis posterior major, while inferiorly, it is attached to the atlas.
4. **Obliquus capitis inferior (Inferior oblique)**: It extends from the axis to the atlas. The greater occipital nerve (C2) emerges below it.
5. Floor of the suboccipital triangle: Posterior arch of the atlas and the posterior atlanto-occipital membrane.
6. Contents: The triangle contains the suboccipital nerve (C1), which innervates the suboccipital muscles and has no cutaneous branch, and the vertebral artery, which lies on the posterior arch of the atlas and then passes through the posterior atlanto-occipital membrane.

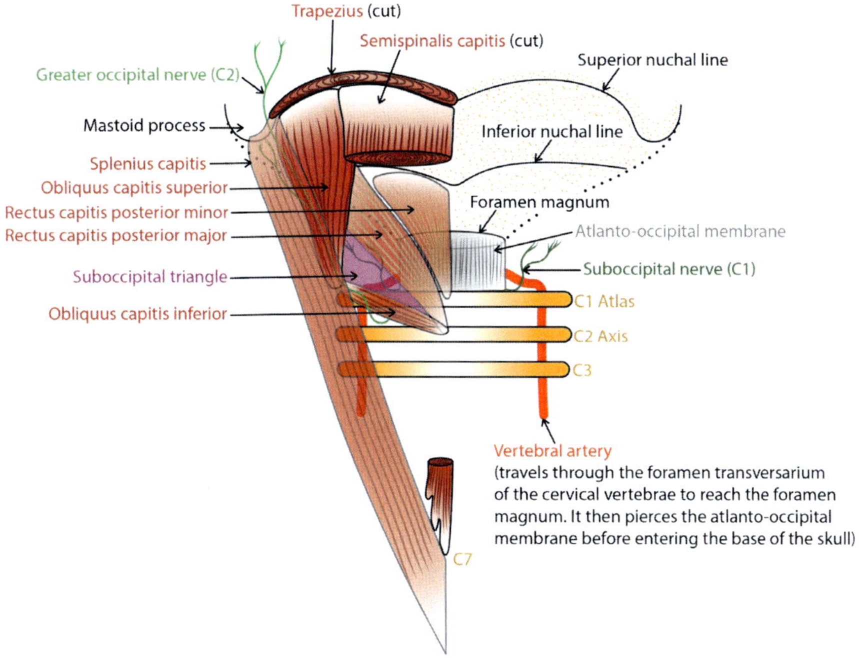

Figure 10.43. Suboccipital triangle. This lies inferior to the occipital bone. It is bounded superiorly by the superior oblique, inferiorly by the inferior oblique, and medially by the rectus capitis major and minor muscles. The triangle is covered or roofed by the semispinalis capitus and trapezius, with the latter being most superficial. The floor is formed by the posterior atlanto-occipital membrane. Winding around the membrane is the suboccipital nerve (C1). Emerging below the inferior oblique is the greater occipital nerve (C2). Arrows indicate the course of the vertebral artery as it ascends along the foramen transversarium. In the suboccipital triangle, it pierces through the posterior atlanto-occipital membrane.

Neck (Back of the Neck) Muscles Over the Sub-Occipital Triangle (Fig. 9.19; Fig. 10.43)

1. **Trapezius**: It elevates, retracts, and rotates the scapula. It is innervated by the spinal accessory nerve (CN XI) with some proprioceptive fibers from C3–4.
2. **Splenius capitis**: It unilaterally flexes laterally and rotates the head to the same side (ipsilateral). It extends the head and neck when both sides contract.
3. **Semispinalis capitis**: It extends the head and neck bilaterally (e.g., looking up to the ceiling). Unilateral contraction rotates the head to the opposite side (contralateral).

4. **Longissimus capitis**: It is positioned laterally in the deep back. Bilateral contraction extends the head, while unilateral contraction rotates it to the same side (ipsilateral).

ERECTOR SPINAE (SACROSPINALIS)

This is a group of back muscles that lie in the "gutter" on both sides of the spines of the vertebral column **(Fig. 9.19)**. They are organized into three main longitudinal columns, which may be interrupted at certain points, and extend from the iliac crest and sacrum up to the suboccipital region. They are antigravity muscles that play important roles in maintaining body posture (straightening the back), balance, coordination, and locomotion. They facilitate extension, rotation, and lateral flexion of the head and trunk. The three longitudinal columns are:

1. **Iliocostalis**: It is composed of the iliocostalis lumborum, iliocostalis thoracis, and iliocostalis cervicis.
2. **Longissimus**: The longest of the erector spinae muscles, consisting of the longissimus thoracis, longissimus cervicis, and longissimus capitis.
3. **Spinalis**: It comprises the spinalis thoracis, spinalis cervicis, and spinalis capitis.
4. Deep back muscles are composed of the following:
   (a) <u>Intertransversarii and interspinalis</u>: They extend between the transverse processes or between the spines of the adjacent vertebrae.
   (b) <u>Rotatores</u>: It lies in the deepest layer, also known as the transversospinalis.
   (c) <u>Multifidus</u>: It is also part of the transversospinalis group, extending from the mammillary process (on the superior articular process) of the lumbar vertebrae to the spinous process above. It is involved in the rotation of the lumbar region.

   <u>Innervation</u>: The muscles are mainly innervated by the posterior rami of the spinal nerves.

CRANIAL NERVES

Olfactory Nerves (I) (Fig. 10.44)

The olfactory epithelium is localized over the superior nasal concha in the nasal cavity.

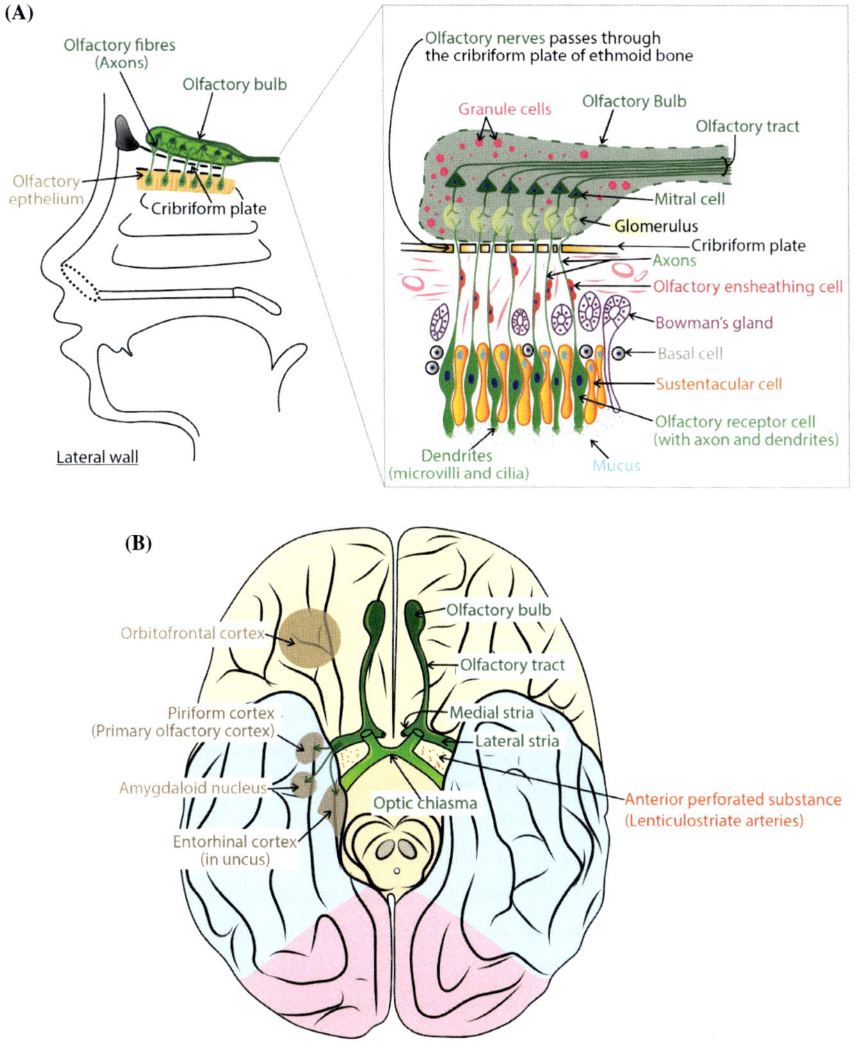

Figure 10.44. Olfactory nerves and their central pathways. (A) The olfactory receptor cells in the olfactory mucosa over the superior nasal concha send their fibers or axons through the cribriform plate (olfactory nerves). The axons synapse with the mitral cells in the olfactory bulb. **(B)** The axons of the mitral cells form the olfactory tract and project to the piriform cortex and amygdaloid nucleus (AN) and entorhinal cortex, and thence to other parts of the brain.

1. The olfactory epithelium consists of the olfactory receptor cells, which are bipolar neurons whose dendrites bear cilia projecting into the overlying mucus layer.

2. Between the sensory receptor cells are the supporting "sustentacular cells" and "basal cells."
3. Bowman's glands, which are serous, release their secretions via their ducts onto the surface of the olfactory epithelium.
4. The axons (nerve fibers) of the sensory receptor cells pass through the cribriform plate. They make synaptic contacts with the dendrites of the "mitral cells" in the olfactory bulb.
5. The axons of the sensory receptor cells are enveloped by olfactory ensheathing cells, which promote nerve growth or regeneration.
6. The axons of the mitral cells project to the primary olfactory cortex (piriform cortex), entorhinal cortex, and amygdaloid nucleus.
7. From the entorhinal cortex, the sensory impulse projects to different areas of the brain, including the thalamus.

N.B. The olfactory nerves, therefore, represent the axons of the olfactory receptor cells.

Applied anatomy

1. In the fracture of the frontal bone (due to an automobile accident) involving the olfactory nerves and olfactory bulb, the victim may suffer olfactory dysfunction — anosmia. In addition, there may be CSF leakage into the nasal cavity — CSF rhinorrhea.
2. It has been reported that COVID-19 damages the basal cells and olfactory ensheathing cells, causing long-term anosmia.

Optic Nerve (II) (Fig. 10.45)

1. The optic nerve arises from the retina.
2. It is composed exclusively of axons of the retinal ganglion cells (RGCs), which leave the retina at the optic disc (optic cup in the central area, also known as a "blind spot").
3. Both optic nerves cross at the "optic chiasma," and continue separately as the optic tracts.
4. Only the RGC axons from the nasal half of the retina cross over to the contralateral optic tract.
5. The RGC axons from the temporal half of the retina remain uncrossed.

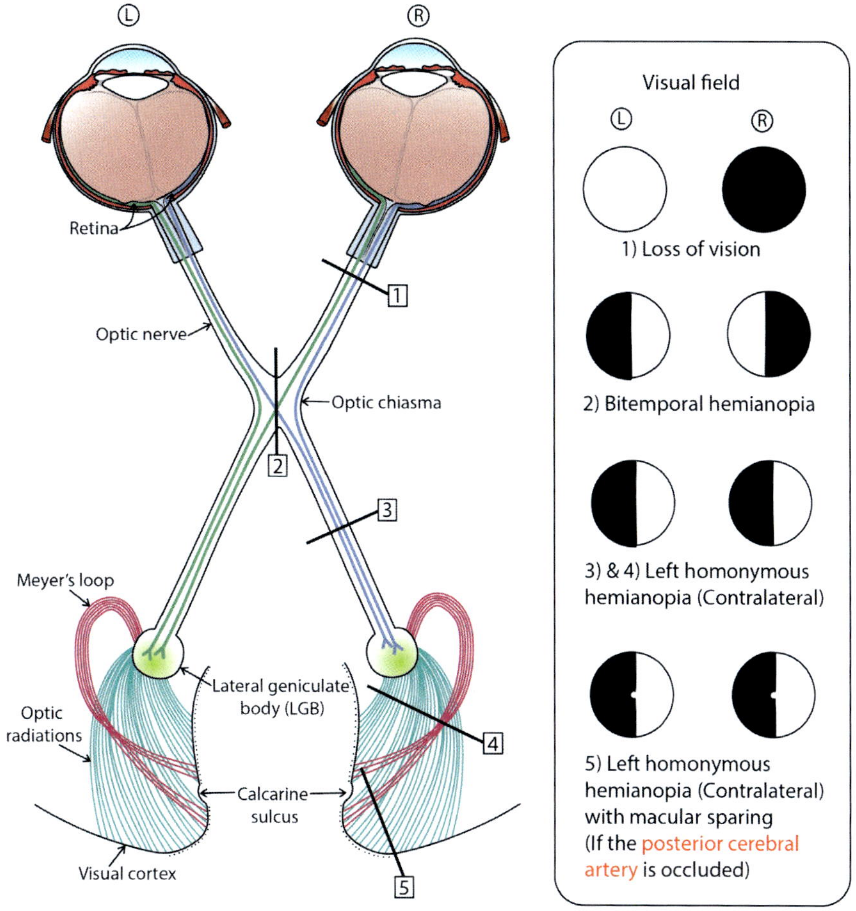

Figure 10.45. Optic nerve and its pathways. The optic nerve arises from the retina. It contains the axons of the retinal ganglion cells. The axons originate from the temporal half of the retina and pass through the optic chiasma without crossing. On the other hand, the axons that originate from the nasal half of the retina cross over to the contralateral side at the optic chiasma. From the optic chiasma, the axons project to the lateral geniculate body (LGB) via the optic tract. From the LGB, the axons of the thalamic neurons project to the ipsilateral visual cortex (calcarine sulcus). Some axons loop to the visual cortex separately via Meyer's loop. If the optic pathway is damaged at 1, 2, 3, and 4 (as indicated), there will be a loss of vision (the affected visual field is blackened), as indicated on the right of the figure. (Refer to the text for more details.)

6. Therefore, each optic tract contains axons from both eyes: crossed axons from the contralateral nasal retina and uncrossed axons from the ipsilateral temporal retina. Functionally, this arrangement allows each optic tract to carry visual information from the contralateral visual field.

7. Axons from RGC synapse with neurons in the lateral geniculate body (LGB) (thalamus). Here, the thalamic neurons project their axons to the visual cortex (occipital lobe) via the optic radiation or via Meyer's loop.
8. Some axons project to the superior colliculus (midbrain) and the pretectal area involved in the visual reflex.
    a. **Pupillary reflex and its pathway**
    The pupillary reflex occurs in response to changes in light intensity, such as bright or dim light. Light enters through the eye and is detected by photoreceptors in the retina. The signal is then transmitted to retinal ganglion cells (RGCs). Axons of the RGCs leave the eye via the optic nerve and project to the pretectal area in the midbrain. Neurons in the pretectal area send bilateral projections to the Edinger–Westphal nucleus (EWN), the parasympathetic component of the oculomotor complex. Preganglionic parasympathetic fibers from the EWN travel with the oculomotor nerve (CN III) (fibers hitch-hike) to reach the ciliary ganglion. Postganglionic parasympathetic fibers (short-ciliary nerves from the ciliary ganglion) innervate the sphincter pupillae and ciliary muscles, causing pupil constriction.
    b. **Accommodation reflex and its pathways**
    The accommodation reflex enables the eyes to focus on near and far objects by adjusting extraocular muscle activity and the shape of the lens.

Pathways involved

Convergence (eye movement): Visual input from the retina travels via the optic nerve to the superior colliculus. Signals are relayed to the oculomotor (III), trochlear (IV), and abducens (VI) nuclei, which control the extraocular muscles. This results in medial rotation (adduction) of both eyes, known as convergence, necessary for near vision (e.g., reading a book).

Lens accommodation: Light from the object passes from the retina through the optic nerve to the pretectal area. Signals are sent to the EWN, whose preganglionic parasympathetic fibers travel with CN III to the ciliary ganglion. Postganglionic fibers innervate the ciliary muscles, which adjust tension on the suspensory ligaments.

Lens shape changes: Rounded lens for near vision; flattened lens for distant vision (e.g., looking at a bus number plate)

Applied anatomy

Lesion of the optic nerve **(*Fig. 10.45*)**

1. Lesion at the right optic nerve: total blindness of the right eye
2. Lesion at the optic chiasma: bitemporal hemianopsia (hemianopia)
3. Lesion at the right optic tract: left homonymous hemianopsia (hemianopia)
4. Lesion at the right optic radiation, e.g., if the PCA is occluded: left homonymous hemianopia with macular sparing (because of the collateral circulation from the MCA).

Oculomotor Nerve (Fig. 10.26)

It arises from the midbrain at the level of the superior colliculus.

The following are brainstem nuclei associated with the nerve:

1. *Oculomotor nucleus (OMN)*: The nerve (composed of axons from the OMN) leaves the brainstem and passes forward in the lateral wall of the cavernous sinus. It enters the orbit through the superior orbital fissure within the common tendinous ring. It innervates the eye muscles, including the superior rectus, levator palpebrae superioris, medial rectus, inferior rectus, and inferior oblique.
2. *Edinger–Westphal nucleus*: This is the parasympathetic component of the nerve. The preganglionic parasympathetic neurons are localized in the EWN dorsomedial to the OMN. The preganglionic fibers (axons) travel along with the motor fibers from the OMN and synapse with the postganglionic neurons in the ciliary ganglion. The postganglionic parasympathetic fibers (short-ciliary nerves from the ciliary ganglion) run forward to supply the ciliary muscles and sphincter pupillae.

Quiz: *Explain why injury to the oculomotor nerve can result in the following?*

1. *Divergent squint (abduction or lateral rotation of the eyeball*
2. *Dilation of the pupil*
3. *Loss of accommodation*
4. *Ptosis (drooping of the upper eyelid)*
5. *Diplopia (double vision)*

Trochlear Nerve (Fig. 10.17; Fig. 10.25)

1. The nerve arises from the midbrain at the level of the inferior colliculus.
2. It is associated with the trochlear nucleus (TN) containing the motor neurons.
3. The nerve fibers or axons of the motor neurons course upward and decussate to the opposite side. Thus, the nerve supplies the contralateral superior oblique muscle.

Applied anatomy

1. Injury to the nerve results in diplopia, which is prominent when the patient is looking downward and laterally on the same side (ipsilateral superior oblique palsy).
2. If the injury is to the TN, the muscle it supplies (superior oblique) on the contralateral side is paralyzed (contralateral superior oblique palsy).

Trigeminal Nerve (V) (Fig. 10.46) (*See also the section on Oral Cavity*)

1. This is the largest cranial nerve, which arises from the pons.
2. The following are brainstem nuclei associated with the nerve: sensory nucleus (mesencephalic nucleus, chief sensory nucleus, and spinal nucleus of V) and the motor nucleus of V.
3. Trigeminal ganglion (semilunar ganglion) is associated with the nerve. It contains sensory ganglion cells, which are comparable to the dorsal root (sensory) ganglion of the spinal nerves.
4. From the ganglion, the trigeminal nerve divides into three divisions: ophthalmic (V_1), maxillary (V_2), and mandibular (V_3).
5. **Ophthalmic division (V_1)**: It exits the cranial cavity through the superior orbital fissure and divides into the frontal (which further divides into supraorbital and supratrochlear nerves), lacrimal, and nasociliary (external nasal, infratrochlear) nerves. These are exclusively sensory to the eye, eyelid, external nose, forehead, and scalp.
6. **Maxillary division (V_2) (Fig. 10.29)**: It is exclusively sensory as well. It exits the cranial fossa through the foramen rotundum. It supplies the upper jaw (maxilla), maxillary sinus and upper teeth, nasal cavity, face, eyelid, etc. For details of its course and distribution, refer to the section on the nasal cavity.

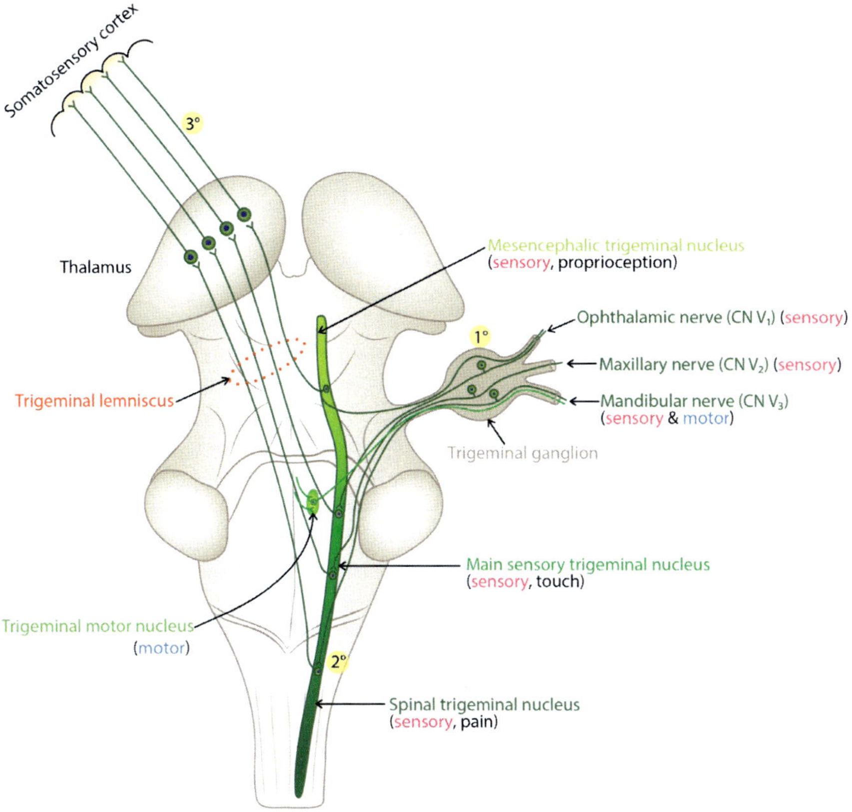

Figure 10.46. Trigeminal (V) nerve. The trigeminal nerve arises from the pons, whose sensory ganglion (trigeminal ganglion) contains the pseudounipolar sensory neurons. The ganglion gives rise to three main nerves: ophthalmic, maxillary, and mandibular nerves. Both the ophthalmic and maxillary divisions are exclusively sensory; the mandibular (blue) also contains axons from the motor nucleus of V. All sensory inputs (pain, temperature, and touch) from the facial areas are transmitted via the trigeminal ganglion cells (first-order sensory neurons). Next, the central afferents of the sensory neurons project to the second-order neurons in the spinal nucleus. The axons from the spinal nucleus neurons cross over to the opposite side and project to the thalamic nucleus (VPM) via the trigeminal lemniscus. The thalamic neurons (third-order) project to the somatosensory cortex.

7. **Mandibular division (V_3) (Fig. 10.33)**: It has both motor and sensory components. It innervates all muscles of mastication, sensory to the temporomandibular joint, lower jaw and teeth, and buccal mucosa and gingiva.

Applied anatomy

All pain sensation from the face is mediated by one of the three divisions of the trigeminal nerve. The sensory neurons mediating these signals have their cell bodies in the trigeminal (semilunar) ganglion, and their central processes project to the spinal trigeminal nucleus in the brainstem. Trigeminal neuralgia may involve one of the three divisions.

Quiz 1: *Trace the pain pathway from an ulcer of the tongue to the brain.*

Quiz 2: *Which nerves need to be numbed prior to the extraction of the lower wisdom tooth?*

Abducent (Abducens) Nerve (*See the section on the Eye*)

1. It arises from the pontomedullary junction near the midline of the brainstem.
2. The abducent nucleus is localized in the pons (floor of the fourth ventricle).
3. The nerve passes forward through the cavernous sinus lateral to the internal carotid artery **(Fig. 10.17)**.
4. It enters the orbit through the superior orbital fissure within the tendinous ring **(Fig. 10.25)**.
5. It is motor to the lateral rectus muscle.

Applied anatomy

Injury to the abducens nerve results in convergent squint and diplopia.

Facial Nerve (VII) (*See also the sections on the Face and the Ear*) (Fig. 10.11; Fig. 10.41)

1. The facial nerve arises from the pontomedullary junction.
2. It consists of motor, parasympathetic, sensory, and special sensory nerve fibers.
3. Motor fibers (originating from facial nucleus): The motor fibers innervate the stapedius muscle in the middle ear, occipitalis via the posterior auricular branch, the posterior belly of the digastric muscle, and the stylohyoid muscle. The main trunk traverses the parotid gland, where it gives five terminal motor branches (temporal, zygomatic, buccal, marginal mandibular, and cervical branches), which innervate muscles of facial expression.

4. Parasympathetic fibers (secretomotor), originating from the superior salivatory nucleus, supply the lacrimal gland (via the greater petrosal nerve → pterygopalatine ganglion) and sublingual and submandibular glands (via the chorda tympani → submandibular ganglion).
5. Special sensory (taste) fibers, originating from the solitary nucleus, innervate the anterior 2/3 of the tongue (via the chorda tympani).
6. Sensory fibers, originating from the spinal trigeminal nucleus, provide cutaneous sensation to the external ear.

Clinical anatomy

Upper and lower motor lesions of the facial nerve (*see also the section on the Face*).

Vestibulocochlear Nerve (*See the section on the Ear*) (Fig. 10.40; Fig. 10.42)

1. The vestibular nerve transmits signals related to balance, angular, and linear acceleration from the vestibular organs: semicircular canals, utricle, and saccule.
2. The cell bodies of sensory neurons are localized in the vestibular ganglion.
3. The central projections are to the vestibular nuclei in the brainstem and then to the cerebellum for the coordination of balance.
4. The cochlear nerve transmits hearing (sound) signals from the organ of Corti. The sensory neurons are in the spiral ganglion, located in the modiolus of the cochlea. The central projections of the cochlear nerve are to the cochlear nuclei in the brainstem. From there, the signals are transmitted to the superior olivary nucleus (ipsilaterally or contralaterally via the trapezoid body) → the inferior colliculus (midbrain) → the medial geniculate body of the thalamus → the primary auditory cortex in the temporal lobe for perception of sound.

Glossopharyngeal Nerve (IX) (Fig. 10.47)

1. The nerve arises from the medulla oblongata in the brainstem and is associated with the following nuclei:
   a. Inferior salivatory nucleus
      — Supplies the parotid gland

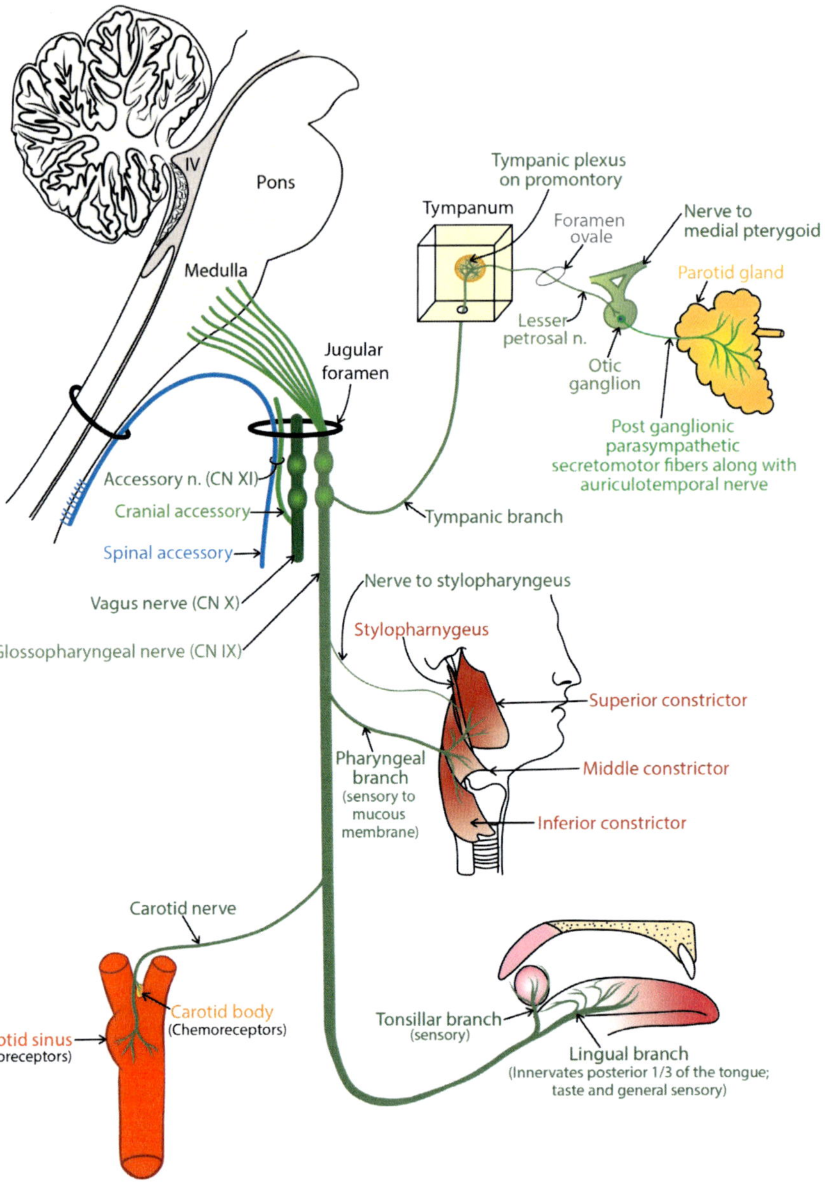

Figure 10.47. Glossopharyngeal nerve. The glossopharyngeal nerve arises from the medulla dorsal to the olive. It leaves the skull through the jugular foramen. Below this are its two sensory ganglia. It gives rise to the following branches: tympanic, stylopharyngeus, pharyngeal, tonsillar, lingual, and carotid. The tympanic branch enters the tympanum to form the tympanic plexus — lesser petrosal nerve — synapse in the otic ganglion — parotid gland. The lingual branch carries general and taste sensations from the posterior one-third of the tongue to the brainstem nuclei. The carotid branch registers the change in blood pressure in the carotid sinus (baroreceptor). (*Refer to the text for more details.*)

b. Nucleus of the tractus solitarius (NTS)
   - Receives the taste signal from the circumvallate papillae
   - Receives signal (blood pressure) from the carotid sinus (baroreceptor).

c. Nucleus ambiguus (NA): stylopharyngeus

d. Spinal nucleus of V
   - Pain sensation from the mucous membrane of the pharynx, e.g., in pharyngitis.

3. There are two sensory ganglia: superior (jugular) ganglion and inferior (petrosal) ganglion.

4. Branches and functions:

   a. **Tympanic branch (Jacobson's nerve)**: It is a recurrent branch that enters the middle ear (tympanum) through the tympanic canaliculus. It then forms the tympanic nerve plexus on the promontory in the middle ear and gives rise to the lesser petrosal nerve, which carries the preganglionic parasympathetic fibers to the otic ganglion. The postganglionic parasympathetic fibers (secretomotor fibers) from the otic ganglion hitch-hike along the auriculotemporal nerve (a branch of the mandibular division of the trigeminal nerve) to supply the parotid gland.

   b. **Pharyngeal branch**: This is general sensory to the mucosa of the pharynx. The cell bodies of these sensory neurons are localized in the inferior sensory ganglion. The central projections are to the spinal nucleus of V.

   c. **Stylopharyngeus**: The motor branch originates from the nucleus ambiguus.

   d. **Tonsillar branch**: This is general sensory to the tonsillar fossa.

   e. **Lingual branch**: This carries general sensory and taste sensations from the posterior one-third of the tongue.

   f. **Carotid nerve branch**: Innervates carotid sinus (baroreceptor) and carotid body (chemoreceptors). The central projections are to the nucleus of the tractus solitarius.

<u>Applied anatomy</u>

Test for an IX nerve lesion: Gag reflex is absent when the back of the tongue is touched.

Quiz: Why do you think a patient with pharyngitis ("sore throat") also complains of "pain in the ear"?

Vagus Nerve (X) (Fig. 10.48)

1. The vagus nerve arises from the medulla oblongata dorsal to the olive along with the CN IX and CN XI nerves.
2. It leaves the cranial fossa through the jugular foramen.
3. It has two sensory ganglia; the lower one is called the "nodose ganglion."
4. It is called the "wandering nerve" because it arises from the brainstem but descends to supply many structures and organs in the neck, thorax, and abdomen, e.g., the heart, lungs, and the digestive tract distally up to the proximal two-thirds of the transverse colon.
5. The following are brainstem nuclei associated with the vagus nerve:
   a. **Dorsal motor nucleus:** It contains the preganglionic parasympathetic neurons supplying the smooth muscles and glands, including those associated with the myenteric nerve plexus (Auerbach's plexus) and submucous (Meissner's) nerve plexus in the small intestines.
   b. **Nucleus tractus solitarius:** It receives sensory inputs from the carotid sinus and carotid body and taste (over the epiglottis).
   c. **Nucleus ambiguus (NA)**: It provides branchial motor fibers to the muscles of the pharynx and larynx (via the vagus nerve).

The following are the main branches of the vagus nerve:

1. Laryngeal branch: Superior laryngeal nerve, which gives rise to the internal laryngeal nerve and external laryngeal nerve. The internal laryngeal nerve is sensory and innervates the mucous membrane of the larynx above the level of the vocal cord. The external laryngeal nerve is motor and innervates the cricothyroid muscle (*see the section on the Larynx*).
2. Pharyngeal branch: This branch carries efferent fibers from the nucleus ambiguus and contributes to the pharyngeal plexus. From this plexus, the fibers innervate the muscles of the pharynx (superior, middle, and inferior constrictors) and soft palate (except the tensor veli palatini).
3. Recurrent laryngeal nerve: It innervates all the intrinsic muscles of the larynx (except for the cricothyroid) and the mucous membrane below the level of the vocal cord.
4. Cardiac, pulmonary, and digestive tract branches.

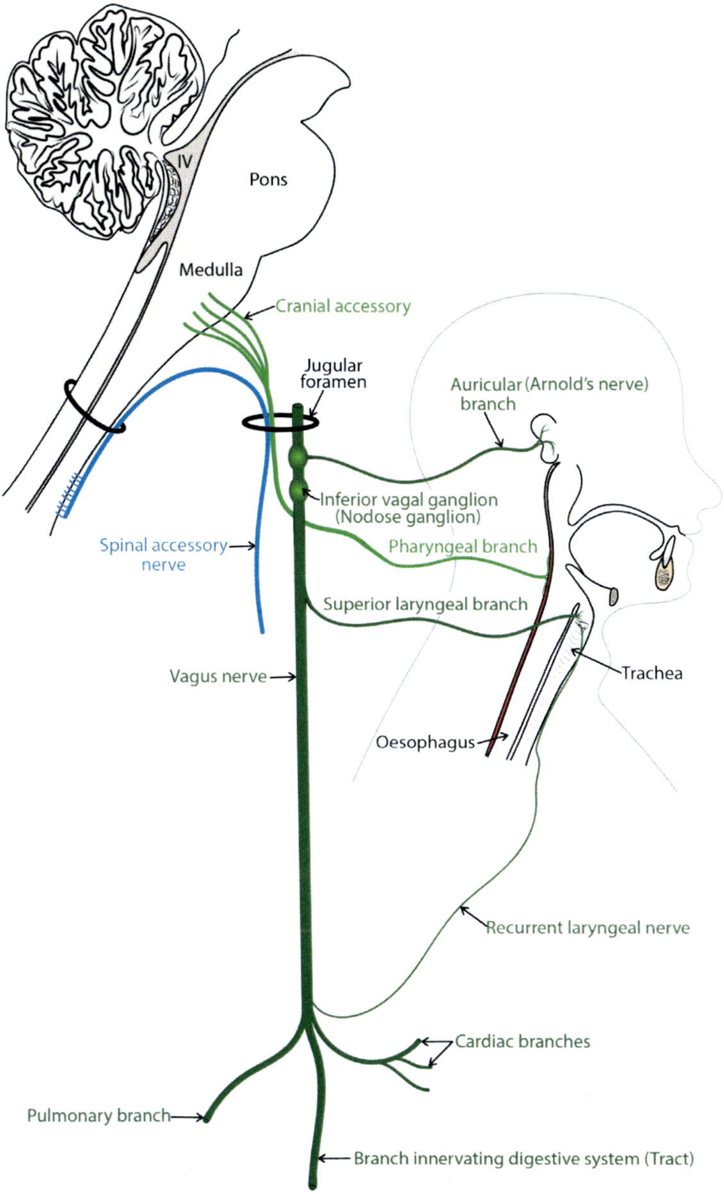

Figure 10.48. Vagus nerve. The vagus nerve arises from the medulla. It exits through the jugular foramen. It has two sensory ganglia (superior and inferior). The nerve is joined by the cranial accessory nerve (CA). The main branches include the pharyngeal branch and laryngeal branch, which supply the pharyngeal and laryngeal muscles. Other branches include the recurrent laryngeal branch, which supplies the intrinsic muscles of the larynx and the mucous membrane. The vagus also supplies the heart (cardiac branch), lungs (pulmonary branch), and the digestive tract till the proximal two-thirds of the transverse colon.

Applied anatomy

Test for a vagus (X) nerve lesion: Ask the patient to say "ahh." The soft palate or uvula is deviated to the intact side.

Accessory Nerve (XI) (Fig. 10.49)

1. The accessory nerve has two components:
   a. *Cranial accessory nerve*: This originates from the NA (in the medulla).
   b. *Spinal accessory nerve*: It originates from the C1–5 ventral horn neurons (motor neurons) of the spinal cord.
2. The spinal accessory nerve ascends through the foramen magnum. It joins with the cranial accessory nerve before they exit together through the jugular foramen as the "accessory nerve" (CN XI).
3. Below the jugular foramen, the cranial part of the accessory nerve joins with the vagus nerve. The fibers (or axons) originally derived from the NA are distributed as the pharyngeal and laryngeal branches supplying the pharyngeal and laryngeal muscles (*see the section on the Vagus Nerve*).
4. The spinal part of the accessory nerve supplies the sternocleidomastoid and trapezius muscles.

N.B. Pharyngeal nerve plexus (Definition): It is formed by the pharyngeal branch of the vagus and the pharyngeal branch of the glossopharyngeal nerve, together with the pharyngeal nerve of the superior cervical ganglion (SCG) (sympathetic ganglion). The "pharyngeal nerve plexus" lies on the lateral walls of the pharynx. Motor fibers of the nerve plexus, originating from NA, innervates the pharyngeal constrictors and elevators. It also innervates the palatoglossus, levator veli palatini, and musculus uvulae. Sensory fibers from the glossopharyngeal nerve innervate the mucous membrane of the pharynx. The sympathetic fibers are primarily vasomotor.

Applied anatomy

Test for a lesion of the spinal accessory nerve: The patient is not able to raise his hand above his head. Explain.

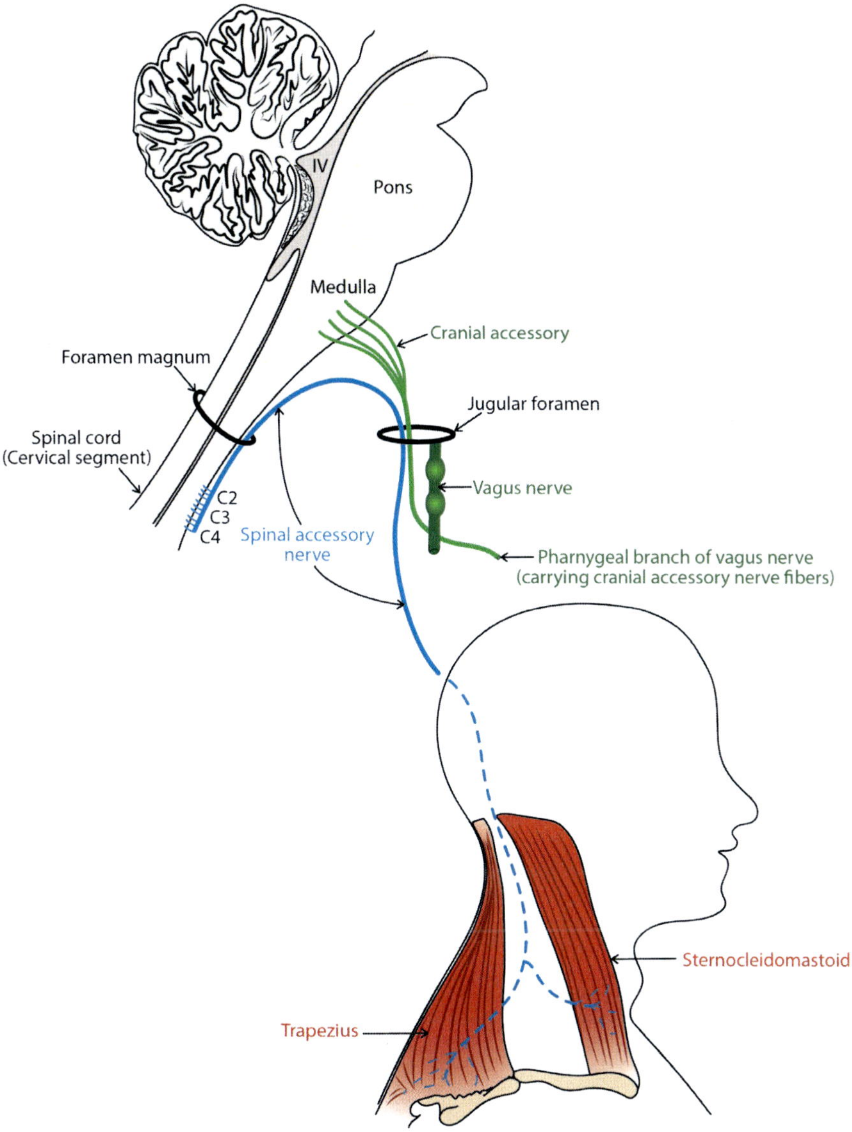

Figure 10.49. Accessory nerve. The nerve arises from the medulla. It has two functional components: cranial accessory and spinal accessory nerves. The cranial accessory joins with the vagus to be distributed by the pharyngeal and laryngeal branches of the vagus. The spinal accessory nerve, exclusively motor, innervates the sternocleidomastoid and trapezius muscles.

Hypoglossal Nerve (XII) (Fig. 10.50)

1. The nerve arises from the medulla oblaongata, ventral to the olive.
2. The motor neurons are localized in the hypoglossal nucleus at the floor of the fourth (IV) ventricle.
3. The nerve exits through the hypoglossal canal.
4. The nerve descends posterior to the internal carotid artery.
5. It then winds around the occipital artery.

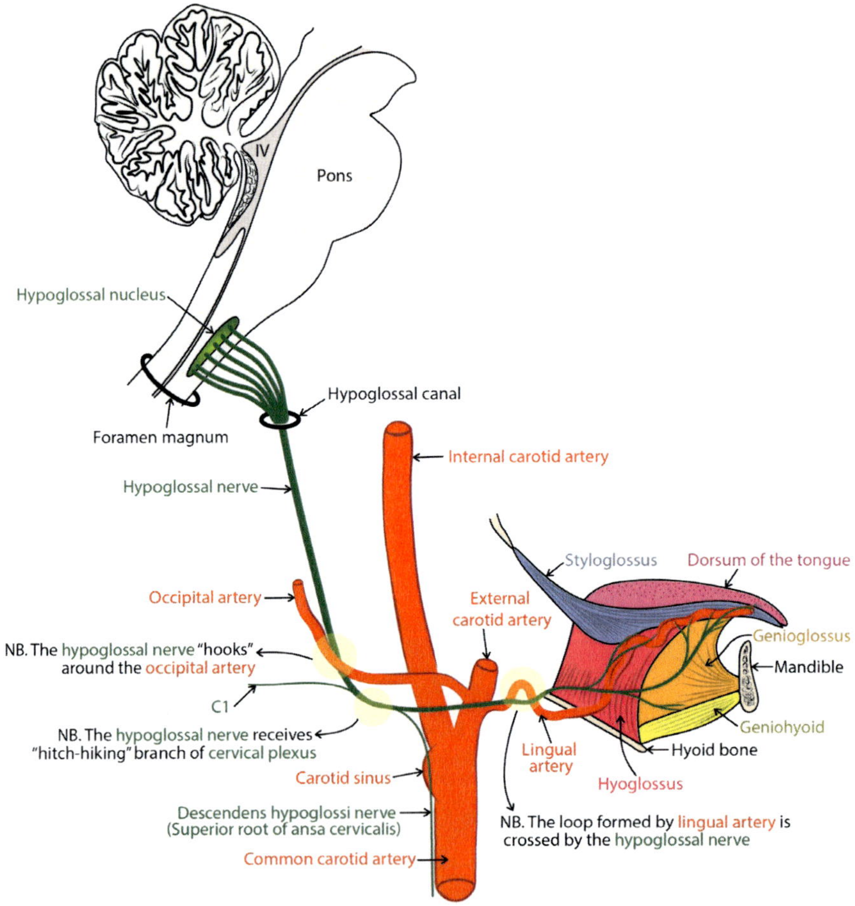

Figure 10.50. Hypoglossal nerve. The nerve arises from the medulla ventral to the olive. It passes through the hypoglossal canal and descends posterior to the internal carotid artery (ICA). It crosses lateral to both the ICA and the external carotid artery (ECA). It then winds around the occipital artery, crossing the loop of the lingual artery and finally supplying the intrinsic and extrinsic muscles of the tongue except the palatoglossus. (*Refer to the text for more details.*)

6. It proceeds forward lateral to the internal and external carotid arteries.
7. It crosses the "loop" of the lingual artery and continues forward, lying lateral to the hyoglossus muscle.
8. It innervates the extrinsic muscles of the tongue, including the genioglossus, hyoglossus, and styloglossus, except the palatoglossus, which is supplied by the pharyngeal branch of the vagus (cranial accessory).
9. It innervates all intrinsic muscles of the tongue.
10. Fibers from the C1 spinal nerve hitch-hike along the hypoglossal nerve as the descendens hypoglossi, contributing to the formation of the ansa cervicalis.

Applied anatomy

Test for a hypoglossal nerve XII lesion: The tongue deviates to the lesion side on protrusion.

SYMPATHETIC INNERVATION OF HEAD AND NECK

The cervical sympathetic trunk and its ganglia provide sympathetic innervation to the head and neck. They lie on the prevertebral muscle (longus capitis) and are adherent to the prevertebral layer of the deep cervical fascia. There are three cervical sympathetic ganglia. Unlike the paravertebral sympathetic ganglia in the thoracic region, the cervical sympathetic ganglia do not have white rami communicantes. The preganglionic sympathetic neurons are localized in the lateral horn of the thoracic 1 and 2 (T1, T2) spinal cord segments. The preganglionic sympathetic fibers (axons) pass through the ventral rootlets of T1–2 spinal cord segments and enter the paravertebral sympathetic chain via the white rami communicantes.

Preganglionic sympathetic fibers destined for the head and neck do not synapse in the thoracic paravertebral ganglia. Instead, they ascend the cervical sympathetic trunk and synapse in the cervical sympathetic ganglia. The postganglionic sympathetic fibers are then distributed via the spinal nerves, cranial nerves, outer walls of arteries (vascular branches), and cardiac nerves.

The following are the three main cervical sympathetic ganglia (**Fig. 10.51**):

1. **Superior cervical ganglion**: It is localized at the level of the C1–2 vertebrae. The following are branches of the ganglion that "hitch-hike" along the carotid arteries or cranial/spinal nerves.

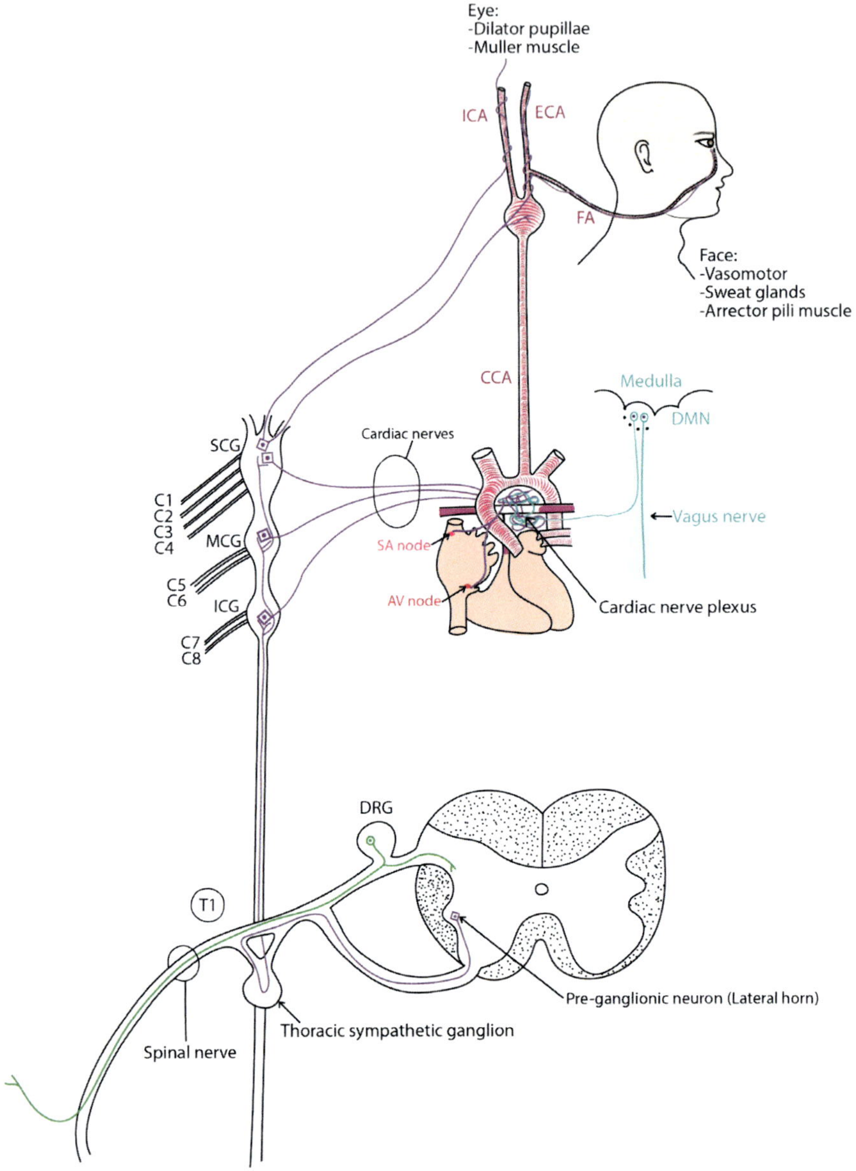

Figure 10.51. Cervical sympathetic ganglia and their distribution. The cervical sympathetic ganglia, namely, the superior cervical ganglion (SCG), the middle cervical ganglion (MCG), and the inferior cervical ganglion (ICG), are connected by the sympathetic trunk. The containing-postganglionic sympathetic neurons are postsynaptic to preganglionic sympathetic neurons localized in the lateral horn of the upper segments of the thoracic spinal cord (T1–2). The preganglionic fibers leave the cord via the ventral rootlets and travel in the spinal nerves. They enter the thoracic sympathetic ganglion but do not make synaptic contacts with the neurons; instead, they ascend through the cervical

a. **Internal carotid artery and branches**: The postganglionic sympathetic fibers accompany the internal carotid artery and its branches. Some fibers pass through the ciliary ganglion and supply the dilator pupillae; other fibers pass through the pterygopalatine ganglion without making any synaptic contacts to supply the mucous glands in the palate, nasal cavity, and pharynx. The "deep petrosal nerve" in the pterygoid canal represents the postganglionic sympathetic fibers, originating from the internal carotid plexus. Note that they do not synapse with neurons in the pterygopalatine ganglion. Most fibers are either vasomotor or secretomotor to the mucous glands in the nasal cavity and palate. Some sympathetic fibers supply the smooth muscle component of the levator palpebrae superioris.

b **External carotid artery and branches**: The postganglionic sympathetic fibers accompanying the arteries supply the sweat glands, arrector pili, vascular smooth muscles, and salivary glands.

c. **Cardiac nerves**: They contribute to the formation of cardiac nerve plexuses, which regulate the sinoatrial (SA) and atrioventricular (AV) nodes.

d. **Cervical spinal nerve branches**: Some postganglionic fibers from the cervical sympathetic ganglia join the ventral rami of C1 and C2 spinal nerves.

e. **Pharyngeal branch**: It contributes to the formation of the pharyngeal nerve plexus. These fibers mainly innervate vascular smooth muscles and glands.

Figure 10.51. (*Continued on facing page*) sympathetic trunk and make synaptic contacts with the postganglionic sympathetic neurons in the respective cervical ganglia (SCG, MCG, ICG). The postganglionic sympathetic fibers (axons) arise from the SCG and accompany the internal carotid artery (ICA) to supply the dilator pupillae and Müller muscle (superior tarsal muscle). Those that accompany the external carotid artery (ECA) and its branches, e.g., the facial artery (FA), supply the vascular smooth muscles, sweat glands, and arrector pili muscles in the face. In addition, there are cardiac nerves to the cardiac plexus in the heart to regulate the sinoatrial (SA) and atrioventricular (AV) nodes; others are distributed by the cervical spinal nerves (C1–4). The MCG also gives rise to cardiac nerves, vascular branches along the inferior thyroid artery (ITA) and spinal nerves (C5–6). The ICG gives rise to cardiac nerves, vascular branches along the vertebral artery (VA) and subclavian artery (SVA), and spinal nerves (C7–8).

2. **Middle cervical ganglion — lies at the level of C6**
   a. **Cervical spinal nerve branches (C3 and C4) — grey rami communicantes**: Postganglionic sympathetic fibers are distributed via the grey rami communicantes to the C3 and C4 spinal nerves, innervating the vascular smooth muscle, sweat glands, and arrector pili in the neck/shoulder.
   b. **Inferior thyroid branch**: Postganglionic sympathetic fibers supply the vascular smooth muscle of the thyroid and adjacent arteries.
   c. **Cardiac nerves — cardiac plexus**: Postganglionic sympathetic fibers contribute to the cardiac nerve plexus, regulating sinoatrial (SA) and atrioventricular (AV) nodes and smooth muscles in large arteries such as the aorta.
3. **Inferior cervical ganglion — lies at the level of C7**
   a. **Cervical spinal nerve branches (C5–8) — through grey rami communicans**: The postganglionic sympathetic nerve fibers innervate the vascular smooth muscle, sweat glands, and arrector pili in the upper limb.
   b. **Subclavian artery and vertebral artery**: The postganglionic sympathetic nerve fibers innervate the sweat glands, vascular smooth muscle in the neck and upper limb.
   c. **Cardiac nerves — cardiac nerve plexus**: It regulates the SA and AV nodes and smooth muscles in the large arteries, e.g., aorta.

Applied anatomy

Quiz 1: *A tumor at the apex of the lung may cause Horner's syndrome (drooping of the upper eyelid, pupil constriction). Explain.*

Quiz 2: *What surgical procedure may be performed to reduce hyperhidrosis (excessive sweating) in the palm?*

Quiz 3: *Why do you think the hand feels warm and dry when the median nerve is damaged?*

Made in the USA
Las Vegas, NV
15 November 2026

ca35e2b6-0ac8-4c68-b936-2a1754d3b018R01